Norms for Fitness, Performance, and Health

Jay Hoffman, PhD

College of New Jersey

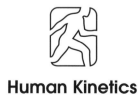

Human Kinetics

Library of Congress Cataloging-in-Publication Data

Hoffman, Jay, 1961-
   Norms for fitness, performance, and health / Jay Hoffman.
     p. ; cm.
   Includes bibliographical references and index.
   ISBN 0-7360-5483-9 (soft cover)
   1. Physical fitness--Measurement. 2. Physical fitness--Evaluation.
  3. Physical fitness--Standards. I. Title.
   [DNLM: 1. Physical Fitness--physiology. 2. Anthropometry--methods.
  3. Body Weights and Measures--statistics & numerical data. 4. Physical
  Endurance. 5. Reference Values. QT 255 H699f 2006]
  QP301.H634 2006
   613.7--dc22

                       2005025909

ISBN-10: 0-7360-5483-9
ISBN-13: 978-0-7360-5483-6

The Web addresses cited in this text were current as of February 8, 2006, unless otherwise noted.

Acquisitions Editor: Michael S. Bahrke, PhD; **Developmental Editor:** Amanda S. Ewing; **Assistant Editors:** Carla Zych and Cory Weber; **Copyeditor:** Jocelyn Engman; **Proofreader:** Sarah Wiseman; **Indexer:** Betty Frizzéll; **Permission Manager:** Carly Breeding; **Graphic Designer:** Robert Reuther; **Graphic Artist:** Dawn Sills; **Photo Manager:** Sarah Ritz; **Cover Designer:** Keith Blomberg; **Photographer (interior):** Sarah Ritz, unless otherwise noted; photos on pages 192-193 by Dan Wendt; **Art Manager:** Kelly Hendren; **Illustrator:** Al Wilborn; **Printer:** Sheridan Books

Printed in the United States of America   10 9 8 7 6 5 4 3 2 1

Human Kinetics
Web site: www.HumanKinetics.com

United States: Human Kinetics
P.O. Box 5076
Champaign, IL 61825-5076
800-747-4457
e-mail: humank@hkusa.com

Canada: Human Kinetics
475 Devonshire Road Unit 100
Windsor, ON N8Y 2L5
800-465-7301 (in Canada only)
e-mail: orders@hkcanada.com

Europe: Human Kinetics
107 Bradford Road
Stanningley
Leeds LS28 6AT, United Kingdom
+44 (0) 113 255 5665
e-mail: hk@hkeurope.com

Australia: Human Kinetics
57A Price Avenue
Lower Mitcham, South Australia 5062
08 8277 1555
e-mail: liaw@hkaustralia.com

New Zealand: Human Kinetics
Division of Sports Distributors NZ Ltd.
P.O. Box 300 226 Albany
North Shore City
Auckland
0064 9 448 1207
e-mail: info@humankinetics.co.nz

For my wife, Yaffa, and children, Raquel, Mattan, and Ariel.
The accomplishment is greater when it can be shared by those
closest to you. Remember that success begins with a dream!

Contents

Preface

Evaluating the health and fitness levels of various populations (both athletic and nonathletic) has become an integral part of the physical education, allied health, and sport science professions. The ability to properly assess athletes has given coaches a greater understanding of how to maximize their players' athletic performances, and as a result the effort toward optimizing training programs has grown immensely over the last few years. Sport scientists have also focused their research in athletic profile development to determine which physical characteristics an athlete needs in order to succeed in a respective sport. Developing an athletic profile for each sport not only helps coaches select their teams but also provides standards for both athletes and coaches for setting training goals. However, fitness evaluation is not limited to the athletic community. The development of standards in a host of health and fitness measurements provides critical tools for health professionals for assessing the health and wellness of recreational and sedentary populations. Physical performance standards have also provided key information for opening the doors to females for positions in both civil service (e.g., police and fire) and military occupations that were traditionally assigned to men.

While numerous fitness and health books are available, *Norms for Fitness, Performance, and Health* differs from these others by providing comprehensive normative data for numerous fitness and health components. It provides the reader with normative fitness and health data for a variety of ages, abilities, occupations, and athletic backgrounds. It builds a basic foundation for understanding the purpose and benefits of fitness and norms. In addition, it briefly reviews relevant statistical procedures and analyses, including inferential statistics, in order to assist the interpretation of descriptive statistics. This text also contains an appendix of 24 test descriptions.

This book will become a standard reference for fitness instructors, physical educators, exercise scientists, coaches, and civil service professionals, providing them with the most comprehensive compilation of normative fitness and health data in existence. Chapters are fortified with figures and tables, making the text more attractive. A unique aspect of this book is its inclusion of performance data for specific civil service populations such as police, fire, and military personnel. In addition, normative data highlight various athletic populations from football, basketball, baseball, and other sports.

The reader will come away with a basic understanding of statistical analysis and fitness and health norm development.

Organization

The book is organized into three parts. Part I discusses the need for fitness and health assessment, briefly discusses the development of a testing protocol, and provides a basic understanding of the statistical interpretation of data. Part II provides normative data for various components of athletic performance and fitness. These chapters briefly discuss the tests available for each fitness component and provide comprehensive normative data from both laboratory and field tests commonly used to assess various age, profession, and sport populations. Gender and ethnic differences are discussed when applicable. Part III provides normative values for various health data, including cardiovascular profiles (i.e., blood pressure, heart rates), lipid profiles (i.e., cholesterol, triglycerides), hematological profiles (i.e., hemoglobin, iron), energy expenditures, and caloric values.

Acknowledgments

I wish to thank a number of people who graciously shared with me the sport performance data that they have collected over the years: Mike Barnes, Bud Bjornara, Mike Brungardt, Kevin Cleary, Josh Cooper, Dr. Avery Faigenbaum, Dr. Jeff Falkel, Michael Falvo, Lorne Goldenberger, John Graham, Allen Hedricks, Mike Nitka, Joe Owens, Dr. Ken Rundell, Dr. Frank Spaniol, John Taylor, Dan Wathen, Steve Wilmont, and Ron Yacyzk.

PART I

Assessment and Analysis

CHAPTER 1

Fitness and Health Assessment

The reasons for assessing health and fitness often differ between a competitive athletic population and a recreationally active or sedentary population. In competitive athletes, developing an *athletic performance profile* requires a detailed battery of testing that thoroughly analyzes all the components comprising athletic performance (i.e., strength, anaerobic power, speed, agility, maximal aerobic capacity and endurance, flexibility, and body composition). Test results can determine the relevance of a fitness component to a particular sport and can direct the appropriate emphasis on that variable in the athlete's training program. In addition, a sport-specific athletic profile can help establish standards for predicting potential success in that sport. Athletes and coaches alike can use these standards as a motivational tool when establishing personal training goals by comparing personal results to normative data from similar athletic populations. Performance testing can also provide baseline data for prescribing individual exercise programs, feedback for evaluating a training program, and information for assessing recovery following injury. This chapter provides information on assessment protocols in both athletic and nonathletic populations.

In the recreationally active or sedentary individual, *health and fitness assessment* assesses the health and wellness of the majority of our popula-tion. Epidemiological studies of the past 40 years have clearly demonstrated the importance of physical activity and its reduction of mortality and morbidity (Paffenbarger, Wing, and Hyde 1978; Paffenbarger, Wing, and Hsieh 1986; Paffenbarger and Hyde, 1980). These studies have consistently shown that a sedentary lifestyle is associated with higher risks of coronary heart disease and all-cause mortality. These studies have been the backbone of a public health initiative to combat physical inactivity and obesity in not only adults but also youth. The United States Department of Health and Human Services (USDHHS) has developed a national strategy to improve the health of Americans. The program, *Healthy People 2010*, focuses on enhancing quality of life, extending the years of healthy life, and eliminating health disparities among Americans (USDHHS 2000). These goals are for all age groups, with the intent that physical activity during adolescence continues into adulthood, resulting in a healthier and more productive society.

Physical fitness testing on recreational athletes provides benefits similar to those seen in the competitive athletic population. The primary difference is that assessment emphasizes health-risk appraisal in the recreational population while it focuses primarily on athletic achievement in the athletic population. Fitness assessments in both populations provide information for exercise prescription and serve as a motivating tool for all individuals.

Factors Affecting Fitness Assessment

In evaluating performance testing, test results may be influenced by several factors relevant within a homogenous group, such as body size, muscle fiber type, and training status of the athlete. In addition, the specificity and relevance of the test to the sport or training program and the validity and reliability of the test are also critical factors that influence evaluation.

BODY SIZE

The influence of an individual's physical size on performance testing is often seen in strength assessment. Absolute strength positively correlates to body size, meaning that bigger individuals are generally stronger than smaller individuals, while correlation between body size and the strength–mass ratio is negative (Hoffman, Maresh, and Armstrong 1992). Thus, expressing strength in relative terms may be more appropriate when comparing individuals of various body sizes. For example, American football linemen should have a greater absolute strength whereas skill-position players (e.g., running backs) should have a greater relative strength.

FIBER TYPE COMPOSITION

For a given muscle size and architecture, the force production, contractile velocity, and fatigue rate vary considerably. This variability primarily relates to the inherent contractile properties of the muscle, which are determined in part by fiber type composition (percentage of fibers that are fast twitch or slow twitch). Fast-twitch fibers are associated with a greater force capability and a faster contraction velocity. Individuals who possess a high percentage of fast-twitch fibers are more likely to succeed in high-intensity activities such as sprinting, basketball, or football than are individuals with a high percentage of slow-twitch fibers. Slow-twitch fibers are associated with a reduced rate of fatigue, a low force capability, and a slow contraction velocity. Individuals with predominantly slow-twitch fibers find success primarily in endurance sports. Although training may transform fiber subtypes (Kraemer et

al. 1995; Staron et al. 1991), scientific evidence for transforming fiber type composition through training does not exist. Therefore, when evaluating the speed or agility of athletes, remember that physiological limitations may affect an athlete's ability to improve speed. Although a slow athlete may become faster, it is highly unlikely that a slow athlete will become fast.

TRAINING STATUS OF ATHLETE

Athletes with greater experience have a smaller potential for achieving performance gains. During the early stages of a training program, performance can significantly improve. As the duration of training increases, the rate of performance improvement declines. As training continues, further changes in performance become difficult, and a plateau will appear to have been reached (see figure 1.1). This plateau may be a genetic ceiling, suggesting that performance improvements at this level are limited to the physiological makeup of the individual.

The effect of pretraining status on strength improvement has been demonstrated in several studies examining the in-season training programs of both collegiate basketball and football players (Hoffman, Maresh et al. 1991; Hoffman and Kang 2003). In the study on basketball players, athletes with previous strength training were compared to athletes with no previous strength training who were considered novice lifters. During the basketball season, no strength improvements were observed in the trained group, while a significant 4% increase in upper-body strength (in a 1RM bench press) was noted in the untrained group (see table 1.1). Although the groups participated in an identical strength-training program, the differ-

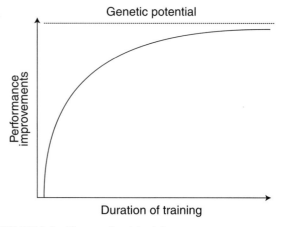

FIGURE 1.1 Theoretical training curve.

Reprinted, by permission, from J. Hoffman, 2002, *Physiological aspects of sport training and performance* (Champaign, IL: Human Kinetics), 74.

TABLE 1.1 Effect of In-Season Resistance Training on Strength in Trained and Untrained College Basketball Players		
Variable	**Trained**	**Untrained**
Bench press (kg)		
Pre	101.6 ± 9.6	92.4 ± 26.0
Post	102.9 ± 11.0	96.2 ± 24.2*
Squat (kg)		
Pre	161.4 ± 16.4	131.1 ± 23.3
Post	150.8 ± 13.1	133.7 ± 20.9

• = significantly different from pretraining levels ($p < .05$).

Adapted from Hoffman et al., 1991, *Journal of Human Muscle Performance* 1:48-55.

ence in strength improvement between the groups appeared to relate to the initial strength training of the athletes.

In the football study, the effect of previous experience in resistance training was also seen. Athletes in their senior year of collegiate football were compared to freshman athletes in their first collegiate season. The freshmen had resistance training from their high school programs, and thus this study compared different levels of training experience. Results showed no differences in gains in upper-body strength (in a 1RM bench press) between the groups, but the strength improvement of the freshman athletes in a 1RM squat (15.1 ± 6.4 kg) was significantly greater than that of the senior athletes (5.5 ± 8.2 kg).

Recognizing an individual's level of experience is also imperative for interpreting performance results. For instance, in a 1 y investigation of elite weightlifters, small increases in strength were observed, though the increases did not reach statistical significance (Hakkinen et al. 1987). Despite no statistically observable change, the athletes and coaches could rate the training program a success because training improvements in elite athletes are so difficult to achieve that even small improvements can be the difference between a medal and no medal. Practical significance should precede statistical significance when interpreting test results in such a situation.

TEST SPECIFICITY AND RELEVANCE

For a test to provide any significant information concerning an individual's performance in the training program, the test must be specific to the training program. When training and testing use a similar exercise (i.e., squats for strength training) and mode (i.e., free weights), test results will more accurately reflect strength improvements. How-

ever, if training and testing are performed with different modes (e.g., machines versus free weights) or exercises (e.g., squats versus leg presses), the actual strength improvement may not be demonstrated. For example, following 10 wk of training on variable-resistance machines, subjects increased leg strength by 27% when tested with a variable-resistance leg press; however, when tested with a dynamic constant resistance exercise, the subjects improved their strength by only 7.5% (Pipes 1978). Conversely, in that same study a group of subjects on an exercise program of dynamic constant resistance showed a 28.9% strength improvement when tested with a dynamic constant resistance exercise but only a 7.5% improvement when tested with a variable-resistance device. In addition, when evaluating athletes each test should relate to the specific sport.

Tests should provide the athlete and coach with information concerning the athlete's ability to succeed in a specific sport. For example, the Wingate anaerobic power test is considered to be the gold standard in laboratory power measurements. However, because it is performed on a cycle ergometer, its relevance to many sports has been questioned. As a result, efforts have been made to develop anaerobic power tests that have a greater relevance to sports consisting of running or jumping.

Validity and Reliability of Testing

One of the most important characteristics of a test is its validity and reliability. Validity is the degree to which a test measures what it is intended to or claims to measure. Various types of validity are used for determining the effectiveness of an assessment:

- Content
- Predictive
- Concurrent
- Construct
- Face

Content validity concerns the degree to which a sample of test items represents the content that the test is designed to measure. For example, a physiology professor tells his class that the final exam will cover material in 15 chapters of the textbook. However, only 60 of the 100 exam questions can actually be found in those chapters. In the best-case scenario, a student in that class can prepare for only 60% of the exam. This test does not have strong content validity. An example involving physical assessment is utilizing an isometric measurement to assess strength in an athlete who participates in a dynamic sport. What validity does isometrically measuring maximal strength hold for assessing athletes playing a dynamic sport? On the other hand, using the squat to assess lower-body strength does have content validity due to the amount of muscle mass the squat recruits, the popularity of the squat in the training programs of most competitive athletes, and the similarity of the squat to movements in many sporting events.

Predictive validity is the degree to which predictions made by an assessment are confirmed by later actions of the subjects. It is a criterion-related validity, meaning that it measures how well a performance assessment measures the ability in another variable. An example of this is the National Football League (NFL) college combine. Each year the top 100 college football players are evaluated by every NFL team. These physical and medical evaluations assist the draft selection of each team. Another example is the standard aptitude test (SAT) used by admissions officers in various United States universities. Similar to the assessments at the NFL combine that are used to predict potential success in the NFL, the SAT scores are used to determine a student's potential for academic success in college.

Concurrent validity is another criterion-related validity. It is determined by relating test scores of a group of subjects to a criterion measure administered at the same time as or shortly after the test. The distinction between predictive and concurrent validity is the time at which the criterion measure is administered. An example of concurrent validity is using a vertical jump test to provide information on peak power.

Construct validity measures the extent to which a particular test can measure a hypothetical construct. For instance, intelligence, anxiety, and creativity are all hypothetical constructs because they are not directly seen but are rather inferred by their observable effects on behavior. Construct validity is not often seen in fitness and performance assessment. However, some researchers have used it to assess endurance runs as tests of aerobic capacity (Jackson et al. 1990) and tests of upper-body strength (Pate et al. 2003).

Face validity concerns the degree to which a test measures what it purports to measure. The other forms (content, predictive, concurrent, and construct) of validity provide evidence that an assess-

ment measures what it purports to measure. Face validity can only provide supplemental information about the other forms of validity, but it can never replace that information. For instance, the 40 yd sprint is universally accepted as a speed measure for football and many other sports, despite there not being a single study that has proven the validity of this sprint test. Since most strength and conditioning and football coaches believe that it is a valid measure of the speed of an athlete, it would be considered to have face validity.

Reliability is the ability of a test to produce consistent and repeatable results. Tests with proven reliability can reflect even slight changes in performance when evaluating a conditioning program. If a test is unreliable, differences in its results may reflect only the variation of the test and not the effectiveness of the training program. For example, if a test is administered to the same individual on two separate occasions and different results are obtained, the differences could be attributed to errors in measurement. When error is high, the reliability of the test is low. To estimate reliability, a correlation coefficient is computed between two sets of measures. This reliability coefficient ranges from 0.00 (no reliability) to 1.00 (perfect reliability) and reflects the extent to which a test is free of error variance. The square of the coefficient provides the amount of shared variance. For instance, a reliability coefficient of 0.70 suggests that 49% of the variance of a test can be explained by the other test. That is, if leg strength had a correlation coefficient of 0.70 to sprint speed, we can state that 49% of the variance in speed can be explained by the strength of the individual. The other 51% may be explained by other factors such as muscle fiber composition, training status, limb length, and body composition. In general, a reliability coefficient of 0.90 is desirable, but a coefficient of 0.80 is acceptable.

Several factors can influence reliability, including the type of test, the test length, and the range of abilities and ability levels of the individuals being tested. Tests of maximal effort appear more reliable than tests of submaximal effort due to the greater variability of submaximal tests. The duration of the test also affects reliability: the longer the duration, the greater the reliability. The ability of the individual taking the test is also an important factor. Younger students are generally less reliable than older students due to differences in motor ability. In assessments of all populations, experienced individuals generally have higher reliabilities than novices. Unfamiliarity with certain movement patterns or skills has a large effect on test reliability. Once the skill is learned, reliability improves. Oftentimes in athletes with little to no experience in a specific test, improvements in performance are rapid. These rapid improvements relate more to a learning effect than to any physiological adaptation.

Results of performance tests may vary due to differences in how testers assess the same test. This variability, known as *intertester reliability*, refers to the objectivity of a test. If a test is truly objective, then regardless of who assesses the skill the results should be similar. However, if scores vary with testers, the variability may be the result of differences in the experiences and abilities of the scorers. For instance, when timing a 40 yd (36.6 m) sprint, testers using handheld stopwatches often see differences when timing the same athlete during the same sprint. This variability may result from differences in the reaction delay between the moment that the athlete crosses the finish line and the moment that the tester presses the start button. Another example of how tester subjectivity can affect test outcome can be seen during the testing of maximal strength. When judging whether an athlete has reached the parallel position during a 1RM squat lift, testers can show differences in leniency (i.e., the magnitude of depth on the downward portion of the lift) that can result in different strength scores. If the coach assessing maximal strength performance at the end of a training program is stricter in judging the parallel position than the coach judging at the beginning of the program, the strength improvement of the athlete may be underestimated.

To minimize intertester variability, several factors should be controlled. The testers (e.g., coaches, physical educators) should be experienced in performing the test to establish a measure of consistency, and the same tester should perform both the pretest and posttest. Other sources for inconsistent results are inattentiveness on the part of the tester, failure to follow standardized procedures for calibrating the testing device, and failure to properly administer tests (Harman et al., 2000).

Test Administration

For accurate assessments, tests need to be administered safely and in an organized fashion. The time of assessment needs to be carefully planned, and the tests should be administered in proper sequence. Finally, all individuals being tested (either recreational or competitive athletes) should clearly understand the purpose of each test.

SAFETY CONSIDERATIONS

All individuals, regardless of the level of competition, should be advised to be medically cleared before participating in any health or performance assessment. Attaining medical clearance determines whether there is any contraindication to participating in an exercise program or a fitness assessment. The guidelines for exercise testing from the American College of Sports Medicine (ACSM), shown in table 1.2, suggest that it is unnecessary

TABLE 1.2 ACSM Guidelines for Exercise Testing and Participation

	APPARENTLY HEALTHY		HIGHER RISK*		
	Younger, ≤ 40 y (men) or ≤ 50 y (women)	Older	No symptoms	Symptoms	With disease**
Medical exam and diagnostic exercise test recommended before:					
moderate exercise	No	No	No	Yes	Yes
vigorous exercise	No	Yes	Yes	Yes	Yes
Physician supervision recommended during:					
submaximal testing	No	No	No	Yes	Yes
maximal testing	No	Yes	Yes	Yes	Yes

A *no* response means that an item is not necessary. A *yes* response means that an item is recommended. Moderate exercise is performed at an intensity ranging from 40% to 60% $\dot{V}O_2$max, while vigorous exercise is performed at an intensity exceeding 60% $\dot{V}O_2$max.

* = person with two or more risk factors (see Cardiovascular Disease Risk Factors on page 8);

** = person with known cardiac, pulmonary, or metabolic disease.

Adapted, by permission, from American College of Sports Medicine (ACSM), 2000, *Guidelines for exercise testing and prescription*, 6th ed. (Philadelphia, PA: Lippincott, Williams & Wilkins), 27.

Cardiovascular Disease Risk Factors

1. Diagnosed hypertension, systolic blood pressure ≥140 mmHg or diastolic blood pressure ≥90 mmHg on at least two separate occasions, or currently on antihypertension medication
2. Total serum cholesterol ≥200 mg/dl or high-density lipoprotein cholesterol <35 mg/dl or low-density lipoprotein cholesterol >100 mg/dl
3. Cigarette smoking
4. Obesity with a body mass index >30 kg/m^2
5. Family history of coronary or other atherosclerotic disease before age 55 in parents or siblings
6. Impaired fasting glucose >110 mg/dl
7. Sedentary lifestyle

Reprinted, by permission, from American College of Sports Medicine, 2000, *ACSM's Guidelines for Exercise Testing and Prescription*, 6th ed. (Philadelphia, PA: Lippincott, Williams & Wilkins), 24.

for asymptomatic, apparently healthy men under age 40 and women under age 50 to have a medical evaluation performed by a physician. In older individuals or individuals at higher risk (individuals with two or more of the cardiovascular disease risk factors shown above), the guidelines recommend that a physician be present during maximal testing but not necessarily present during submaximal testing if the individual is asymptomatic.

TIME OF ASSESSMENT

Tests for assessing the effectiveness of a training program should be administered before and after the program. Often, testing precedes the onset of a competitive season and provides information on the physical preparedness of the athletes. Novice individuals being evaluated before the onset of a fitness program should be provided with sufficient time to learn how to perform each test. Doing this allows a more accurate assessment, which provides a more effective exercise prescription. Figure 1.2 shows examples of possible testing dates for a strength or power sport at various times of the year and the primary purposes of these testing times.

TESTING BATTERY

Test selection is generally based on the relevance that a fitness component has for a particular sport or on the importance that each component has in screening health and appraising risk for coronary heart disease. For the athlete, a typical testing

Sample Testing Battery for a College Football Team

1. Anthropometry
   - Body mass
   - Body fat analysis
2. Strength assessment
   - 1RM bench press
   - 1RM squat
3. Power assessment
   - Vertical jump
   - Wingate anaerobic power test
4. Speed and agility assessment
   - 40 yd (36.6 m) sprint
   - T-drill
5. Anaerobic conditioning assessment
   - 300 yd (274.3 m) shuttle

battery may include strength tests for the upper and lower body, power tests, speed and agility tests, cardiovascular endurance tests, body composition tests, and flexibility tests (see sample shown above). For the recreational athlete who

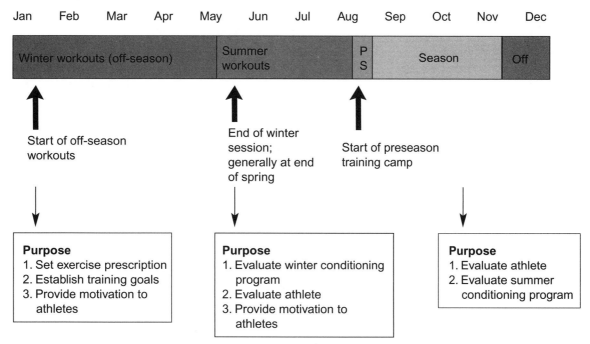

FIGURE 1.2   Examples of testing times for a strength or power sport.

Sample Assessment Program for a Recreational Athlete

1. Anthropometry
   - Body mass
   - Body fat analysis
2. Strength assessment
   - 6RM bench press
   - 6RM leg press
3. Flexibility assessment
   - Sit and reach
4. Cardiovascular endurance assessment
   - 1.5 mi (2.41 km) run

is primarily interested in health assessment, the testing battery may be quite different from that seen for the competitive athlete. An example of an assessment program for a recreational athlete can be seen above.

TESTING SEQUENCE

One of the most important concerns for the practitioner (e.g., coach or physical educator) is the order in which to perform the testing battery. In general, the least fatiguing tests should be performed first. Tests that require high-skill movements, such as agility measurements, should be performed before fatiguing tests. Any performance test that fatigues the athlete will confound the results of subsequent tests. For example, endurance exercise preceding strength training appears to significantly decrease strength expression (Leveritt and Abernathy 1999). However, no detrimental effects on endurance performance have been noted when strength testing is performed first. Thus, the more fatiguing tests (e.g., 300 yd or 274.3 km shuttle, line drill, 1.5 mi or 2.41 km run) should be performed last.

Many factors influence the testing sequence: the number of individuals being tested, the duration of the testing (i.e., 2 h, 1 d, or 2 d), and the number of coaches available to assist testing. In the ideal scenario, every athlete performs the same testing sequence, and if testing is performed over an extended time (i.e., over 2 d), the most fatiguing tests are performed last. However, due to time constraints the ideal testing situation may not be realistic. When testing a large group (i.e., a football team), several testing stations may need to be operating simultaneously. Athletes rotate through various stations within the set time for testing to be completed. Some athletes may perform a 40 yd (36.6 m) sprint followed by strength measurements, while others may perform strength tests followed by sprint and agility assessments. If proper rest is provided (at least 5 min between stations in order to restore the phosphagen energy system) (Harris et al. 1976), and endurance and shuttle runs (the most fatiguing tests) are still performed at the end of the testing battery, such a scenario is still likely to yield accurate results.

DELINEATION OF RESULTS

Once testing is completed, the information attained must be interpreted for the individual, and when appropriate, for the coach as well. How the results are interpreted relates to the goals of the testing program. If health assessment and disease risk are the primary goals of the fitness assessment, interpretation should be made in that light. Results for a competitive athlete can be compared to those of previous tests to evaluate her progress in the team's conditioning program, or results can be compared to those of other members of the team. Results can be compared to those of other athletes playing the same sport and position in order to evaluate an athlete's potential. Results can also be

used to prescribe exercise, develop training goals, and motivate athletes.

Summary

- Assessing the health and fitness levels of various populations is an integral part of the physical education, allied health, and sport science professions.
- The benefits of health and fitness assessment include creating athletic performance profiles and evaluating the health and wellness of the majority of our population.
- Several factors affect fitness assessment, including the body size, fiber type composition, and training status of the person being assessed as well as the specificity and relevance of the test.
- The validity and reliability of the testing must be determined in order for the testing to be meaningful.
- Test administration must be safe and well organized

CHAPTER 2

Interpretation of Normative Data

For assessment programs to have any meaning, the data collected must be evaluated and interpreted. *Data* are simply the results of measurement (Vincent 2005). Since the data collected during physical assessment are generally quantitative (i.e., are expressed in amounts or proportions and are not subject to evaluator judgment), they are called *quantitative data*. In contrast, data that require subjective judgment are referred to as *qualitative data*. For the data to have any substantial meaning, they must be treated through statistics. *Statistics* is a branch of applied mathematics concerned with the collection and interpretation of quantitative data and the use of probability theory to estimate population parameters. The *evaluation* of the statistical analysis gives meaning and value to the assessment.

This chapter describes basic statistical procedures to help the reader determine which statistical procedure is most appropriate for a particular question and provides the most meaningful interpretation of the data collected. This chapter does not detail the mathematical concepts used in developing an analysis. Readers interested in the development of these procedures should explore these concepts in statistics textbooks. This chapter emphasizes experimentation and hypothesis testing, descriptive statistics, correlation analysis, and basic inferential statistics.

Data Classification

In a testing battery used for assessment, each component of fitness that is tested is a *variable.* Variables can be classified as either discrete or continuous. A *discrete variable* is limited to whole numbers. For instance, the number of runs scored in a baseball game can only be expressed as a whole number. A team can score 3 runs but can never score 3.5 runs. Similarly, heart rates are expressed as beats per minute, as whole numbers or complete beats, and not as partial beats. In contrast, *continuous variables* can assume any value. Power output can be reported as a whole number but may also be measured to the tenth, hundredth, or thousandth decimal place, depending upon the sensitivity of the instrument being used for the measurement. The expression of time also depends on the sensitivity of the measuring instrument.

Data collected on variables can be categorized into four measurement scales. These scales provide for a more accurate interpretation of results and assist in determining an appropriate statistical analysis. A *nominal scale* is a set of mutually exclusive categories. Each category represents one aspect of an attribute being measured. Each score can represent only one category, and the ordering of the numbers has little to no meaning. Gender classification (male or female), experience status (experienced or novice), and simple yes or no questions are examples of data collected with a nominal scale. An *ordinal scale,* also referred to as a *rank-order scale,* is determined by ranking a set of objects according to specific characteristics. However, the scores between ranks have little meaning. For instance, in the National Collegiate Athletic Association (NCAA) ranking of the top 20 basketball teams, the number one team may be better than the 20th team; however, the difference in ranking does not imply that the top-ranked team is 20 times better than the 20th team. An *interval scale* has equal units, or intervals, arranged in a meaningful order. However, since there is no point of absolute zero on this scale, one point is not 2 or 3 times greater than another point. An example of an interval scale is temperature. Since there is no zero point (temperatures can be below 0°), it is inappropriate to state that 30° is twice as warm as 15°. It is appropriate to state that 30° is warmer. In a *ratio scale,* a zero score represents the absence of an attribute. Thus, the ordering of the numbers has meaning. A score of 80 is twice as big as a score of 40. Ratio scales are frequently used in measuring sport skills such as maximal strength, power, and speed.

Experimentation

In discussing statistical analysis, it is difficult to ignore its importance in research and experimentation. There are three primary categories of research. *Descriptive research* describes the characteristics of a population. It will likely be the category used for individuals performing fitness assessments. *Causal research* compares the relationship between two variables. For instance, investigators may compare anaerobic power to sprint speed in 200 m sprinters or may assess the relation of strength to team rank in football. *Experimental research* is concerned with the effects of manipulating variables. For example, an investigator may study the effect that protein supplementation has on lean-tissue accruement. As part of the research design, one set of subjects is given the actual supplement while another group is given a placebo. A placebo looks and tastes like the supplement but is inert, meaning that it does not contain any of the active ingredients of the supplement.

Hypothesis Testing

Most coaches or physical educators who use performance assessments on their students or athletes will not concern themselves with hypotheses. However, for the exercise scientist the hypothesis is the basis of a research project. A hypothesis usually predicts relationships or differences between groups. However, when hypotheses are tested statistically, it is usually stated that there is no relationship or difference between the groups. This is the *null hypothesis,* and the statistical analysis is performed to determine the probability that the results stated are true. If the probability that the results are true is large, then the null hypothesis is accepted. If the probability is small, the null hypothesis is rejected and the conclusion of the study states that there was a difference between the groups. When existing literature suggests that a difference does exist between the groups, investigators may use a *directional hypothesis.* Then the statistical analysis determines the probability that the results stated are true and that the directional hypothesis can be accepted (meaning that there is a difference between the groups) or rejected (meaning that there is no difference between the groups).

To determine whether to accept or reject a hypothesis, the researcher needs to establish a *level of confidence* or *level of significance.* In general, most researchers reject the null hypothesis if the probability against it is $\leq 5\%$. This is often reported as p (the probability that the hypothesis is false and that there is a significant difference) $\leq .05$. However, a more conservative $(p \leq .01)$ or liberal $(p \leq .10)$ probability level can also be used. There are two types of errors that can be made when accepting or rejecting the research hypothesis. A *Type I error* is committed when the hypothesis is true but is erroneously rejected. For instance, a Type I error occurs when the researcher incorrectly accepts the null hypothesis when differences actually exist. A *Type II error* is committed when the null hypothesis is accepted but should be rejected. That is, the researcher fails to detect an existing difference. Table 2.1 demonstrates the conditions in which Type I and II errors can be made.

Making a Type I error, or concluding that a difference exists when in reality it does not, can be quite dangerous. For instance, if a researcher examining a new drug for hypertension concludes that this new medication is superior to the more traditional drug when in reality there is no differ-

TABLE 2.1 Type I and II Errors		
	REALITY	
	Null hypothesis is true	**Null hypothesis is false**
Accept null	No error, conclusion is correct	Type II error, conclusion is incorrect
Reject null	Type I error, conclusion is incorrect	No error, conclusion is correct

Reprinted, by permission, from W.J. Vincent, 2005, *Statistics in kinesiology*, 3rd ed. (Champaign, IL: Human Kinetics), 143.

ence between the new and old drugs, hypertensive individuals may be at risk if prescribed this new medication. On the other hand, the conclusion that there is no difference between the two medications when in fact there is such a difference may prevent hypertensive individuals from being treated with a more effective medication. The Type II error may be less dangerous than the Type I, but it still prevents individuals from receiving a drug they can benefit from.

Descriptive Statistics

Descriptive statistics describe the basic features of the data, whether they are collected in a research investigation or during an assessment of a sport team. They are the basis for the quantitative analysis of data. The most common measures of descriptive statistics are the *measures of central tendency*. These measures are the most common score *(mode)*, the middle score *(median)*, and the average score *(mean)*.

The mode is the score that appears the most frequently. It can easily be found by inspecting the raw data. Once the data are tabulated by a frequency distribution, the most common score is the mode. In table 2.2, the resting heart rates of a physical education class are listed. The heart rate that occurs with the greatest frequency is 60 (appearing 8 times). Therefore, 60 is the mode.

The median is the score associated with the 50th percentile. In table 2.2, 29 resting heart rates are reported. Since the 50th percentile represents the 15th score, one can scan the cumulative frequency column to locate the 15th score and observe that the corresponding resting heart rate is 62. Thus, 62 is the median.

The mean is the average score of the class' resting heart rate. To calculate the mean, the resting heart rates are added (56 + 56 + 58 + 58 + 60 + 60 . . . + 72) and then divided by the total number of measurements (29). In the data in table 2.2, the average, or mean, resting heart rate is 62. The

TABLE 2.2 Resting Heart Rates of a Physical Education Class		
Resting heart rate (beats/min)	**Frequency**	**Cumulative frequency**
56	2	2
58	2	4
60	8	12
62	7	19
64	5	24
66	2	26
68	1	27
70	1	28
72	1	29

formula for the mean $(\bar{X})$ of a variable (X) is

$\bar{X} = \Sigma X / n$.

One of the advantages of creating a frequency distribution table is that upon scanning the scores one can identify any outliers. An *outlier* is a value in a data set that lies outside the limits of a typical score. An outlier, especially one in a relatively small sample, can greatly affect the sensitivity of the measure. For instance, if we measure an additional student, find that his resting heart rate is 120, and add that result to the groups' heart rates, the median and mode do not change. However, the mean becomes 64. This outlier would have an even greater effect in a data set including fewer heart rates.

When data are normally distributed, the mode, median, and mean are the same or close together (see figure 2.1). Figure 2.1a shows the *normal curve*, the most commonly reported curve in statistics. It is also referred to as the *Gaussian curve* or *bell-shaped curve* and is characterized by a symmetrical distribution of data about the center of the curve. In a normal curve the mean, mode, and median are the same. When the data are skewed, so that a disproportionate number of data points lies near one end of the scale, the scale is not normally distributed and is said to be *positively* or *negatively* skewed. In a positively skewed distribution most of the scores fall in the lower portion of the scale. This could mean that most of the people did not do well on an exam or that most people scored low on a specific assessment. In a positively skewed distribution the measures of central tendency proceed from left to right (mode, median, and mean). In a negatively skewed distribution most of the scores fall in the higher portion of the scale, suggesting that most of the people did well on a test or scored high on an assessment. In a negatively skewed distribution the order of central tendency is mean, median, and mode. Positively and negatively skewed distributions can be seen in figure 2.1, *b* and *c*.

In deciding which measure of central tendency to use, in a normal distribution the mean, mode, and median should give similar results. However, when scores are badly skewed in either direction and data are on an ordinal scale, Vincent (2005) recommends using the median. The mode may be appropriate when only a rough estimate of the measures of central tendency is needed. When data are presented on a ratio or interval scale, the mean is recommended, especially for making further calculations (i.e., standard deviations or standardized scores) (Vincent 2005).

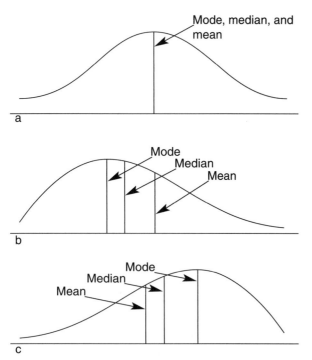

FIGURE 2.1 *(a)* Normal, *(b)* positive, and *(c)* negative distributions.

VARIABILITY MEASURES

Variability quantitatively measures the degree to which scores in a distribution deviate from the mean. The measures of central tendency provide the central tendency of the raw data. However, the data can be clustered around the mean or spread out. The measures of central tendency are unable to provide any information concerning the extent of the deviation.

The *range* is the simplest measure of spread. It equals the difference between the largest and the smallest values of a data set. Because of its simplicity, the range can be useful; however, it is very sensitive to extreme scores since it is based on only two values. Like the mode, it provides only a rough estimate since extreme scores can skew it. The range should almost never be used as the only measure of spread, but it can be used to supplement other measures of spread such as variance and standard deviation. The range of the data listed in table 2.2 is 56 to 72.

In examining the deviation of a score from the mean, it is logical to subtract the mean from each score $(X - \bar{X})$. However, in a normal distribution where half of the scores are below and half are above the mean, simply subtracting the mean from each score results in a zero variance, suggesting that there is no variability in the data set. Thus, to obtain a deviation that accurately describes the variance about the mean, the deviation is squared. This statistic is s^2, or V, and is known as the *variance*. Variance is the average of the sum of the squared deviations around the mean (Hinkle et al., 1988). However, variance may not be the ideal statistic for describing the dispersion of scores around the mean. Because it is the result of squaring the deviation scores, variance is generally disproportionate to the mean and hence is difficult to interpret. To transform variance into a statistic that is more easily understood, its square root is taken in order to convert it to a *standard deviation*. The standard deviation is more useful than the variance because it is computed in the units of the actual test. An example of the differences between variance and standard deviation can be seen in table 2.3. The mean of the scores is 28, and the variance (26.7) has little meaning compared to the mean, but since the standard deviation (5.2) is in the units of the actual test it is easier to understand and interpret. Standard deviation is the most common method for reporting the variability of a data set.

A small standard deviation indicates that the scores of a data set are closer to the mean, while

TABLE 2.3 Variance and Standard Deviation ($\bar{X}$ = 28)		
X	**D**	**D²**
20	–8	64
22	–6	36
24	–4	16
26	–2	4
28	0	0
30	2	4
32	4	16
34	6	36
36	8	64
$\Sigma \bar{X}$ = 252	ΣD = 0	ΣD^2 = 240
Variance = $\Sigma D^2 / n$ = 240 / 9 = 26.7		
Standard deviation = $\Sigma D^2 / n$ = 26.7 = 5.2		

X = score; D = difference.

a large standard deviation indicates scores that are spread out from the mean. In addition, the standard deviation allows scores to be interpreted relative to each variable. For instance, when examining football players' times for a 40 yd (36.6 m) sprint, scores may range from 4.2 to 5.74 s, with a mean of 4.95 s and a standard deviation of 0.32 s; however, when examining a 2 km run, scores may range from 6:58 to 15:30 min, with a mean of 9:49 min and a standard deviation of 1:06 min. The standard deviation in both of these variables relates to the performance time expressed for each measure and is in proper proportion to the mean, making it easy to interpret.

PERCENTILES

One of the more useful statistics used by coaches and physical educators to interpret data is the calculation of percentiles. *Percentiles* represent the fraction, or percent, in a distribution at or below which a given percentage of scores is found. For example, individual results from a 1RM bench press can be reported as a percentage of the results for the group being tested or as a percentage to standards set by the sport science literature. Percentiles can serve as a motivational tool by comparing athletes to their peers (e.g., team members) or to normative data for their respective sports. In addition, percentiles help coaches and educators accurately assess their athletes or students. Percentiles can be computed by hand but are easily generated by most statistical packages. Readers interested in the formulas used to compute percentiles by hand should consult a statistics textbook.

Percentiles are standard scores derived from raw data. Data on a 1RM squat from a Division III college football team are shown in figure 2.2. It is difficult to evaluate a single raw score of a player who can squat 405 lb (183.7 kg). However, when percentiles are used to compare this score to those for the rest of the players, the coach can see that this player performed better than 70% of the others.

An interesting phenomenon often occurs when evaluating performance with a percentile scale. Numerous sports physiology textbooks have suggested that during the early stages of a training program, the rate of performance improvement is quite large, and then it reduces until it eventually plateaus (Hoffman 2002; Fleck and Kraemer 2004). A freshman football player increasing his squat strength from 315 to 365 lb (142.9-165.6 kg) by his sophomore season showed a 15.9% improvement in strength but a 20% improvement on the percentile scale. A more experienced and stronger player whose initial 1RM squat was 450 lb (204.1 kg) had a similar absolute increase in squat strength (50 lb or 22.7 kg). However, this improvement was only a 12% increase on the percentile scale. Despite similar strength improvements, the more experienced and stronger athlete had a lower relative gain in percentile rank. Athletes whose strength levels are at the top of the scale will likely find it far more challenging to make further improvements as their strength levels may be close to their genetic ceilings (Hoffman 2002; Fleck and Kraemer 1997). Coaches and educators need to recognize the outstanding effort made by such athletes and understand that the closer the athlete is to the top of a performance scale, the more difficult it is for the athlete to improve.

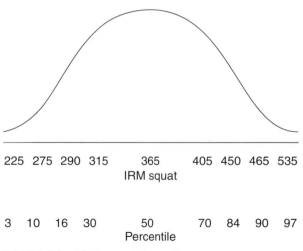

| 225 | 275 | 290 | 315 | | 365 | | 405 | 450 | 465 | 535 |

IRM squat

| 3 | 10 | 16 | 30 | | 50 | | 70 | 84 | 90 | 97 |

Percentile

FIGURE 2.2 1RM squat strength.

Z SCORES

Percentile ranks are one method for comparing raw scores. Another method is expressing the raw score in standard deviation units. This transformation describes the position of a single score in terms of the mean and standard deviation. This standard score is a *Z score*. A *Z* score of 0 indicates that the raw score equals the mean. A *Z* score above 0 indicates that the raw score is greater than the mean, while a negative *Z* score indicates a raw score that is less than the mean. The formula for computing a *Z* score is

$$Z \text{ score} = (X - \bar{X}) / SD,$$

where *X* is the raw score, $\bar{X}$ is the mean, and *SD* is the standard deviation.

For example, the mean 1RM squat for the Division III college football team reported in figure 2.2 is 367 lb (166.5 kg), with a standard deviation of 79 lb (35.8kg). What are the corresponding *Z* scores for players whose 1RM squats were 350, 400, and 525 lb (158.8, 181.4, and 238.1 kg)?

$Z \text{ score} = (350 - 367) / 79 = -17 / 79 = -0.22$

$Z \text{ score} = (400 - 367) / 79 = 33 / 79 = 0.42$

$Z \text{ score} = (525 - 367) / 79 = 158 / 79 = 2.0$

The first player had a negative score, indicating that his results were below the mean maximal squat strength of the team, while the other two players had scores that were above the mean.

The shape of the distribution of standard scores is always identical to that of the original distribution of raw scores. In addition, the mean of the distribution of *Z* scores is always 0, regardless of the mean of the raw scores.

Z scores can be used to compare scores of different distributions. For instance, if a coach wants to award the most outstanding athlete on the team, how could she objectively differentiate a player who is faster and jumps higher from a player who is stronger in the squat and bench press? One possible method is to convert all the raw scores to *Z* scores. The coach can then sum the *Z* scores and award the player with the highest total score. Table 2.4 shows the raw scores of eight college football players who were tested for strength (1RM bench press and 1RM squat), power (vertical jump), speed (40 yd or 36.6 m sprint), and agility (T-drill). Table 2.5 shows the conversion of the raw scores to *Z* scores and shows the combined *Z* score for each player. From the data in table 2.4 one can easily determine that Ellis has the highest overall *Z* score and should win the coach's award.

TABLE 2.4 Raw Scores of Strength, Power, Speed, and Agility of Selected College Football Players

	1RM bench press (kg)	1RM squat (kg)	Vertical jump (cm)	40 yd (36.6 m) sprint (s)	T-drill (s)
$\bar{X} \pm SD$	142 ± 20.1	167 ± 35.9	65.4 ± 8.3	4.95 ± 0.33	9.4 ± 0.51
Mark	140	150	67	4.90	8.9
Ellis	150	190	79	4.48	8.4
Steve	160	230	58	5.30	9.7
Stan	130	180	76	4.45	8.2
Matt	185	240	69	5.03	9.2

TABLE 2.5 Z Scores of Strength, Power, Speed, and Agility of Selected College Football Players

	1RM bench press	1RM squat	Vertical jump	40 yd (36.6 m) sprint	T-drill	Total Z score
Mark	-0.10	-0.47	0.19	0.15	0.98	0.75
Ellis	0.40	0.64	1.64	1.42	1.96	6.06
Steve	0.90	1.75	-0.89	-1.06	-0.59	0.11
Stan	-0.60	0.36	1.28	1.52	2.35	4.91
Matt	2.14	2.03	0.43	-0.24	0.39	4.75

However, when computing the Z score for variables in which a lower score indicates better performance (i.e., speed and endurance performance), the mean and raw score need to be reversed. The formula is

$Z \text{ score} = (\bar{X} - X) / SD.$

When the Z score is known, the percentage of area between the mean and Z score can be computed. In figure 2.3 the area under the curve is used to determine the percentage of scores lying between the mean and a given Z score. Table 2.6 provides the areas under the normal curve between the mean and the Z scores. To determine the proportion of this area, look down the column for the appropriate Z score, scan across to the column "Area from $\bar{X}$ to Z" (on the right) and record the percentage of scores listed. In a normal distribution 68.26% of the total scores lie between a Z score of –1 and +1 (34.13% between –1 and 0 and 34.13% between 0 and +1). This makes sense considering that most scores in a normal distribution lie close to the mean.

Table 2.6 can also be used to determine the percentage rank of a particular individual. For instance, if the coach is interested in the percentage rank of Ellis' time for a 40 yd (36.6 m) sprint (see tables 2.4 and 2.5), he can take the Z score (1.96) and determine that the area under the curve between the mean and a Z of 1.96 is .4750. Since .5000 of the area is below Z = 0, and since .5000 + .4750 = .9750, the total area below a Z of 1.96 is .9750, which means that the percentile rank of the score is 97.50%.

T SCORE

For some people, the Z score may be difficult to manage and report. When raw scores below the mean are converted to Z scores they become negative numbers, and parents of students, athletes, or others may not like to hear of a negative score. It may be easier for individuals to hear a different standard score.

A T score is a standard score that has a mean of 50 and standard deviations reported in intervals of 10. To compute a T score the Z score needs to be calculated first. A Z score is transformed into a T score with the following formula:

$T \text{ score} = 10 \, (Z \text{ score}) + 50.$

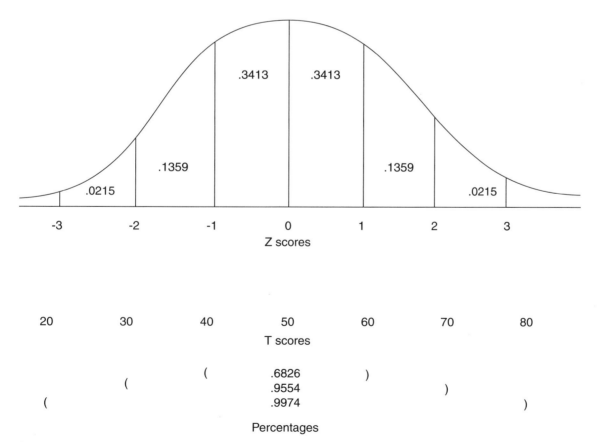

FIGURE 2.3   Percentage of area under the normal curve for selected Z scores.

TABLE 2.6 Areas Under the Normal Curve Between $\bar{X}$ and Z

Z	Area from $\bar{X}$ to Z	Z	Area from $\bar{X}$ to Z	Z	Area from $\bar{X}$ to Z	Z	Area from $\bar{X}$ to Z	Z	Area from $\bar{X}$ to Z
>0.00	.0000	0.41	.1628	0.82	.2967	1.23	.3925	1.64	.4505
0.01	.0040	0.42	.1664	0.83	.2995	1.24	.3944	1.65	.4515
0.02	.0080	0.43	.1700	0.84	.3023	1.25	.3962	1.66	.4525
0.03	.0120	0.44	.1736	0.85	.3051	1.26	.3980	1.67	.4535
0.04	.0160	0.45	.1772	0.86	.3078	1.27	.3997	1.68	.4545
0.05	.0199	0.46	.1808	0.87	.3106	1.28	.4015	1.69	.4554
0.06	.0239	0.47	.1844	0.88	.3133	1.29	.4032	1.70	.4564
0.07	.0279	0.48	.1879	0.89	.3159	1.30	.4049	1.71	.4573
0.08	.0319	0.49	.1915	0.90	.3186	1.31	.4066	1.72	.4582
0.09	.0359	0.50	.1950	0.91	.3212	1.32	.4082	1.73	.4591
0.10	.0398	0.51	.1985	0.92	.3238	1.33	.4099	1.74	.4599
0.11	.0438	0.52	.2019	0.93	.3264	1.34	.4115	1.75	.4608
0.12	.0478	0.53	.2054	0.94	.3289	1.35	.4131	1.76	.4617
0.13	.0517	0.54	.2088	0.95	.3315	1.36	.4147	1.77	.4625
0.14	.0557	0.55	.2123	0.96	.3340	1.37	.4162	1.78	.4633
0.15	.0596	0.56	.2157	0.97	.3365	1.38	.4177	1.79	.4641
0.16	.0636	0.57	.2190	0.98	.3389	1.39	.4192	1.80	.4649
0.17	.0675	0.58	.2224	0.99	.3413	1.40	.4207	1.81	.4656
0.18	.0714	0.59	.2257	1.00	.3438	1.41	.4222	1.82	.4664
0.19	.0753	0.60	.2291	1.01	.3461	1.42	.4236	1.83	.4671
0.20	.0793	0.61	.2324	1.02	.3485	1.43	.4251	1.84	.4678
0.21	.0832	0.62	.2357	1.03	.3508	1.44	.4265	1.85	.4686
0.22	.0871	0.63	.2389	1.04	.3531	1.45	.4279	1.86	.4693
0.23	.0910	0.64	.2422	1.05	.3554	1.46	.4292	1.87	.4699
0.24	.0948	0.65	.2454	1.06	.3577	1.47	.4306	1.88	.4706
0.25	.0987	0.66	.2486	1.07	.3599	1.48	.4319	1.89	.4713
0.26	.1026	0.67	.2517	1.08	.3621	1.49	.4332	1.90	.4719
0.27	.1064	0.68	.2549	1.09	.3643	1.50	.4345	1.91	.4726
0.28	.1103	0.69	.2580	1.10	.3665	1.51	.4357	1.92	.4732
0.29	.1141	0.70	.2611	1.11	.3686	1.52	.4370	1.93	.4738
0.30	.1179	0.71	.2642	1.12	.3708	1.53	.4382	1.94	.4744
0.31	.1217	0.72	.2673	1.13	.3729	1.54	.4394	1.95	.4750
0.32	.1255	0.73	.2704	1.14	.3749	1.55	.4406	1.96	.4756
0.33	.1293	0.74	.2734	1.15	.3770	1.56	.4418	1.97	.4761
0.34	.1331	0.75	.2764	1.16	.3790	1.57	.4429	1.98	.4767
0.35	.1368	0.76	.2794	1.17	.3810	1.58	.4441	1.99	.4772
0.36	.1443	0.77	.2823	1.18	.3830	1.59	.4452	2.00	.4778
0.37	.1480	0.78	.2852	1.19	.3849	1.60	.4463	2.01	.4783
0.38	.1517	0.79	.2881	1.20	.3869	1.61	.4474	2.02	.4788
0.39	.1554	0.80	.2910	1.21	.3888	1.62	.4484	2.03	.4793
0.40	.1591	0.81	.2939	1.22	.3907	1.63	.4495	2.04	.4798

Z	Area from $\bar{X}$ to Z	Z	Area from $\bar{X}$ to Z	Z	Area from $\bar{X}$ to Z	Z	Area from $\bar{X}$ to Z	Z	Area from $\bar{X}$ to Z
2.05	.4803	2.38	.4916	2.71	.4967	3.04	.4989	3.37	.4996
2.06	.4808	2.39	.4918	2.72	.4968	3.05	.4989	3.38	.4996
2.07	.4812	2.40	.4920	2.73	.4969	3.06	.4989	3.39	.4997
2.08	.4817	2.41	.4922	2.74	.4970	3.07	.4990	3.40	.4997
2.09	.4821	2.42	.4925	2.75	.4971	3.08	.4990	3.41	.4997
2.10	.4826	2.43	.4927	2.76	.4972	3.09	.4991	3.42	.4997
2.11	.4830	2.44	.4929	2.77	.4973	3.10	.4991	3.43	.4997
2.12	.4834	2.45	.4931	2.78	.4974	3.11	.4991	3.44	.4997
2.13	.4838	2.46	.4932	2.79	.4974	3.12	.4991	3.45	.4997
2.14	.4842	2.47	.4934	2.80	.4975	3.13	.4992	3.46	.4997
2.15	.4846	2.48	.4936	2.81	.4976	3.14	.4992	3.47	.4997
2.16	.4850	2.49	.4938	2.82	.4977	3.15	.4992	3.48	.4997
2.17	.4854	2.50	.4940	2.83	.4977	3.16	.4992	3.49	.4998
2.18	.4857	2.51	.4941	2.84	.4978	3.17	.4993	3.50	.4998
2.19	.4861	2.52	.4943	2.85	.4979	3.18	.4993	3.51	.4998
2.20	.4864	2.53	.4945	2.86	.4979	3.19	.4993	3.52	.4998
2.21	.4868	2.54	.4946	2.87	.4980	3.20	.4993	3.53	.4998
2.22	.4871	2.55	.4948	2.88	.4981	3.21	.4994	3.54	.4998
2.23	.4875	2.56	.4949	2.89	.4981	3.22	.4994	3.55	.4998
2.24	.4878	2.57	.4951	2.90	.4982	3.23	.4994	3.56	.4998
2.25	.4881	2.58	.4952	2.91	.4982	3.24	.4994	3.57	.4998
2.26	.4884	2.59	.4953	2.92	.4983	3.25	.4994	3.58	.4998
2.27	.4887	2.60	.4955	2.93	.4984	3.26	.4995	3.59	.4998
2.28	.4890	2.61	.4956	2.94	.4984	3.27	.4995	3.60	.4998
2.29	.4893	2.62	.4957	2.95	.4985	3.28	.4995	3.61	.4998
2.30	.4896	2.63	.4959	2.96	.4985	3.29	.4995	3.62	.4998
2.31	.4898	2.64	.4960	2.97	.4986	3.30	.4995	3.63	.4998
2.32	.4901	2.65	.4961	2.98	.4987	3.31	.4995	3.64	.4998
2.33	.4904	2.66	.4962	2.99	.4987	3.32	.4995	3.65	.4998
2.34	.4906	2.67	.4963	3.00	.4987	3.33	.4995	3.66	.4998
2.35	.4909	2.68	.4964	3.01	.4987	3.34	.4995	3.67	.4998
2.36	.4911	2.69	.4965	3.02	.4988	3.35	.4996	3.68	.4998
2.37	.4913	2.70	.4966	3.03	.4988	3.36	.4996	3.69	.4999

Thus, Z scores of 1.2, 0.48, and −1.4 would be transformed as such:

$T = 10 (1.2) + 50 = 62,$

$T = 10 (0.48) + 50 = 54.8,$

$T = 10 (-1.4) + 50 = 36.$

The relationships among Z scores, T scores, and percentiles are shown in figure 2.3.

Correlation

The relationship between two variables is a commonly used method of analysis in research, especially in the life sciences. For instance, a researcher investigating the effects of resistance training on both speed and strength may wish to know if the scores of these two dependent variables are related. That is, if scores in one variable improve, are improvements in the scores of the other variable related? Thus a *correlation* can be defined as a quantitative index that describes the extent to which two variables are related to, or associated with, each other. This quantitative index is known as a *correlation coefficient* and is a value between –1.00 and + 1.00. The correlation coefficient used most often in the life sciences is the *Pearson product-moment correlation coefficient,* symbolized by *r.* It was developed by the English statistician Karl Pearson (1857-1936).

The sign of the correlation coefficient indicates the direction of the relationship. A negative sign indicates that the scores are inversely related, meaning that as one score increases the other decreases. An example of a negative relationship is the relationship between improvement in lower-body strength and sprint speed. As an athlete increases lower-body strength, the improved strength may result in a faster sprint time. Since improved sprint speed is expressed as a reduction in sprint time, the increased strength and decreased time are inversely, or negatively, related. A positive correlation coefficient indicates that as one of the measured variables increases the other increases as well. Figure 2.4 uses scatter plots to illustrate the varying degrees of relationship between two variables.

In these scatter plots the data points are clustered around a line. This *line of best fit* provides the best linear estimate of the relationship between the two variables. The *slope* of the line indicates the general direction of the relationship. In a positive relationship the line of best fit has a positive slope and goes from the lower left corner to the upper right corner. If the line of best fit goes from the upper left corner to the lower right corner, it has a negative slope.

The magnitude of the correlation coefficient (i.e., how close the value is to 1) indicates the strength of the relationship. As the correlation coefficient approaches 1, the data points in a scatter plot approach the line of best fit. In a perfect correlation ($r = 1$), all the data points appear on the line. Most relationships between variables do not approach 1. Thus, the correlation coefficient must be interpreted in regard to the meaning of the relationship between the two variables. Table 2.7 provides criteria for interpreting the correlation coefficient.

The correlation coefficient not only measures the relationship between two variables but also

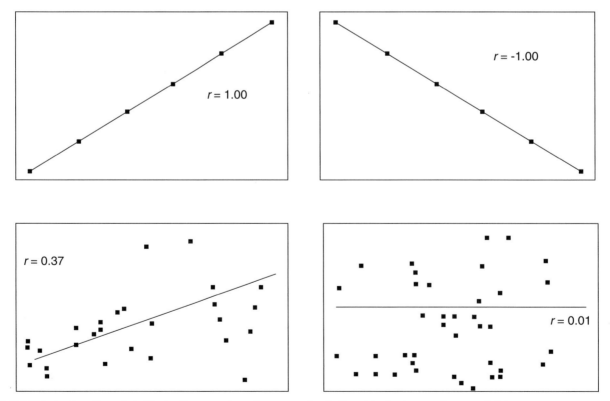

FIGURE 2.4 Scatter plots illustrating varying degrees of relationship between two variables.

TABLE 2.7 Interpretation of the Correlation Coefficient	
Range of correlation coefficient	**Interpretation**
0.90-1.00 (–0.90 to –1.00)	Very high positive (negative) correlation
0.70-0.90 (–0.70 to –0.90)	High positive (negative) correlation
0.50-0.70 (–0.50 to –0.70)	Moderate positive (negative) correlation
0.30-0.50 (–0.30 to –0.50)	Low positive (negative) correlation
0.00-0.30 (0.00 to –0.30)	Little, if any, correlation

Hinkle, Dennis E., William Wiersma, and Stephen G. Jurs, *Applied Statistics for the Behavioral Sciences*, Second Edition. Copyright © 1988 by Houghton Mifflin Company. Used with permission.

indicates the proportion of individual differences in one variable that can be associated with the individual differences in another variable (Hinkle et al. 1988). For example, an exercise scientist studying the relationship between strength and muscle size reports a correlation of 0.70 between 1RM squat strength and the cross-sectional area of the upper thigh. The magnitude of the correlation demonstrates a high positive correlation between these two variables. However, factors other than muscle size, such as training experience and fiber type composition, affect the expression of muscular strength.

The square of the correlation coefficient (r^2) equals the proportion of the total variance in one variable that can be associated with the variance in another variable. The square of the correlation coefficient (r^2) is the *coefficient of determination*. In the previous example $(r = 0.70, r^2 = 0.49)$, 49% of the variance in the cross-sectional area of the muscle is associated with the variance in leg strength. The coefficient of determination can also be illustrated by overlapping circles (see figure 2.5). Each circle represents one variable, with the overlap representing the proportion of shared variance.

When the scores of either one or both variables being correlated are ranks, using the Pearson cor-

relation coefficient is inappropriate. The *Spearman ρ coefficient* is the statistical analysis used to determine the relationship between ranked variables. For example, an exercise scientist investigating the relationship of team strength and speed to team rank in the NCAA Division I top 20 football teams needs to use the Spearman coefficient to determine the relationship between strength and speed and NCAA rank.

Inferential Statistics

Inferential statistics draws inferences about a population from a sample of the population. Experimental researchers manipulate a treatment variable and examine the resulting effects on specific dependent variables. For example, a research team wishes to examine the effects of protein supplementation on gains in lean body mass. In setting up the design protocol of the study the research team needs to decide which population to examine. All athletes? Specifically strength or power athletes? Regardless of the chosen population, it is impossible to study the entire population. Therefore, the researchers select a random sample of the chosen population and infer from the group studied what would occur if they had used the entire population.

The initial step in inferential statistics is to state the null or directional hypothesis. Once the hypothesis is developed, the researcher selects a level of significance. The level of significance is the probability that defines how rare or unlikely the sample data must be before the researcher can reject the hypothesis (Huck, Cormier, and Bounds 1974). Once the level of significance is selected, the researcher computes the calculated value, obtains the critical value, and finally decides whether to reject or accept the hypothesis.

As mentioned earlier, if the null hypothesis is rejected then the difference between the groups reflects a true difference between the population

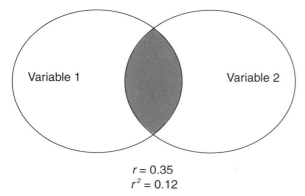

$r = 0.35$
$r^2 = 0.12$

FIGURE 2.5 The degree of shared variance between two variables.

means. A *test of statistical significance* determines whether to accept or reject the hypothesis. This test depends on numerous factors relating to the study design and the number of study groups. Exercise scientists use several statistical analyses, descriptions of which go beyond the scope of this text. The reader is highly recommended to consult with a statistics textbook for further details concerning these statistical analyses. However, brief explanations of common tests of significance are given in the remainder of this chapter.

t TESTS

The *t* test is a statistical analysis used most often in comparing the means of two groups. The means, variances, and sample sizes of the two groups are entered into a formula that produces a *t* value. The *t* value is compared to a critical value for *t* that relates to the *degrees of freedom* (the number of values in a data set less the number of restrictions placed on the values) and to the level of significance. Critical values for *t* are listed in a table found in practically any statistics textbook. A partial table of critical *t* values is seen in table 2.8. If the calculated *t* value exceeds the critical value of *t* found in the table, the researcher can conclude that a significant difference exists between the two sample means. For example, a researcher wanting to determine the effects of resistance training on bone mineral density selects two groups of subjects. The degrees of freedom for this study (*n* [number of total subjects] –1) is 20. The researcher selects $p \leq .05$ as the level of significance. The first group has, on average, 6 y of experience in resistance training, while the second group has no such experience. Both groups are tested for bone mineral density on a dual X ray absorptiometry unit. The researcher uses a *t* test to analyze the difference in the means, and the calculated *t* value is 2.54. By examining the critical values listed in table 2.8, the researcher determines that the calculated *t* value exceeds the critical value (2.086). The researcher concludes that there is a significant difference in bone mineral content between the groups.

For the *t* test to be valid several assumptions must be met:

- The population from which the sample is drawn is normally distributed.
- The subjects are randomly selected.
- The variances of the group are similar (there is *homogeneity of variance*).
- The data are on an interval or a ratio scale.

There are two specific types of *t* tests. The first is a paired, or dependent, *t* test, in which one group of subjects is measured under two different conditions. For instance, when examining subjects before and after a training program, the effectiveness of the program (e.g., whether performance gains are observed) is assessed through a paired *t* test. The second type of *t* test is the unpaired, or independent, *t* test. This test examines the mean difference between two groups of subjects. An unpaired *t* test is used when comparing bone density in experienced and novice weightlifters.

TABLE 2.8 Critical Values of the *t* Test (Two-Tailed Test)		
	LEVEL OF SIGNIFICANCE	
Degrees of freedom	**0.05**	**0.01**
2	4.303	9.925
4	2.776	4.604
8	2.306	3.355
10	2.228	3.169
15	2.131	2.947
20	2.086	2.845
30	2.042	2.750
40	2.021	2.704
60	2.000	2.660
120	1.980	2.617

Adapted, by permission, from E.S. Pearson and H.O. Hartley (Eds.), 1966, *Biometrika Tables for Statisticians, Vol I.*, 3rd ed. (London: Biometrika Trustees).

ONE-WAY ANALYSIS OF VARIANCE

When there are three or more sets of data, the *t* test is no longer appropriate. Instead, the *one-way analysis of variance (one-way ANOVA)* is the more appropriate statistical analysis. It is an extension of the *t* test, but rather than comparing the means of two groups it compares the variability of the group means *(between-group variability)* and the variability of the scores within the groups *(within-group variability)*. This comparison produces a value known as the *F ratio*. If the between-group variability exceeds the within-group variability, the F ratio is high and the researcher can conclude that one of the group means differs. This assessment of hypothesis validity is similar to that discussed for the *t* test. The primary differences are that an F ratio is calculated instead of a *t* value and that when the critical value is exceeded, instead of concluding that there is a significant difference between the means, the researcher can only know that at least one of the means was significantly different from the others.

Once a significant F ratio is determined, the researcher needs to ascertain where the differences exist. Several analytical procedures, referred to as *post-hoc analyses,* have been developed to do this. Post-hoc analyses use varying statistical techniques to locate statistical differences. These procedures range from liberal to conservative. A more liberal technique makes it easier to determine significant differences, while a more conservative technique makes it more difficult. The more liberal the test, the greater the risk for a Type I error.

REPEATED MEASURES ANOVA

A common research design in exercise science is examining two or more treatment groups over time. *Repeated measures ANOVA* is the inferential technique used to determine whether the mean scores on one or more factors significantly differ from each other and whether these various factors interact significantly with each other. For example, a researcher investigating the effect of creatine monohydrate on anaerobic power performance and recovery randomly assigns subjects to either an experimental group (given the study supplement) or a control group (given a placebo). All subjects are tested before, during, and after 10 wk of supplementation. The statistical analysis that this researcher uses is a repeated measures 2 (groups) × 3 (times) ANOVA. Similar to the one-way ANOVA, an F ratio is computed and if it is significant, post-hoc analyses are performed to determine where significant differences exist.

Summary

- The coach's or physical educator's understanding of basic statistical procedures is important for properly interpreting physical and health assessments.
- Descriptive statistics provide measures of central tendency, percentile ranks, and standardized scores. They describe the characteristics of a population.
- Variability measures such as standard deviation determine how scores deviate from the mean.
- Standard scores such as *Z* scores and *T* scores allow comparisons of scores from different distributions.
- Correlational analysis describes the extent to which two variables are related to or associated with each other.
- Inferential statistics such as *t* tests and analyses of variance help researchers examine how manipulating one or several treatment variables affects specific dependent variables.

PART II

Fitness and Performance Norms

CHAPTER 3

Muscular Strength

Muscular strength refers to the force that a muscle or muscle group can exert in a single maximal effort (Harman, Garhammer, and Pandorf 2000). It is a common fitness measure for assessing the strength or power athlete. Maximal strength can be quantified through directly assessing the maximal weight an individual can lift in a specific exercise (i.e., bench press or squat), the amount of force generated in an isometric contraction, or the amount of torque generated during an isokinetic contraction. The most popular method of assessing strength in competitive athletes is the maximal strength testing of exercises that are common to an athlete's training program. Maximal strength can be measured directly by recording the maximal load an athlete can lift one time or indirectly by having the athlete lift a submaximal weight for as many repetitions as possible. The efficacy of these methods is discussed in this chapter. In addition, other modes of strength assessment are explained, and normative and descriptive data of strength assessment for various subject populations are presented.

Strength Testing

As discussed in chapter 1, there are several purposes underlying assessment programs, including determining the effectiveness of a training program, comparing individuals to population norms, and predicting potential sport performance. To maximize the effectiveness of the strength test, the test should use an exercise that is part of the individual's training program and a movement pattern and muscle mass similar to that routinely recruited during sport performance (Hoffman, Maresh, and Armstrong 1992). Strength testing generally involves multijoint exercises that use a large muscle mass. It generally assesses both upper- and lower-body strength. Typically, the exercises recruit the greatest amount of muscle mass possible for a particular body part. For instance, the bench press is commonly accepted as the ideal measure for upper-body strength because of the large muscle mass it recruits and its popularity in training programs. The lower body tends to show more variability in any chosen exercise, but the choice is generally between the squat and the leg press. Both exercises recruit a similar muscle mass (hip extensors and knee flexors), but the squat has a greater sport-specific movement pattern that makes it a more appropriate lower-body strength test for many athletic populations.

Strength testing can also use an exercise that recruits a smaller muscle mass of an isolated joint action. Force outputs from an isometric contraction assessed by a dynamometer or an isokinetic testing device are used to determine specific muscle or joint strength. For example, comparing muscle groups from bilateral limbs (i.e., right knee flexors versus left knee flexors) or from agonist and antagonist muscle groups (i.e., knee flexors versus knee extensors) may find a potential weakness that can predispose the athlete to injury.

ISOMETRIC TESTING

An isometric contraction measures force produced without joint movement. Any force assessed through such a device (e.g., handgrip dynamometer) is specific to the joint angle measured. Although the ease in data assessment for and the reliability of isometric testing have been established for both male and female populations in various age groups (Bemben et al. 1992; Christ et al. 1994), the usefulness of such testing has been questioned. Wilson and colleagues (1995) have shown that isometric testing does not relate to dynamic performance in male competitive athletes. Considering that most athletic events are dynamic, the information provided by an isometric force measurement does appear limited. Still, various sport scientists, athletic trainers, and physical therapists use such testing to evaluate both injured and healthy athletes.

A popular isometric testing device is the handgrip dynamometer (see figure 3.1). It is often used in athletic populations in which grip plays an important role (i.e., in baseball and tennis players). Grip strength is generally measured with a commercially available handgrip dynamometer. Both the dominant and nondominant hands are measured. The arm is held straight at the side with the elbow in a fully extended position, or the elbow is held at a 90° angle. Following two maximal efforts, the higher score is recorded in kg. Descriptive data on grip strength for various athletic populations are shown in table 3.1. Table 3.2 provides normative percentile data for right and left grip strength in recreationally active boys and girls between the ages of 7 and 12. Previous studies have shown no significant strength differences between genders at these age groups (Blimkie 1989; Faigenbaum, Milliken, and Westcott 2003). Table

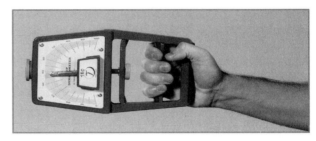

FIGURE 3.1   Handgrip dynamometer.

TABLE 3.1 Descriptive Data for the Handgrip Dynamometer (in kg)				
Population	Gender	Dominant hand	Nondominant hand	Source
Baseball				
13 y	M	26.1 ± 6.6		Unpublished data
14 y	M	32.3 ± 7.2		Unpublished data
15 y	M	37.3 ± 6.7		Unpublished data
16 y	M	40.7 ± 6.5		Unpublished data
17 y	M	43.4 ± 7.3		Unpublished data
NAIA	M	45.2 ± 8.4	45.6 ± 6.8	Unpublished data
NCAA DII	M	57.0 ± 6.7		Hughes, Lyons, and Mayo 2004
Boxing				
Middleweight Italian amateurs	M	58.2 ± 6.9		Guidetti, Musulin, and Baldari 2002
Softball				
Masters	F	37.3 ± 6.9	38.4 ± 6.0	Terbizan et al. 1996
Tennis				
Ranked junior players (11.6 ± 0.6 y)	M	22.0 ± 5.8	18.4 ± 5.1	Roetart et al. 1992
Collegiate	F	36.6 ± 4.0	33.3 ± 2.2	Kraemer et al. 2003
Competitive (30.2 ± 5.8 y)	M	27.7 ± 2.7	22.2 ± 2.8	Ellenbecker 1991

TABLE 3.2 Percentile Ranks for Handgrip Strength (kg) in Recreationally Active Children

% rank	7-8 Y		9-10 Y		11-12 Y	
	Right hand	Left hand	Right hand	Left hand	Right hand	Left hand
90	19.5	20.0	22.0	22.0	29.7	27.5
80	18.0	18.5	21.5	20.0	27.3	24.6
70	17.5	17.8	20.0	19.1	24.9	22.5
60	17.0	16.0	20.0	18.4	22.2	22.0
50	16.0	15.5	19.0	18.0	22.0	20.0
40	15.0	14.5	18.0	17.0	21.5	19.0
30	13.5	13.0	17.0	16.0	21.0	19.0
20	13.5	12.0	16.0	15.5	20.0	17.4
10	12.0	12.0	15.0	15.0	18.0	16.4
$\bar{X}$	16.0	15.5	18.9	18.0	23.0	21.2
SD	3.2	3.0	3.0	2.7	3.9	4.2
n	54	54	102	102	46	46

TABLE 3.3 Normative Values of Dominant Grip Strength (kg) in Adults

	20-29 Y		30-39 Y		40-49 Y		50-59 Y		60-69 Y	
	M	F	M	F	M	F	M	F	M	F
Excellent	>54	>36	>53	>36	>51	>35	>49	>33	>49	>33
Good	51-54	33-36	50-53	34-36	48-51	33-35	46-49	31-33	46-49	31-33
Average	43-50	26-32	43-49	28-33	41-47	27-32	39-45	25-30	39-45	25-30
Fair	39-42	22-25	39-42	25-27	37-40	24-26	35-38	22-24	35-38	22-24
Poor	<39	<22	<39	<25	<37	<24	<35	<22	<35	<22

Adapted, by permission, from L.R. Gettman, 1993, Fitness testing. In *ACSM's resource manual for guidelines for exercise testing and prescription*, 2nd ed., edited by J.L. Durstine, et al. (Philadelphia, PA: Lippincott, Williams & Wilkins), 229-246.

3.3 provides normative values for dominant grip strength in adults.

ISOKINETIC TESTING

Isokinetic testing devices measure joint movement at a constant velocity. The device meets the force exerted by a moving body segment during an isokinetic contraction with an equal and opposite resistance that constantly alters as the body segment moves through its full range of motion. The force exerted by the body segment to rotate about its axis is referred to as torque, which is expressed in newton-meters (N·m). The test–retest reliability of isokinetic devices is well established (Farrel and Richards 1986). Since isokinetic testing only evaluates a single joint unilateral movement, its role in strength evaluation is primarily evaluating peak torque outputs about specific joints and the athlete's potential for muscle injury from a bilateral deficit or a muscle imbalance (Hoffman, Maresh, and Armstrong 1992).

Peak torque is a reliable indicator of muscle function in both healthy and injured joints. Torque outputs of specific muscle groups surrounding a joint measure the integrity and stability of the joint. Since measuring all muscle joints is not efficient, generally the joint in which the primary movement in sport occurs or the joint at the highest risk for injury is assessed. The knee joint is the one most frequently measured in both competitive and recreational athletic populations. The velocity tested ranges from slow (60°/s) to moderate (180°/s) to fast (300°/s). When testing at a single velocity, the moderate speed of contraction is generally used. Table 3.4 provides peak torque outputs in various athletic populations.

		60°/S		180°/S		300°/S		
Population	**Gender**	**Flex**	**Ext**	**Flex**	**Ext**	**Flex**	**Ext**	**Source**
Basketball								
NCAA DI	M	165.4 ± 26.2	178.1 ± 32.9	133.2 ± 21.2	135.3 ± 29.7	101.1 ± 30.7	96.9 ± 34.0	Hoffman, Fry et al. 1991
Canadian national	F	125.9 ± 22.7	200.5 ± 30.3					Smith and Thomas 1991
Greek professional	M	187.7 ± 44.6	287.2 ± 62.9	127.3 ± 29.2	151.7 ± 37.5			Theoharopoulos et al. 2000
Kickboxing								
Canadian elite	M		220.0					Zabukovec and Tiidus 1995
Soccer								
Youth club, 16.4 ± 1.1 y	F	88.0 ± 25	156.1 ± 35					Nyland et al. 1997
Youth club, 15.7 ± 0.7 y	M	119.1 ± 21.7	201.0 ± 32					Kraemer et al. 2004
NCAA DI	M	152.0 ± 9.3	240.3 ± 11.1					
Speed skating								
Canadian elite	F			99.0 ± 11.6	130.2 ± 15.3			Smith and Roberts 1991
	M			145.5 ± 26.2	195.9 ± 18.4			
Wrestling								
High school	M			115.6 ± 28.7	211.3 ± 43.3	57.6 ± 14.0	76.4 ± 6.8	Housh et al. 1997
NCAA DI	M	156.9 ± 9.9	256.2 ± 12.1			98.6 ± 7.0	100.8 ± 6.8	Kraemer et al. 2001
Volleyball								
NCAA DI	F	77.8 ± 10.3	153.3 ± 26.2	59.2 ± 9.1	115.8 ± 21.0	48.5 ± 8.1	88.8 ± 19.4	Fry et al. 1991

TABLE 3.4   Peak Torque Output (N·m) for Knee Extension and Flexion in Athletic Populations

Flex = flexion; Ext = extension. 60°/s = 1.05 rad/s; 180°/s = 3.14 rad/s; 300°/s = 5.24 rad/s.

Peak torque measures are frequently utilized in bilateral comparisons and to establish a ratio between agonist and antagonist muscle groups. The hamstring-to-quadriceps ratio (H:Q) is the most prevalent agonist-to-antagonist relationship reported for the lower body. A 6:10 strength is accepted as the normal H:Q (Hoffman, Maresh, and Armstrong 1992). However, 2:3 (Fry and Powell 1987) and 3:4 (Knapik et al. 1991) have also been reported as acceptable. The H:Q can also be reported as a percentage. That is, a 2:3 H:Q can be reported as the hamstring muscle group being 67% as strong as the quadriceps. Large variation is often seen in the H:Q among athletes participating in different sports and among different testing velocities. Reported ratios range from 51% in female college volleyball athletes to greater than 100% in NCAA Division I basketball players (see table 3.5). This wide variation likely reflects the specific demands of each sport as well as the specific speed of contraction.

Differences in the H:Q may be a function of resistance training. A lower H:Q observed at slow contraction velocities may reflect the type of strength training employed. For example, the squat may disproportionately increase knee extensor strength at a slow velocity (i.e., 60°/s), reducing the H:Q (Fry and Powell 1987). In addition, the type of athlete being tested also influences the H:Q. Athletes involved in high-intensity anaerobic activities such as basketball, football, and ice hockey have greater knee flexor strength, which

TABLE 3.5 Hamstring-to-Quadriceps Ratios (%) of Athletic Populations

Population	Gender	60°/s	180°/s	300°/s	Source
Basketball					
NCAA DI	M	93	98	104	Hoffman, Fry et al. 1991
Canadian national	F	63			Smith and Thomas 1991
Greek professional	M	65	84		Theoharopoulos et al. 2000
Football					
High school	M				Parker et al. 1983
15 y			80		
16 y			75		
17 y			78		
NCAA DII	M		78	89	Housh et al. 1988
Ice hockey					
Canadian national	M		76		Smith et al. 1982
Professional	M		86		
Soccer					
Youth club					Nyland et al. 1997
16.4 ± 1.1 y	F	56			
15.7 ± 0.7	M	59			
NCAA DI	M	63			Kraemer et al. 2004
Swedish national	M		74		Oberg et al. 1986
U.S. national	M	56			Mangine et al. 1990
Speed skating					
Canadian elite	F		76		Smith and Roberts 1991
	M		74		
Sprinting					
NCAA DI	M	55	63	66	Anderson et al. 1991
Wrestling					
High school	M			55	Housh et al. 1997
NCAA DI	M	61			Kraemer et al. 2001
Volleyball					
NCAA DI	F	51	51	55	Fry et al. 1991

60°/s = 1.05 rad/s; 180°/s = 3.14 rad/s; 300°/s = 5.24 rad/s.

results in a high H:Q at all contraction speeds (Hoffman, Fry et al. 1991; Housh et al. 1988; Smith et al. 1982). Table 3.5 provides H:Q data in various athletic populations.

Isokinetic testing at different velocities of muscle contraction has merit; however, testing at fast velocities in the lower limb may have added importance considering the greater power of the knee flexors (hamstring muscle group) at fast speeds (Read and Bellamy 1990). Knapik and colleagues (1991) reported that female athletes with an H:Q less than 75% at 180°/s were 1.6 times more likely to experience injury than athletes with stronger knee flexors. However, the same study

indicated that the H:Q may not independently predict injury when bilateral comparisons are also considered.

Initial studies examining differences in bilateral strength reported that ratios greater than 10% in the knee flexors enhanced the likelihood of muscle injury (Burkett 1970). However, subsequent studies have suggested that strength deficits between bilateral muscle groups may reach 15% before the injury rate significantly increases (Knapik et al. 1991). In athletes with strength imbalances greater than 15%, the incidence of muscle injury has been reported as 2.6 times greater (Knapik et al. 1991). Still, others have been unable to conclusively determine that a bilateral deficit is a significant predictor of injury in the lower leg (Worrell et al. 1991). Although bilateral deficits in the lower extremity that exceed 10% to 15% may raise concern, normative strength balances are still uncertain.

In some athletes bilateral deficits are seen in muscles of the shoulder, elbow, and wrist due to activity patterns that rely predominantly on unilateral arm action (e.g., patterns in tennis or in baseball pitching) (Cook et al. 1987; Ellenbecker 1991). Strength differences in the upper limb have approached 20% in tennis athletes and baseball pitchers. These large bilateral differences may be compounded by the non-weight-bearing requirements of the upper-body musculature. Whether this large difference affects performance negatively or increases the risk for injury is not fully understood.

In athletes who rely on unilateral arm action during performance, significant differences in agonist and antagonist strength balance (e.g., in shoulder internal and external rotators) have been reported (Cook et al. 1987; Ellenbecker 1991; McMaster, Long, and Caiozzo 1991). These imbalances have been attributed to the emphasized shoulder adduction and internal rotation of these activities (tennis, baseball pitching, or water polo) and are characterized by weakness in the external rotators and by significantly stronger internal rotators in the dominant shoulder. Since the external rotators stabilize the shoulder joint, any imbalance may potentiate injury in athletes who have laxity in the shoulder capsule (McMaster, Long, and Caiozzo 1991).

DYNAMIC CONSTANT RESISTANCE

Using dynamic constant resistance exercises (e.g., bench press and squat) is the most common form of strength testing among athletes, primarily because these exercises simulate actual sport movement and recruit a large muscle mass. In addition, most athletes use dynamic constant resistance exercises as part of their resistance training programs. The

controversy frequently encountered in testing maximal strength is whether to test for a 1-repetition maximum (1RM) or to test for the number of repetitions that can be performed with a submaximal load. Often the reason for choosing the submaximal test is to save time. In general, a 1RM is achieved within 3 to 5 attempts. When testing a large group of athletes (such as a football team), time becomes a critical element. For instance, with a team of 60 the total sets performed may range from 180 to more than 300. Depending on the number of testing stations, testing can become a daunting task. The risk of injury from a maximal lift may also be a potential drawback for using the 1RM.

Several studies have shown that using submaximal loads to predict maximal strength is highly valid (with correlation coefficients >0.90) (Landers 1985; Mayhew, Ball, and Bowen 1992; Mayhew et al. 1999). Many teams in the National Football League (NFL) routinely use submaximal testing to estimate the maximal strength of their players. However, several studies have also reported that the number of repetitions performed at selected percentages of the 1RM varies among different exercises and that the variance within an exercise is also quite large (Hoeger et al. 1987, 1990). Table 3.6 provides several published formulas for predicting a 1RM. However, most of these equations significantly underestimate or overestimate maximal strength performance in strength-trained athletes (Ware et al. 1995). The NFL 225 lb (102.1 kg) bench press test for maximal upper-body strength has been reported to be accurate as long as fewer than 10 repetitions are performed (Mayhew et al. 1999). If more than 10 repetitions are performed the test loses its validity and underestimates actual strength. Table 3.7 provides percentiles of the NFL 225 lb (102.1 kg) bench press test and the predicted 1RM values for prospective NFL players participating in the NFL combine.

An additional concern in using 1RM tests to assess maximal strength is increasing the risk for injury. However, no published reports have

TABLE 3.6 Equations for Predicting the 1RM Strength Test	
Equation	Source
Repetition weight / (1.0278 − 0.0278 (reps))	Brzycki 1993
(0.033) (reps) (repetition weight) + repetition weight	Epley 1985
(100) (repetition weight) / (101.3 − 2.67123(reps))	Landers 1985
(100) (repetition weight) / (52.2 + 41.9 $e^{-0.055 \text{ (reps)}}$)	Mayhew, Ball, and Bowen 1992
(100) (repetition weight) / (48.8 + 53.8 $e^{-0.075 \text{ (reps)}}$)	Wathen 1994

TABLE 3.7 Percentiles for the Bench Press and the Predicted 1RM for Players in the NFL Combine

	DB			DL			LB		
		PRED 1RM			PRED 1RM			PRED 1RM	
% rank	Reps	lb	kg	Reps	lb	kg	Reps	lb	kg
90	18.0	345	157	28.1	416	189	29.3	423	192
80	17.0	340	155	26.0	400	182	27.0	405	184
70	15.0	325	148	25.0	395	180	26.0	400	182
60	14.0	320	145	24.0	385	175	25.2	396	180
50	13.0	315	143	23.0	380	173	22.5	378	172
40	12.0	305	139	21.6	371	169	21.6	372	169
30	10.0	295	134	20.0	360	164	19.1	356	162
20	10.0	295	134	18.8	353	160	15.4	329	150
10	8.0	280	127	17.0	340	155	13.7	319	145
$\bar{X}$	13.2	315	143	22.8	378	172	22.2	375	170
SD	4.1	28	13	4.4	29	13	5.7	38	17
n	62			68			26		

	OL			RB			TE		
		PRED 1RM			PRED 1RM			PRED 1RM	
% rank	Reps	lb	kg	Reps	lb	kg	Reps	lb	kg
90	30.0	430	195	23.0	380	173	27.4	411	187
80	27.0	405	184	20.0	360	164	24.2	389	177
70	25.6	398	181	19.0	355	161	22.4	377	171
60	24.0	385	175	18.0	345	157	20.4	363	165
50	23.0	380	173	18.0	345	157	19.0	355	161
40	22.0	375	170	17.0	340	155	18.0	345	157
30	21.0	365	166	16.0	335	152	18.0	345	157
20	20.0	360	164	15.0	325	148	17.4	342	155
10	17.0	340	155	14.0	320	145	13.8	320	145
$\bar{X}$	23.3	382	174	17.9	346	157	20.1	361	164
SD	5.1	35	16	3.3	22	10	4.2	28	13
n	97			67			11		

Pred 1RM = predicted 1RM; DB = defensive back; DL = defensive line; LB = linebacker; OL = offensive line; RB = running back; TE = tight end.
Data from 1999 NFL player combine.

determined whether a greater risk of injury exists when properly performing a 1RM test than when performing a submaximal test. Using safety precautions (i.e., spotters, proper technique, and qualified supervision) minimizes the possibility for injury. In addition, the resistance selected during a 1RM is generally based on the training experience of the athlete. That is, from the training history of the athlete both the athlete and the coach should have an idea of what the maximum strength in a particular exercise should be. When competitive athletes undergo submaximal testing and perform a maximal number of repetitions with an absolute resistance, the last repetition is an RM. Regardless of whether it's an 8RM, a 14RM, or even a 25RM, the athlete performs an RM with a potentially fatigued muscle. A fatigued muscle may be more susceptible to injury due to changes in neuromuscular recruitment patterns or to muscle and tendon stress. Thus, when testing a strength-trained athlete the risk of injury may be lower when performing a 1RM than when performing a maximal number of repetitions with a submaximal load. A protocol for assessing a 1RM follows:

1. Perform a warm-up set of 10 repetitions at a resistance that equals approximately 50% of the expected 1RM.
2. Perform another warm-up set of 5 repetitions at a resistance that equals approximately 75% of the expected 1RM.
3. Rest 3 to 5 min.
4. Perform 1 repetition with a resistance that equals approximately 90% to 95% of the expected 1RM.
5. Rest 3 to 5 min.
6. Attempt a 1RM lift.
7. Rest 3 to 5 min.
8. If the 1RM lift was successful, increase the resistance and attempt a new 1RM.
9. Continue this protocol until failure.

The bench press, squat, and power clean are widely used dynamic constant resistance tests for upper-body strength, lower-body strength, and explosive power, respectively. These tests have been demonstrated to have strong test–retest reliability (with $r > 0.90$) (Hoffman et al. 1990, Hoffman, Fry et al.1991). For some populations (e.g., children and deconditioned or novice adults) it may be preferable to test for strength in a controlled environment using exercise machines. Utilizing exercise machines does not reduce either the reliability or the validity of the strength test as long as the exercise is part of the training program of the individual. However, machines may not be appropriate for an athletic population considering their lack of specificity to dynamic, sport-specific movements.

📖 For descriptions and photos of the bench press, squat, and power clean, please see pages 190-193 in the appendix.

Considering that strength testing is a common assessment tool of many athletic programs it is surprising that there are limited normative data on general populations and little or no data on various athletic populations. Tables 3.8, 3.9, and 3.10 provide normative values (relative to body weight) for the bench press, squat, and leg press in various age groups in the general population. Table 3.11 provides strength–mass ratios of selected exercises in college-aged men and women. Table 3.12 shows percentile ranks for children performing 1RMs on both the chest press and leg press machines. These data combine both boys and girls. As mentioned earlier, studies have shown no significant gender differences in these age groups (Blimkie 1989; Faigenbaum, Milliken, and Westcott 2003).

The percentile values for the 1RM bench press, squat, and power clean in high school and college football players can be seen in table 3.13. Tables 3.14 and 3.15 provide the percentile values for these exercises in NCAA Division I female and male athletes. Information for descriptive strength measurements on various athletic populations is limited in the sport science literature. Table 3.16 provides strength measurements of various male and female athletic populations. When possible, position-specific strength measurements for different sports are reported.

TABLE 3.8 Normative Values for Relative Bench Press Strength (1RM / body mass) in a General Population

% rank	20-29 Y M	20-29 Y F	30-39 Y M	30-39 Y F	40-49 Y M	40-49 Y F	50-59 Y M	50-59 Y F	60+ Y M	60+ Y F
90	1.48	0.54	1.24	0.49	1.10	0.46	0.97	0.40	0.89	0.41
80	1.32	0.49	1.12	0.45	1.00	0.40	0.90	0.37	0.82	0.38
70	1.22	0.42	1.04	0.42	0.93	0.38	0.84	0.35	0.77	0.36
60	1.14	0.41	0.98	0.41	0.88	0.37	0.79	0.33	0.72	0.32
50	1.06	0.40	0.93	0.38	0.84	0.34	0.75	0.31	0.68	0.30
40	0.99	0.37	0.88	0.37	0.80	0.32	0.71	0.28	0.66	0.29
30	0.93	0.35	0.83	0.34	0.76	0.30	0.68	0.26	0.63	0.28
20	0.88	0.33	0.78	0.32	0.72	0.27	0.63	0.23	0.57	0.26
10	0.80	0.30	0.71	0.27	0.65	0.23	0.57	0.19	0.53	0.25

Adapted from V.H. Heyward, 2002, *Advanced fitness assessment & exercise prescription*, 4th ed. (Champaign, IL: Human Kinetics), 119. Data from The Cooper Institute, Dallas, TX, 1994.

TABLE 3.9 Normative Values for Relative Squat Strength (1RM / body mass) in a General Population

	20-29 Y		30-39 Y		40-49 Y		50-59 Y		60+ Y	
	M	F	M	F	M	F	M	F	M	F
Excellent	>2.07	>1.62	>1.87	>1.41	>1.75	>1.31	>1.65	>1.25	>1.55	>1.14
Good	2.00	1.54	1.80	1.35	1.70	1.26	1.60	1.13	1.50	1.08
Average	1.83	1.35	1.63	1.20	1.56	1.12	1.46	0.99	1.37	0.92
Fair	1.65	1.26	1.55	1.13	1.50	1.06	1.40	0.86	1.31	0.85
Poor	<1.65	<1.26	<1.55	<1.13	<1.50	<1.06	<1.40	<0.86	<1.31	<0.85

Adapted, by permission, from L.R. Gettman, 1993, Fitness testing. In *ACSM's resource manual for guidelines for exercise testing and prescription*, 2nd ed., edited by J.L. Durstine, et al. (Philadelphia, PA: Lippincott, Williams & Wilkins), 229-246.

TABLE 3.10 Normative Values for Relative Leg Press Strength (1RM / body mass) in a General Population

	20-29 Y		30-39 Y		40-49 Y		50-59 Y		60+ Y	
% rank	M	F	M	F	M	F	M	F	M	F
90	2.27	2.05	2.07	1.73	1.92	1.63	1.80	1.51	1.73	1.40
80	2.13	1.66	1.93	1.50	1.82	1.46	1.71	1.30	1.62	1.25
70	2.05	1.42	1.85	1.47	1.74	1.35	1.64	1.24	1.56	1.18
60	1.97	1.36	1.77	1.32	1.68	1.26	1.58	1.18	1.49	1.15
50	1.91	1.32	1.71	1.26	1.62	1.19	1.52	1.09	1.43	1.08
40	1.83	1.25	1.65	1.21	1.57	1.12	1.46	1.03	1.38	1.04
30	1.74	1.23	1.59	1.16	1.51	1.03	1.39	0.95	1.30	0.98
20	1.63	1.13	1.52	1.09	1.44	0.94	1.32	0.86	1.25	0.94
10	1.51	1.02	1.43	0.94	1.35	0.76	1.22	0.75	1.16	0.84

Adapted from V.H. Heyward, 2002, *Advanced fitness assessment & exercise prescription*, 4th ed. (Champaign, IL: Human Kinetics), 120. Data from The Cooper Institute, Dallas, TX, 1994.

TABLE 3.11 Strength–Mass Ratios for Selected 1RM Tests in College-Aged Men and Women

	BENCH PRESS		LAT PULL-DOWN		LEG PRESS		LEG EXTENSION		LEG CURL		ARM CURL	
Points	M	F	M	F	M	F	M	F	M	F	M	F
10	1.50	0.90	1.20	0.85	3.00	2.70	0.80	0.70	0.70	0.60	0.70	0.50
9	1.40	0.85	1.15	0.80	2.80	2.50	0.75	0.65	0.65	0.55	0.65	0.45
8	1.30	0.80	1.10	0.75	2.60	2.30	0.70	0.60	0.60	0.52	0.60	0.42
7	1.20	0.70	1.05	0.73	2.40	2.10	0.65	0.55	0.55	0.50	0.55	0.38
6	1.10	0.65	1.00	0.70	2.20	2.00	0.60	0.52	0.50	0.45	0.50	0.35
5	1.00	0.60	0.95	0.65	2.00	1.80	0.55	0.50	0.45	0.40	0.45	0.32
4	0.90	0.55	0.90	0.63	1.80	1.60	0.50	0.45	0.40	0.35	0.40	0.28
3	0.80	0.50	0.85	0.60	1.60	1.40	0.45	0.40	0.35	0.30	0.35	0.25
2	0.70	0.45	0.80	0.55	1.40	1.20	0.40	0.35	0.30	0.25	0.30	0.21
1	0.60	0.35	0.75	0.50	1.20	1.00	0.35	0.30	0.25	0.20	0.25	0.18

To determine the strength fitness category, add up the points equivalent for each test:

Total points	Strength fitness category
48-60	Excellent
37-47	Good
25-36	Average
13-24	Fair
0-12	Poor

Adapted, by permission, from V.H. Heyward, 2002, *Advanced fitness assessment & exercise prescription*, 4th ed. (Champaign, IL: Human Kinetics), 298-299. Data courtesy of Hydra-Fitness (Belton, TX).

TABLE 3.12 Percentile Ranks for 1RM Chest Press and Leg Press in Recreationally Active Children

% rank	7-8 Y LEG PRESS lb	kg	CHEST PRESS lb	kg	9-10 Y LEG PRESS lb	kg	CHEST PRESS lb	kg	11-12 Y LEG PRESS lb	kg	CHEST PRESS lb	kg
90	193	88	63	29	203	92	81	37	232	105	114	52
80	170	77	56	25	155	70	66	30	187	85	95	43
70	159	72	49	22	147	67	58	27	180	82	80	37
60	155	70	41	19	140	64	54	24	173	78	71	32
50	147	67	38	17	132	60	51	23	163	74	65	30
40	120	55	35	16	115	52	49	22	142	65	55	25
30	115	52	31	14	105	48	45	20	135	61	52	24
20	97	44	28	13	95	43	41	18	121	55	44	20
10	91	41	25	11	80	36	33	15	109	49	39	18
$\bar{X}$	139	63	41	19	133	60	56	25	162	74	70	32
SD	38	17	15	7	45	20	22	10	43	19	29	13
n	54	54	58	58	102	102	126	126	46	46	65	65

TABLE 3.13 Percentile Values of the 1RM Bench Press, Squat, and Power Clean in High School and College Football Players

	HIGH SCHOOL 14-15 Y BP lb	kg	SQT lb	kg	PC lb	kg	HIGH SCHOOL 16-18 Y BP lb	kg	SQT lb	kg	PC lb	kg
90	243	110	385	175	213	97	275	125	465	211	250	114
80	210	95	344	156	195	89	250	114	425	193	235	107
70	195	89	325	148	190	86	235	107	405	184	225	102
60	185	84	305	139	183	83	225	102	365	166	223	101
50	170	77	295	134	173	79	215	98	335	152	208	95
40	165	75	275	125	165	75	205	93	315	143	200	91
30	155	70	255	116	161	73	195	89	295	134	183	83
20	145	66	236	107	153	70	175	80	275	125	165	75
10	125	57	205	93	141	64	160	73	250	114	145	66
$\bar{X}$	179	81	294	134	176	80	214	97	348	158	204	93
SD	45	20	73	33	32	15	44	20	88	40	43	20
n	214		170		180		339		249		284	

	NCAA DIII BP lb	kg	SQT lb	kg	NCAA DI BP lb	kg	SQT lb	kg	PC lb	kg
90	365	166	470	214	370	168	500	227	300	136
80	325	148	425	193	345	157	455	207	280	127
70	307	140	405	184	325	148	430	195	270	123
60	295	134	385	175	315	143	405	184	261	119
50	280	127	365	166	300	136	395	180	252	115
40	273	124	365	166	285	130	375	170	242	110
30	255	116	335	152	270	123	355	161	232	105

	NCAA DIII				NCAA DI					
	BP		SQT		BP		SQT		PC	
	lb	kg	lb	kg	lb	kg	lb	kg	lb	kg
20	245	111	315	143	255	116	330	150	220	100
10	225	102	283	129	240	109	300	136	205	93
$\bar{X}$	287	130	375	170	301	137	395	180	252	115
SD	57	26	75	34	53	24	77	35	38	17
n	591		588		1,189		1,074		1,017	

BP = bench press; SQT = squat; PC = power clean.

TABLE 3.14 Percentile Values of the 1RM Bench Press, Squat, and Power Clean in NCAA Division I Female Collegiate Athletes

	BASKETBALL						SOFTBALL					
	BP		SQT		PC		BP		SQT		PC	
% rank	lb	kg	lb	Kg	lb	kg	lb	kg	lb	kg	lb	kg
90	124	56	178	81	130	59	117	53	184	84	122	55
80	119	54	160	73	124	56	108	49	170	77	115	52
70	115	52	147	67	117	53	104	47	148	67	106	48
60	112	51	135	61	112	51	99	45	139	63	100	45
50	106	48	129	59	110	50	95	43	126	57	94	43
40	102	46	115	52	103	47	90	41	120	55	93	42
30	96	44	112	51	96	44	85	39	112	51	88	40
20	88	40	101	46	88	40	80	36	94	43	80	36
10	82	37	81	37	77	35	69	31	76	35	71	32
$\bar{X}$	105	48	130	59	106	48	94	43	130	59	97	44
SD	18	8	42	19	20	9	18	8	42	19	20	9
n	120		86		85		105		97		80	

	SWIMMING				VOLLEYBALL			
	BP		SQT		BP		SQT	
% rank	lb	kg	lb	kg	lb	kg	lb	kg
90	116	53	145	66	113	51	185	84
80	109	50	135	61	108	49	171	78
70	106	48	129	59	104	47	165	75
60	101	46	120	55	100	45	153	70
50	97	44	116	53	98	45	143	65
40	94	43	112	51	96	44	136	62
30	93	42	104	47	90	41	126	57
20	88	40	101	46	85	39	112	51
10	78	35	97	44	79	36	98	45
$\bar{X}$	98	45	118	54	97	44	144	65
SD	15	7	19	9	14	6	33	15
n	42		35		67		62	

BP = bench press; SQT = squat; PC = power clean.

TABLE 3.15 Percentile Values of the 1RM Bench Press, Squat, and Power Clean (lb) in NCAA Division I Male Baseball and Basketball Athletes

	BASEBALL						BASKETBALL					
	BP		SQT		PC		BP		SQT		PC	
% rank	lb	kg	lb	kg	lb	kg	lb	kg	lb	kg	lb	kg
90	273	124	365	166	265	120	269	122	315	143	250	114
80	260	118	324	147	239	109	250	114	305	139	235	107
70	247	112	310	141	225	102	240	109	295	134	230	105
60	239	109	293	133	216	98	230	105	280	127	220	100
50	225	102	270	123	206	94	225	102	265	120	215	98
40	218	99	265	120	200	91	216	98	245	111	205	93
30	203	92	247	112	190	86	210	95	225	102	195	89
20	194	88	237	107	182	83	195	89	195	89	180	82
10	175	80	218	99	162	74	185	84	166	75	162	74
$\bar{X}$	227	103	281	128	210	95	225	102	251	114	209	95
SD	41	19	57	26	36	16	33		57	26	34	15
n	170		176		149		142		131		122	

BP = bench press; SQT = squat; PC = power clean.

TABLE 3.16 Descriptive Strength Data for Various Athletic Populations

Population	Gender	BENCH PRESS		SQUAT		POWER CLEAN		Source
		lb	kg	lb	kg	lb	kg	
Baseball								
NCAA DIII	M	216 ± 47	96 ± 21	272 ± 67	124 ± 30			Unpublished data
Basketball								
NCAA DI	M	227 ± 42	103 ± 19	334 ± 81	152 ± 37	218 ± 33	99 ± 15	Latin, Berg, and Baechle 1994
G		222 ± 40	101 ± 18	332 ± 79	151 ± 36	209 ± 29	95 ± 13	
F		229 ± 48	104 ± 22	356 ± 84	162 ± 38	231 ± 37	105 ± 17	
C		229 ± 37	104 ± 17	304 ± 70	138 ± 32	220 ± 31	100 ± 14	
Canoe and kayak								
U.S. national	F	133 ± 25	60 ± 11					Unpublished data
	M	253 ± 38	115 ± 17					
Football								
NCAA DI	M	363 ± 59	165 ± 27	510 ± 90	232 ± 41	306 ± 42	139 ± 19	Garstecki, Latin, and Cuppett 2004
DL		396 ± 53	180 ± 24	543 ± 77	247 ± 35	323 ± 37	147 ± 17	
LB		352 ± 53	160 ± 24	530 ± 81	241 ± 37	317 ± 35	144 ± 16	
DB		312 ± 37	142 ± 17	458 ± 88	208 ± 40	279 ± 44	127 ± 20	
QB		359 ± 48	163 ± 22	440 ± 99	200 ± 45	275 ± 42	125 ± 19	
RB		385 ± 53	175 ± 24	513 ± 73	233 ± 33	304 ± 33	138 ± 15	
WR		332 ± 59	151 ± 27	453 ± 88	206 ± 40	282 ± 33	128 ± 15	
OL		383 ± 62	174 ± 28	552 ± 75	251 ± 34	315 ± 35	143 ± 16	
TE		378 ± 37	172 ± 17	510 ± 81	232 ± 37	310 ± 31	141 ± 14	

Population	Gender	BENCH PRESS		SQUAT		POWER CLEAN		Source
		lb	kg	lb	kg	lb	kg	
Football								
NCAA DII	M	321 ± 57	146 ± 26	449 ± 90	204 ± 41	277 ± 46	126 ± 21	Garstecki, Latin, and Cuppett 2004
DL		356 ± 46	162 ± 21	482 ± 79	219 ± 36	293 ± 48	133 ± 22	
LB		321 ± 48	146 ± 22	460 ± 84	209 ± 38	290 ± 51	132 ± 23	
DB		277 ± 40	126 ± 18	389 ± 84	177 ± 38	255 ± 42	116 ± 19	
QB		284 ± 51	129 ± 23	394 ± 88	179 ± 40	264 ± 42	120 ± 19	
RB		323 ± 44	147 ± 20	473 ± 88	215 ± 40	279 ± 48	127 ± 22	
WR		271 ± 44	123 ± 20	383 ± 77	174 ± 35	273 ± 37	124 ± 17	
OL		352 ± 55	160 ± 25	488 ± 79	222 ± 36	290 ± 37	132 ± 17	
TE		317 ± 35	144 ± 16	447 ± 64	203 ± 29	271 ± 42	123 ± 19	
Ice hockey								
Minor league	M	209 ± 23	95 ± 10	270 ± 43	123 ± 20			Unpublished data
NHL	M	244 ± 48	111 ± 22	270 ± 34	123 ± 15			Unpublished data
Rugby								
Australian and English professional	M							Meir et al. 2001
Forwards		271 ± 26	123 ± 12					
Backs		251 ± 37	114 ± 17					
Soccer								
NCAA DIII	F	103 ± 13	47 ± 6	186 ± 23	85 ± 10	104 ± 11	47 ± 5	Unpublished data
	M	205 ± 24	93 ± 11	286 ± 27	130 ± 12	165 ± 20	75 ± 9	
Norwegian elite	M	176 ± 33	80 ± 15	330 ± 42	150 ± 19			Wisloff, Helgerud, and Hoff 1998
Team handball								
Norwegian 2nd division	F	121 ± 4	55 ± 2					Hoff and Almasbakk 1995
Track and field								
NCAA DIII	F	123 ± 27	56 ± 12	214 ± 37	97 ± 17			Unpublished data
Volleyball								
NCAA DIII	F	121 ± 15	55 ± 7	209 ± 28	95 ± 13	124 ± 14	56 ± 6	Unpublished data
NCAA DI	F	103 ± 18	47 ± 8	180 ± 26	82 ± 12	112 ± 15	51 ± 7	Fry et al. 1991

C = centers; F = forwards; G = guards; DB = defensive back; DL = defensive line; LB = linebacker; OL = offensive line; QB = quarterback; RB = running back; TE = tight end; WR = wide receiver.

Summary

- Isometric, isokinetic, and dynamic constant resistance exercises can be used to evaluate strength in both general and athletic populations.
- Isokinetic assessment allows coaches and trainers to evaluate agonist and antagonist ratios and bilateral deficits, both of which may indicate risk for muscle injury.
- Dynamic constant resistance exercises assess strength in the athletic population.
- Exercises selected for assessment should be part of the individual's normal exercise routine.
- Both submaximal and maximal tests evaluate strength. However, a test requiring a maximal number of repetitions with a submaximal resistance loses its validity to predict maximal strength if the number of repetitions exceeds 10.

CHAPTER 4

Muscular Endurance

Muscular endurance refers to the ability of a muscle or group of muscles to repeatedly move against a submaximal resistance. Typical endurance tests require an individual to perform as many repetitions as possible in a specific time frame. Examples of endurance tests include the maximum number of pull-ups, push-ups, or sit-ups performed in 1 or 2 min. Performing as many repetitions as possible with a fixed resistance is another muscular endurance test. The National Football League (NFL) 225 lb (102.1 kg) bench press test (see chapter 3) is a muscular endurance test. Tests that count the number of repetitions performed are dynamic. Muscular endurance can also be assessed through static tests. These tests record the amount of time that a muscle contraction is maintained. An example of a static test is the flexed-arm hang.

Muscular Endurance Tests

Muscular endurance tests are specific to a muscle or muscle group. To properly assess muscular endurance, selected tests should measure the upper, mid-, and lower body (Nieman 1999). In this section, frequently used muscular endurance tests are described.

BENT-KNEE SIT-UP

The bent-knee sit-up measures muscular endurance of the midbody, providing information on sport performance and possibly on the health of the lower back. Abdominal weakness may cause back problems as a result of an imbalance between the lower back and abdominal musculature. Hand positioning may vary in the sit-up test. Some fitness organizations recommend crossing the arms on the chest, while others recommend placing the fingers next to the ears or interlocking them behind the neck. Generally, the individual performs as many sit-ups as possible in 1 min. However, some assessments require the individual to perform as many sit-ups as possible in 2 min. Table 4.1 provides normative data for adults in the 1 min sit-up test. Normative values for youth can be seen in table 4.2.

📄 For a description with photos of how to perform the bent-knee sit-up, please see page 194 in the appendix.

TABLE 4.1 YMCA Norms for the Sit-Up Test in Adults

Percentile	18-25 Y M	18-25 Y F	26-35 Y M	26-35 Y F	36-45 Y M	36-45 Y F	46-55 Y M	46-55 Y F	56-65 Y M	56-65 Y F	>65 Y M	>65 Y F
90	77	68	62	54	60	54	61	48	56	44	50	34
80	66	61	56	46	52	44	53	40	49	38	40	32
70	57	57	52	41	45	38	51	36	46	32	35	29
60	52	51	44	37	43	35	44	33	41	27	31	26
50	46	44	38	34	36	31	39	31	36	24	27	22
40	41	38	36	32	32	28	33	28	32	22	24	20
30	37	34	33	28	29	23	29	25	28	18	22	16
20	33	32	30	24	25	20	24	21	24	12	19	11
10	27	25	21	20	21	16	16	13	20	8	12	9

Values represent number of repetitions.

Reprinted from J.T. Cramer and J.W. Coburn, 2004, Fitness testing protocols and norms. In *NSCA's essentials of personal training*, edited by R.W. Earle and T.R. Baechle (Champaign, IL: Human Kinetics), 258; adapted from *YMCA fitness testing and assessment manual*, 4th edition, 2000, with permission of YMCA of the USA, 101 N. Wacker Drive, Chicago, IL 60606.

TABLE 4.2 Bent-Knee Sit-Ups Performed in 1 Min by Youth

Percentile	AGE (Y) 6	7	8	9	10	11	12	13	14	15	16	17+
Boys												
90	37	38	42	44	48	49	53	55	58	59	58	57
80	31	34	38	40	43	45	48	51	54	55	53	53
70	26	31	36	37	40	42	45	48	51	51	50	50
60	24	30	34	34	38	39	43	45	48	49	48	46
50	22	28	31	32	35	37	40	42	45	45	45	44
40	20	25	29	30	33	35	38	40	42	43	42	41
30	17	22	26	27	30	32	35	38	40	40	40	40
20	14	20	23	24	28	29	32	34	37	36	37	36
10	10	15	18	20	23	25	27	30	33	32	31	32
Girls												
90	33	36	40	41	42	44	47	50	49	51	49	47
80	31	32	36	38	38	40	43	44	45	46	43	41
70	28	30	33	35	35	37	40	42	42	41	40	38
60	25	27	30	32	32	35	38	40	40	39	37	36
50	23	25	29	30	30	32	35	37	37	36	35	34
40	20	23	27	29	28	30	32	35	35	34	33	31
30	19	21	24	26	26	28	30	31	32	31	30	30
20	16	19	22	23	23	25	27	28	30	28	27	25
10	11	15	18	19	19	20	23	23	25	23	23	22

Adapted, by permission, from Presidents Council for Physical Fitness, *Presidents Challenge Normative Data Spreadsheet* (Online). Available: www.presidentschallenge.org.

PARTIAL CURL-UP

Some facilities prefer to test muscle endurance of the abdominal musculature with a partial curl-up. This test, also known as abdominal crunches, reduces hip flexor muscle recruitment, thus reducing the strain on the lower back. Normative values for adults in the partial curl-up can be seen in table 4.3. Normative values for children are in table 4.4.

📖 For a description with photos of how to perform the partial curl-up, please see page 194 in the appendix.

TABLE 4.3 Percentiles by Age and Gender for Partial Curl-Up

| | AGE (Y) | | | | | | | | | |
| | 20-29 | | 30-39 | | 40-49 | | 50-59 | | 60-69 | |
Percentile	M	F	M	F	M	F	M	F	M	F
90	75	70	75	55	75	50	74	48	53	50
80	56	45	69	43	75	42	60	30	33	30
70	41	37	46	34	67	33	45	23	26	24
60	31	32	36	28	51	28	35	16	19	19
50	27	27	31	21	39	25	27	9	16	13
40	23	21	26	15	31	20	23	2	9	9
30	20	17	19	12	26	14	19	0	6	3
20	13	12	13	0	21	5	13	0	0	0
10	4	5	0	0	13	0	0	0	0	0

Reprinted, by permission, from American College of Sports Medicine, 2000, *ACSM's guidelines for exercise testing and prescription*, 6th ed. (Philadelphia, PA: Lippincott, Williams & Wilkins), 86. Data from *Canadian Standardized Test of Fitness and Operations Manual*, 3rd ed., Public Health Agency of Canada, 1986. Adapted and reproduced with permission of the Minister of Public Works and Govenment Services Canada, 2006.

TABLE 4.4 Partial Curl-Up for Youth

| | AGE (Y) | | | | | | | | | | | |
Percentile	6	7	8	9	10	11	12	13	14	15	16	17+
Boys												
90	23	27	31	41	38	49	100	60	77	100	79	82
80	20	23	27	33	35	40	58	55	58	70	61	63
70	15	20	25	27	29	35	48	48	52	60	48	50
60	12	16	20	23	27	29	36	42	48	50	40	47
50	10	13	17	20	24	26	32	39	40	45	37	42
40	9	12	15	18	20	22	31	35	33	40	34	39
30	8	10	13	15	19	21	27	31	30	32	30	31
20	7	9	11	14	14	18	24	30	28	29	28	28
10	5	7	9	11	10	13	18	21	24	22	23	24
Girls												
90	23	27	31	41	36	44	56	63	51	45	50	60
80	20	23	27	33	29	40	49	52	44	37	41	50
70	15	20	25	27	27	37	40	46	40	35	32	48
60	12	16	20	23	25	32	34	41	33	30	27	42
50	10	13	17	20	24	27	30	40	30	26	26	40
40	9	12	15	18	21	24	26	36	28	25	23	33
30	8	10	13	15	19	21	24	32	25	22	20	30
20	7	9	11	14	17	18	21	27	21	19	19	28
10	5	7	9	11	12	18	16	20	16	13	15	24

Adapted, by permission, from Presidents Council for Physical Fitness, *Presidents Challenge Normative Data Spreadsheet* (Online). Available: www.presidentschallenge.org.

PULL-UP AND CHIN-UP

The pull-up and chin-up measure muscular endurance in the arms (elbow flexors) and shoulder girdle (adductors). A performance evaluation of college men can be seen in table 4.5. Percentile ranks for pull-ups and chin-ups performed by youth are shown in tables 4.6 and 4.7, respectively.

📖 For a description with photos of how to perform the pull-up and chin-up, please see page 195 in the appendix.

TABLE 4.5 Pull-Ups in College Men

Classification	Number of pull-ups
Excellent	15+
Good	12-14
Average	8-11
Fair	5-7
Poor	0-4

Adapted from B.L. Johnson and J.K. Nelson, 1979, *Practical measurement for evaluation in physical education* (Minneapolis, MN: Burgess Publishing Co.).

TABLE 4.6 Pull-Ups in Youth

Percentile	AGE (Y)											
	6	7	8	9	10	11	12	13	14	15	16	17+
Boys												
90	3	5	6	6	7	7	8	9	11	12	12	15
80	1	4	4	5	5	5	6	7	9	10	10	12
70	1	2	3	4	4	4	5	5	7	9	9	10
60	0	2	2	3	3	3	3	4	6	7	8	10
50	0	1	1	2	2	2	2	3	5	6	7	8
40	0	1	1	1	1	1	1	2	4	5	6	7
30	0	0	0	0	1	0	1	1	3	4	5	5
20	0	0	0	0	0	0	0	0	1	2	4	4
10	0	0	0	0	0	0	0	0	0	1	2	2
Girls												
90	3	3	3	3	3	3	3	2	3	2	2	2
80	1	1	2	2	2	2	2	1	1	1	1	1
70	1	1	1	1	1	1	1	0	1	1	1	1
60	0	0	0	0	1	0	0	0	0	0	0	0
50	0	0	0	0	0	0	0	0	0	0	0	0
40	0	0	0	0	0	0	0	0	0	0	0	0
30	0	0	0	0	0	0	0	0	0	0	0	0
20	0	0	0	0	0	0	0	0	0	0	0	0
10	0	0	0	0	0	0	0	0	0	0	0	0

This table is adapted with permission from *The Journal of Physical Education, Recreation & Dance*, 1985, 44-90. JOPERD is a publication of the American Alliance for Health, Physical Education, Recreation, and Dance, 1900 Association Dr., Reston, VA 20191.

					AGE (Y)				
Percentile	**10**	**11**	**12**	**13**	**14**	**15**	**16**	**17**	**18**
Boys									
90	8	8	8	10	12	14	14	15	16
80	5	5	6	8	9	11	12	13	14
70	4	4	5	7	8	10	12	12	13
60	2	3	4	5	6	8	10	10	11
50	1	2	3	4	5	7	9	9	10
40	1	1	2	3	4	6	8	8	9
30	0	0	1	1	3	5	6	6	7
20	0	0	0	0	1	3	5	4	5
10	0	0	0	0	0	1	2	2	3
Girls									
90	3	3	2	2	2	2	2	2	2
80	2	1	1	1	1	1	1	1	1
70	1	1	1	0	1	1	1	1	1
60	0	0	0	0	0	0	0	0	0
50	0	0	0	0	0	0	0	0	0
40	0	0	0	0	0	0	0	0	0
30	0	0	0	0	0	0	0	0	0
20	0	0	0	0	0	0	0	0	0
10	0	0	0	0	0	0	0	0	0

TABLE 4.7   Chin-Ups in Youth

This table is adapted with permission from *The Journal of Physical Education, Recreation & Dance*, 1985, 44-90. *JOPERD* is a publication of the American Alliance for Health, Physical Education, Recreation, and Dance, 1900 Association Dr., Reston, VA 20191.

PUSH-UP

The push-up assesses endurance of the upper-body musculature (pectoralis major, anterior deltoids, and triceps). The push-up can be administered differently or similarly for males and females. Tables 4.8 and 4.9 provide normative data for push-ups performed to exhaustion by males and females and by youth, respectively.

For a description with photos of how to perform the push-up (traditional and modified), please see page 196 in the appendix.

TABLE 4.8   Push-Up Norms for Men and Women

	AGE (Y)									
	20-29		**30-39**		**40-49**		**50-59**		**60+**	
Percentile	**M**	**F**	**M**	**F**	**M**	**F**	**M**	**F**	**M**	**F**
90	57	42	46	36	36	28	30	25	26	17
80	47	36	39	31	30	24	25	21	23	15
70	41	32	34	28	26	20	21	19	21	14
60	37	30	30	24	24	18	19	17	18	12
50	33	26	27	21	21	15	15	13	15	8
40	29	23	24	19	18	13	13	12	10	5
30	26	20	20	15	15	10	10	9	8	3
20	22	17	17	11	11	6	9	6	6	2
10	18	12	13	8	9	2	6	1	4	0

Modified push-ups were used for women. Data are reported as total number of repetitions completed until exhaustion.

Adapted from D.C. Nieman, 1999, *Exercise testing & prescription: A health related approach*, 4th ed (Mountain View, CA: Mayfield Publishing), with permission of The McGraw-Hill Companies.

	AGE (Y)											
Percentile	**6**	**7**	**8**	**9**	**10**	**11**	**12**	**13**	**14**	**15**	**16**	**17+**
Boys												
90	11	17	19	20	25	30	34	41	41	44	46	56
80	9	13	15	17	21	26	30	35	37	40	41	50
70	7	11	13	15	18	23	25	31	30	35	36	44
60	7	9	11	13	16	19	20	28	25	32	32	41
50	7	8	9	12	14	15	18	24	24	30	30	37
40	5	7	8	10	12	14	15	20	21	27	28	34
30	4	5	7	8	11	10	13	16	18	25	25	30
20	3	4	6	7	10	8	10	12	15	21	23	25
10	2	3	4	5	7	3	7	9	11	18	20	21
Girls												
90	11	17	19	20	21	20	21	22	21	23	26	28
80	9	13	15	17	19	18	20	17	19	20	22	22
70	7	11	13	15	17	17	15	15	12	18	19	19
60	6	9	11	13	14	15	11	13	10	16	15	17
50	6	8	9	12	13	11	10	11	10	15	12	16
40	5	7	8	10	10	8	8	10	8	13	12	15
30	4	5	7	8	9	7	5	7	5	11	10	12
20	3	4	6	7	8	6	3	5	5	10	5	9
10	2	3	4	5	4	2	1	3	2	5	3	5

TABLE 4.9 Push-Up Norms for Youth

Adapted, by permission, from Presidents Council for Physical Fitness, *Presidents Challenge Normative Data Spreadsheet* (Online). Available: www.presidentschallenge.org.

FLEXED-ARM HANG

The flexed-arm hang assesses forearm and elbow flexor endurance. It is used to evaluate youth and female soldiers in some branches of the military. Normative values for the flexed-arm hang can be seen in table 4.10.

For a description of how to perform the flexed-arm hang, please see page 196 in the appendix.

PARALLEL BAR DIPS

Parallel bar dips assess endurance of the upper-body musculature (pectoralis major and minor, triceps, and deltoids).

For a description with photos of how to perform parallel bar dips, please see page 197 in the appendix.

YMCA BENCH PRESS TEST

The YMCA bench press test is another assessment for endurance of the upper-body musculature (pectoralis major, anterior deltoids, and triceps). All members of a gender use the same resistance for this test. Table 4.11 provides normative values for the YMCA bench press.

For a description of how to perform the YMCA bench press test, please see page 197 in the appendix.

TABLE 4.10 Flexed-Arm Hang Standards for Youth

Percentile	AGE (Y)											
	6	7	8	9	10	11	12	13	14	15	16	17+
Boys												
90	16	23	28	28	38	37	36	37	61	62	61	56
80	12	17	18	20	25	26	25	29	40	49	46	45
70	9	13	15	16	20	19	19	22	31	40	39	39
60	8	10	12	12	15	15	15	18	25	35	33	35
50	6	8	10	10	12	11	12	14	20	30	28	30
40	5	6	8	8	8	9	9	10	15	25	22	26
30	3	4	5	5	6	6	6	8	11	20	18	20
20	2	3	3	3	3	4	4	5	8	14	12	15
10	1	1	1	2	1	1	1	2	3	8	7	8
Girls												
90	15	21	21	23	29	25	27	28	31	34	30	29
80	11	14	15	16	19	16	16	19	21	23	21	20
70	9	11	11	12	14	13	13	14	16	15	16	15
60	6	8	10	10	11	9	10	10	11	10	10	11
50	5	6	8	8	8	7	7	8	9	7	7	7
40	4	5	6	6	6	5	5	5	6	5	5	5
30	3	4	4	4	4	4	3	4	4	4	3	4
20	1	2	3	2	2	2	1	1	2	2	2	2
10	0	0	0	0	0	0	0	0	0	1	0	1

Time listed in seconds.

Adapted, by permission, from Presidents Council for Physical Fitness, *Presidents Challenge Normative Data Spreadsheet* (Online). Available: www.presidentschallenge.org.

TABLE 4.11 YMCA Bench Press Norms

% rank	18-25 Y		26-35 Y		36-45 Y		46-55 Y		56-65 Y		>65 Y	
	M	F	M	F	M	F	M	F	M	F	M	F
95	42	42	40	40	34	32	28	30	24	30	20	22
75	30	28	26	25	24	21	20	20	14	16	10	12
50	22	20	20	17	17	13	12	11	8	9	6	6
25	13	12	12	9	10	8	6	5	4	3	2	2
5	2	2	2	1	2	1	1	0	0	0	0	0

Number of repetitions in 1 min using 80 lb (36.3 kg) for men and 35 lb (15.9 kg) for women.

Adapted from *YMCA Fitness Testing and Assessment Manual*, 4th edition, 2000, with permission of YMCA of the USA, 101 N. Wacker Drive, Chicago, IL 60606.

Muscular Endurance Tests
for Civil Service and Military Personnel

Muscular endurance tests such as timed sit-ups, push-ups, and pull-ups are often part of the selection process or fitness assessment of law enforcement, public safety (i.e., firefighter), and military personnel. These tests measure physical fitness to confirm that these individuals are able to successfully perform their tasks. Information concerning endurance testing of police and firefighters is quite limited. Tables 4.12 and 4.13 provide the percentile scores of law enforcement personnel and the standard passing scores for police personnel, respectively. The standard passing scores for sit-ups and push-ups across age and gender in table 4.13 are consistent with physical fitness requirements reported by a host of police departments around the United States.

Muscular endurance tests performed by firefighters are shown in table 4.14. In this study (Findley et al. 1995), 159 male firefighters (32.7 ± 5.8 y) with 7 y of firefighting experience were examined. Although this study measures fitness in these individuals, it does not indicate which performance variables best relate to firefighting performance. However, recent research has shown that muscular endurance (e.g., pull-ups) can predict success in specific physical firefighting tasks (Williford et al. 1999). Minimum standards in muscular endurance for U.S. Army, Navy, Air Force, and Marines personnel can be seen in table 4.15. These measurements are reported across age and gender. Table 4.16 provides a classification for the physical readiness of U.S. Navy personnel.

TABLE 4.12 Percentile Scores of Law Enforcement Personnel

Category	PERCENTILE								
	90	80	70	60	50	40	30	20	10
Sit-ups in 1 min	60	44	40	37	34	31	28	25	20
Push-ups in 1 min	56	47	40	35	31	29	24	19	13

Data from R.J. Hoffman and T.R. Collingwood, 2005, *Fit for Duty*, 2nd ed. (Champaign, IL: Human Kinetics), 39.

TABLE 4.13 Standard Passing Scores for Sit-Ups and Push-Ups for Police Department Personnel

Category	AGE (Y)							
	20-29		30-39		40-49		50-59	
	M	F	M	F	M	F	M	F
Sit-ups in 1 min	38	32	35	25	29	20	24	14
Push-ups until exhaustion	29	15	24	11	18	9	13	9

Data compiled from various police forces around the United States.

TABLE 4.14 Muscle Endurance Performance in Male Firefighters

	AGE (Y)		
Parameter	20-29	30-39	40-49
Sit-ups in 2 min	62.8 ± 16.5	54.1 ± 17.2	50.6 ± 13.6
Push-ups to fatigue	37.2 ± 11.9	35.3 ± 15.4	32.0 ± 13.5

TABLE 4.15 Minimum Standards for Muscle Endurance in American Military Personnel, Adjusted for Age and Gender

	PUSH-UPS IN 2 MIN		SIT-UPS IN 2 MIN	
Age	M	F	M	F
Army				
17-21	42	19	53	53
22-26	40	17	50	50
27-31	39	17	45	45
32-36	36	15	42	42
37-41	34	13	38	38
42-46	30	12	32	32
47-51	25	10	30	30
52-56	20	9	28	28
57-61	18	8	27	27
62+	16	7	26	26
Army basic training				
17-21	35	13	47	47
22-26	31	11	43	43
27-31	30	10	36	36
32-36	26	9	34	34
Navy				
17-19	42	19	50	50
20-29	37	16	46	46
30-39	31	11	40	40
40-49	24	7	35	35
50+	19	2	29	29
Navy basic training				
17-19	51	24	62	62
20-29	47	21	58	58
30-39	41	17	51	51

	PUSH-UPS IN 2 MIN		CRUNCHES IN 2 MIN	
Age	M	F	M	F
Air Force				
<24	42	19	53	53
25-29	40	17	50	50
30-34	36	15	42	42
35-39	34	13	38	38
40-44	30	12	32	32
45-49	25	10	30	30
50-54	20	9	28	28
55-59	18	8	27	27
Air Force basic training				
All	30	14	45	38

	PULL-UPS (M) AND FLEXED-ARM HANGS (F)		CRUNCHES IN 2 MIN	
Age	M	F	M	F
Marines				
17-26	3	15 s	50	50
27-39	3	15 s	45	45
40-45	3	15 s	45	45
46+	3	15 s	40	40
Marines basic training				
Same as active force				

	TABLE 4.16 Physical Readiness Classification for Naval Personnel (Muscle Endurance Assessments)									
	AGE AND GENDER									
	17-19 Y		**20-29 Y**		**30-39 Y**		**40-49 Y**		**50+ Y**	
Category	**M**	**F**	**M**	**F**	**M**	**F**	**M**	**F**	**M**	**F**
Sit-ups in 2 min										
Outstanding	88	86	84	84	75	74	73	72	68	67
Excellent	72	67	68	61	54	54	48	48	45	45
Good	60	52	50	45	40	39	35	34	33	32
Satisfactory	45	40	40	33	32	27	29	24	27	22
Push-ups in 2 min										
Outstanding	62	36	52	29	45	23	41	22	38	21
Excellent	57	31	48	24	41	19	37	18	35	17
Good	51	24	42	17	36	11	32	11	30	10
Satisfactory	38	18	29	11	23	5	20	5	19	5

Adapted from J.A. Hodgdon, 1999, "A history of the U.S. Navy physical readiness program from 1976 to 1999," *Technical Document Number 99-6F* (Washington, DC: Office of Naval Research).

Muscular Endurance Tests for Athletes

Muscular endurance tests are not commonly used among athletic populations. Relative to other fitness components, data on muscular endurance in athletes are limited. Table 4.17 provides muscular endurance measurements in high school athletes, while table 4.18 provides muscular endurance measurements in collegiate, professional, and national athletes.

TABLE 4.17 Muscle Endurance Assessment in High School and Youth Athletes						
Sport	**Age (y)**	**Gender**	**Pull-ups**	**Push-ups**	**Sit-ups**	**Source**
Basketball	14-15	M	5.2 ± 3.0		41.5 ± 8.9	Unpublished data
	16-17	M	6.1 ± 3.1		44.1 ± 7.5	
Field hockey	14-15	F		19.3 ± 7.4	42.1 ± 9.6	Unpublished data
	16-17	F		20.0 ± 6.7	40.3 ± 7.7	
Gymnastics	14.9 ± 3.0	M		42.0 ± 11.0	49.0 ± 10.0	Rivera, Rivera-Brown, and Frontera 1998
	14.8 ± 1.1	F		39.0 ± 4.0	44.0 ± 8.0	
Ice hockey	12.2 ± 2.1	F		29.2 ± 11.1	33.2 ± 8.8	Bracko and George 2001
Soccer	14-15	M		23.9 ± 10.2	45.7 ± 7.1	Unpublished data
	16-17	M		35.7 ± 9.5	50.1 ± 7.2	
Swimming	14-15	F		16.5 ± 9.4	43.6 ± 6.9	Unpublished data
	16-17	F		23.5 ± 9.8	46.2 ± 8.9	
	14-15	M		41.5 ± 20.9	49.8 ± 3.3	
	16-17	M		42.0 ± 7.3	43.3 ± 5.3	
Tennis	11.6 ± 0.6	M		26.6 ± 9.0		Roetart et al. 1992

All data are reported $\bar{X} \pm SD$.

Sport	Gender	Sit-ups	Pull-ups	Push-ups	Dips	Source
TABLE 4.18 Muscle Endurance Assessment in Collegiate, Professional, and National Athletes						

Sport	Gender	Sit-ups	Pull-ups	Push-ups	Dips	Source
Baseball—Puerto Rican national team	M	45.9 ± 7.3		32.7 ± 12.0		Rivera, Rivera-Brown, and Frontera 1998
Basketball—NBA	M	56.9 ± 13.3	8.8 ± 4.5		23.5 ± 9.2	Unpublished data
Canoe/Kayak—U.S. national team	F M	72.9 ± 11.4* 83.4 ± 17.6*	17.3 ± 11.1# 44.7 ± 15.7#			Unpublished data
Football—NCAA DIAA	M		17.2 ± 9.3		32.3 ± 10.8	Unpublished data
Judo—Puerto Rican national team	M F	57.4 ± 8.9 49.3 ± 10.8		61.2 ± 19.0 72.5 ± 19.1		Rivera, Rivera-Brown, and Frontera 1998
Volleyball—NCAA DI	F	52.7 ± 7.6				Fry et al. 1991

* = number of sit-ups in 2 min; # = number of chin-ups in 2 min.

Summary

⊃ Muscular endurance tests evaluate the ability of a muscle or group of muscles to repeatedly move against a submaximal resistance.

⊃ Typical muscular endurance tests require an individual to perform as many repetitions as possible within a specific time frame.

⊃ Many muscular endurance tests use an individual's body mass as the primary resistance.

⊃ Modifying the exercise allows individuals who have difficulty lifting their body mass to be evaluated.

⊃ Muscular endurance tests are frequently utilized by civil service (e.g., police and firefighter) and military personnel to evaluate their physical readiness to perform their duties.

CHAPTER 5

Anaerobic Power

Anaerobic power refers to the ability to perform high-intensity exercise from a fraction of a second to several minutes. Typically, tests of maximal effort in cycling, running, and jumping are used to assess this energy system. Efforts lasting up to 10 s are generally reported as *anaerobic power*, while efforts lasting longer than 10 s are generally termed *anaerobic capacity* (Inbar, Bar-Or, and Skinner 1996; Komi et al. 1977; Sargeant, Hoinville, and Young 1981; Volkov, Shirkovets, and Borilkevich 1975). *Peak power* is the highest power output attained during a test, and *mean power* refers to the average power output of the test. Peak power has often been reported as the highest output produced within 3 or 5 s; however, recent technological advances report peak power on a second-to-second basis. A fatigue rate assesses the ability of the individual to maintain power output during the test.

Anaerobic tests vary in style and sophistication. This is partly why it has been difficult to establish normative standards for athletic populations. Many athletic teams lack an exercise physiology laboratory, which limits their use of the more accurate assessment devices and requires a greater reliance on field measurements. This chapter describes commonly used laboratory and field measurements of anaerobic power and, when possible, provides both normative and descriptive values for these tests in specific populations.

Laboratory Measures of Anaerobic Power

A variety of laboratory tests have been used to assess anaerobic power, including the following:

- Sprints on a motorized treadmill (Cunningham and Falkner 1969; Falk et al. 1996; Funato, Yanagiya, and Fukunaga 2001)
- Repeated jumps on a force plate or contact mat (Bosco, Mognoni, and Luhtanen 1983)
- Maximal effort cycling against various breaking forces, with test durations ranging from 7 to 120 s (Ayalon, Inbar, and Bar-Or 1974; Katch et al. 1977; Sargeant, Hoinville, and Young 1981)

Other laboratory tests used for assessing anaerobic power have included using isokinetic devices (using single movements for peak power and multiple repetitions for anaerobic fatigue) (Thorstensson and Karlson 1976) and performing sprints on a vertical elevation (Margaria, Aghemo, and Rovelli 1966).

The laboratory anaerobic test most commonly used today is the Wingate anaerobic power test (WAnT) (Bar-Or 1987). It is 30 s of cycling or arm-cranking at maximal effort against a resistance relative to the subject's body weight. The WAnT was first developed at the Wingate Institute in Israel (Ayalon, Inbar, and Bar-Or 1974). Of the anaerobic power tests available for laboratory use, the WAnT has the most extensive research base, and its test–retest reliability consistently exceeds $r > 0.90$ (Bar-Or 1987).

📄 For a description of how to perform a Wingate anaerobic power test, please see page 198 in the appendix.

The WAnT assesses an individual's peak power, mean power, and fatigue index. Peak power is the highest mechanical power output achieved at any stage of the test. Most laboratories report it as the highest power output achieved over 5 s; however, some laboratories use a 3 s or shorter interval. Peak power represents the explosive capability of the athlete's lower body. Mean power is the average power output during the 30 s, and it assesses the athlete's anaerobic endurance, or ability to maintain a high power output over a long duration. The fatigue index is often determined by dividing the lowest 5 s power segment (generally the last 5 s of the test) by peak power. Although it is not clear whether the fatigue index is a good indicator of anaerobic fitness, the index correlates well with the percentage of fast-twitch fibers (Bar-Or et al. 1980). Typically a greater fatigue index is seen in athletes with a greater percentage of fast-twitch fibers. Athletes who are endurance trained gener-

ally have a lower fatigue index. Figure 5.1 depicts a typical performance diagram produced from a 30 s WAnT. Table 5.1 shows the percentile ranks for the WAnT of physically active, college-aged individuals, and table 5.2 provides descriptive data on the WAnT from various athletic populations.

The WAnT has become known as a lower-body measure of anaerobic power; however, alterations to the bicycle have permitted upper-body measurements as well. Table 5.3 provides typical values for upper-body Wingate power tests in untrained Israeli men and women from data collected at the Wingate Institute. Although the WAnT is acknowledged as the gold standard of laboratory anaerobic power measurements, it has not achieved widespread acceptance among coaches as a performance test for their athletes. This may relate to questions concerning specificity for muscle and activity pattern as well as to accessibility to laboratories with WAnT capabilities. For example, anaerobic power assessment may be more specific to a basketball player if performed as a vertical jump test. Vertical jump tests generally require the athlete to repeat countermovement jumps on a force plate or contact mat. The flight time (moment subject breaks contact from the mat until moment subject lands and remakes contact) of each jump is recorded. The flight time is used to calculate the change in the athlete's center of gravity (Bosco, Mognoni, and Luhtanen 1983). From body weight

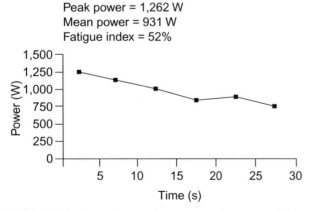

Peak power = 1,262 W
Mean power = 931 W
Fatigue index = 52%

FIGURE 5.1   Sample performance diagram of the Wingate anaerobic power test.

TABLE 5.1   Percentile Ranks for the Wingate Anaerobic Power Test in Physically Active College-Aged Males and Females

Percentile	MALES		FEMALES	
	(W)	(W · kg⁻¹)	(W)	(W · kg⁻¹)
90	662	8.2	470	7.3
80	618	8.0	419	7.0
70	600	7.9	410	6.8
60	577	7.6	391	6.6
50	565	7.4	381	6.4
40	548	7.1	367	6.1
30	530	7.0	353	6.0
20	496	6.6	337	5.7
10	471	6.0	306	5.3

Wingate test performed on a Monark cycle ergometer using a resistance of 0.075 kg · kg body mass⁻¹. Males and females were 18-28 y. For males, $n = 60$; for females $n = 69$.

TABLE 5.2 Descriptive Data for the Wingate Anaerobic Power Test in Athletic Populations

Population	Gender	PEAK POWER (W)	PEAK POWER (W · kg⁻¹)	MEAN POWER (W)	MEAN POWER (W · kg⁻¹)	Device and resistance	Source
		(W)	(W · kg⁻¹)	(W)	(W · kg⁻¹)		
Basketball							
NCAA DI	F	663 ± 98	9.5 ± 1.4	498 ± 51	7.2 ± 0.7	Bodyguard	LaMonte et al. 1999
Guards		629 ± 79	10.2 ±1.2	477 ± 45	7.7 ± 0.7		
Forwards		693 ± 106	9.4 ± 1.3	516 ± 49	7.1 ± 0.8		
Centers		668 ± 78	8.3 ± 1.2	502 ± 58	6.3 ± 0.7		
Israel national	M		14.4 ± 1.7		9.1 ± 1.2	Fleish (0.052 kg · kg body mass)	Hoffman et al. 1999
Bobsled							
U.S. national	M	1005 ± 90	10.8 ± 0.5	796 ± 60	8.6 ± 0.9	Bodyguard	Osbeck, Maiorca, and Rundell 1996
Football							
NCAA DI	M	1,189 ± 130	12.2 ± 1.7	874 ± 102	9.1 ± 1.5	Monark (0.083 kg · kg body mass)	Seiler et al. 1990
Backs		1,130 ± 126	13.2 ± 1.1	836 ± 91	10.0 ± 0.9		
Linebackers		1,298 ± 83	12.6 ± 0.9	928 ± 102	9.4 ± 1.1		
Linemen		1,223 ± 123	10.4 ± 1.5	879 ± 103	7.5 ± 1.3		
NCAA DIII	M	1,894 ± 140		1,296 ± 66		Lode Excalibur (1.1 Nm · kg body mass)	Hoffman et al. 2004
Hockey							
U.S. hockey	F	785		729			Unpublished data
Kickboxing							
Elite	M	1,360	18.8	761	10.5	Monark	Zabukovec and Tiidus 1995
Middle-distance running							
Competitive French	M	842 ± 123	13 ± 2.0	578 ± 64	9.0 ± 1.0	Monark	Granier et al. 1995
Soccer							
Youth	M					Monark (0.075 kg · kg body mass)	Vanderford et al. 2004
U-14			9.3 ± 0.2		8.0 ± 0.2		
U-15			10.0 ± 0.3		8.1 ± 0.2		
U-16			10.5 ± 0.2		8.7 ± 0.2		
U.S. national	M				8.1 ± 0.9	Monark (0.075 kg · kg body mass)	Mangine et al. 1990
Softball							
Masters	F	406 ± 56					Terbizan et al. 1996
Speed skating							
Elite Canadians	F		12.3 ± 0.5		9.7 ± 0.2	Monark (0.092 + 0.112 kp · kg body mass)	Smith and Roberts 1991
	M		16.6 ± 0.9		12.7 ± 0.5		
Sprinting (competitive)							
Belgians	M	1,021 ± 139	14.2 ± 1.4			Monark	Crielaard and Pirnay 1981
French	M	924 ± 105	14 ± 1.0	662 ± 61	10 ± 1.0	Monark	Granier et al. 1995
Tennis							
NCAA	F	699 ± 130				Monark (0.075 kg · kg body mass)	Kraemer et al. 2003

TABLE 5.3 Typical Values (in W) for the Upper-Body Wingate Anaerobic Power Test in Healthy, Untrained Males and Females

Category	<10	10-12	12-14	14-16	16-18	18-25	25-35	>35
				AGE (Y)				
Peak power in males								
Excellent	205	192	473	473	575	658	565	589
Very good	164	171	389	411	484	556	501	510
Good	143	159	343	379	438	507	469	471
Average	122	148	298	348	393	458	437	433
Below average	101	137	253	316	347	409	405	394
Poor	80	126	207	284	301	360	373	356
Very poor	60	115	162	252	256	311	341	317
$\bar{X}$	112	143	275	332	370	433	421	413
SD	42	22	91	63	91	98	64	77
Peak power in females								
Excellent	201	176	214					
Very good	152	159	199					
Good	135	141	184					
Average	119	124	170					
Below average	102	106	155					
Poor	86	89	140					
Very poor	53	55	110					
$\bar{X}$	127	133	177					
SD	33	35	30					
Mean power in males								
Excellent	161	159	333	380	409	477	415	454
Very good	136	142	276	321	349	403	375	395
Good	118	133	248	293	318	366	355	366
Average	100	124	220	264	288	329	335	337
Below average	83	116	192	236	258	292	315	308
Poor	65	107	165	207	227	255	294	279
Very poor	47	98	137	179	197	218	274	249
$\bar{X}$	91	120	206	250	273	310	325	322
SD	35	17	55	37	61	74	40	58
Mean power in females								
Excellent	153	158	194					
Very good	130	137	165					
Good	118	126	151					
Average	107	116	137					
Below average	96	105	122					
Poor	84	94	108					
Very poor	73	83	93					
$\bar{X}$	101	110	129					
SD	23	21	29					

Adapted, by permission, from O. Inbar, O. Bar-Or and J.S. Skinner, 1996, *Wingate anaerobic test* (Champaign, IL: Human Kinetics), 82, 84, 91, 92.

and the calculated jump height, mechanical work is calculated. Finally, anaerobic power is determined from mechanical work and the length of contact time between jumps. A vertical jump anaerobic power test appears to be more sport specific, especially for sports such as basketball and volleyball (Hoffman et al. 2000).

The Margaria-Kalmen stair sprint test has been used since the 1960s to measure anaerobic power. Its popularity in testing athletes, though, does not equal that seen in the WAnT and jump tests. This test requires a staircase with 9 or more steps, each at least 7 in. (17.5 cm) high, and a 20 ft (6 m) strip of flat area for the beginning of a sprint. In addition, it requires an electronic timing system with a start and stop switch placed on the 3rd and 9th steps. Normative data for this assessment can be seen in table 5.4.

📄 For a description of how to perform the Margaria-Kalmen test, please see page 198 in the appendix.

TABLE 5.4 Normative Values (in W) for the Margaria-Kalmen Stair Sprint Test

| | AGE AND GENDER | | | | | | | | | |
| | 15-20 Y | | 20-30 Y | | 30-40 Y | | 40-50 Y | | 50+ Y | |
Category	M	F	M	F	M	F	M	F	M	F
Excellent	2,197	1,789	2,059	1,648	1,648	1,226	1,226	961	961	736
Good	1,840	1,487	1,722	1,379	1,379	1,036	1,036	810	809	604
Average	1,839	1,486	1,721	1,378	1,378	1,035	1,035	809	808	603
Fair	1,466	1,182	1,368	1,094	1,094	829	829	642	641	476
Poor	1,108	902	1,040	834	834	637	637	490	490	373

Adapted from E. Fox, R. Bowers and M. Foss, 1993, *The physiological basis for exercise and sport*, 5th ed. (Dubuque, IA: Wm C. Brown), 676, with permission of The McGraw-Hill Companies; based on data from J. Kalamen, 1968, *Measurement of maximum muscular power in man*, Doctoral Dissertation, The Ohio State University, and R. Margaria, I. Aghemo and E. Rovelli, 1966, "Measurement of muscular power (anaerobic) in man," *J Appl Physiol*, 21:1662-1664.

Field Tests
for Anaerobic Power

When testing large groups, administrative concerns (equipment availability and the fact that subjects must be tested one at a time) may preclude the previously mentioned tests from being widely adopted. As a result, many coaches have searched for field-based assessments similar to those attained from laboratory measurements.

STANDING LONG JUMP

The standing long jump is a common field test used by coaches and physical educators to assess leg power. It is easy to administer and requires only a space approximately 15 ft (4.6 m) long and 5 ft (1.5 m) wide.

📄 For a description of how to perform the standing long jump, please see page 199 in the appendix.

The percentile ranks for the standing long jump among elite male and female athletes can be seen in table 5.5. Table 5.6 provides rankings in 15- and 16-year-olds, and table 5.7 provides the percentile rankings of collegiate football players participating in the National Football League (NFL) combine.

TABLE 5.5 Percentile Ranks for Standing Long Jump in Elite Male and Female Athletes

	MALES		FEMALES	
% rank	in.	cm	in.	cm
90	148	375	124	315
80	133	339	115	293
70	122	309	110	279
60	116	294	104	264
50	110	279	98	249
40	104	264	92	234
30	98	249	86	219
20	92	234	80	204
10	86	219	74	189

Adapted, by permission, from D.A. Chu, 1996, *Explosive power and strength* (Champaign, IL: Human Kinetics), 171.

TABLE 5.6 Rankings for Standing Long Jump in 15- and 16-Year-Old Male and Female Athletes

Category	MALES		FEMALES	
	in.	cm	in.	cm
Excellent	79	201	65	166
Above average	73	186	61	156
Average	69	176	57	146
Below average	65	165	53	135
Poor	<65	<165	<53	<135

Adapted, by permission, from D.A. Chu, 1996, *Explosive power and strength* (Champaign, IL: Human Kinetics), 171.

TABLE 5.7 Standing Long Jump Heights for College Football Players Participating in the NFL Combine

	DB		DL		LB		OL	
% rank	in.	cm	in.	cm	in.	cm	in.	cm
90	127.0	322.6	120.8	306.8	125.0	317.5	108.9	276.6
80	122.0	309.9	118.8	301.8	122.0	309.9	105.8	268.7
70	121.7	309.1	117.2	297.7	117.5	298.5	104.0	264.2
60	120.0	304.8	116.6	296.2	117.0	297.2	101.6	258.1
50	120.0	304.8	115.0	292.1	116.0	294.6	100.0	254.0
40	117.8	299.2	115.0	292.1	114.0	289.6	98.4	249.9
30	116.0	294.6	112.6	286.0	112.5	285.8	97.0	246.4
20	115.0	292.1	110.2	279.9	111.0	281.9	94.0	238.8
10	113.0	287.0	107.2	272.3	106.0	269.2	89.1	226.3
$\bar{X}$	119.5	303.5	114.8	291.6	115.8	294.1	99.7	253.2
SD	5.6	14.2	4.5	11.4	6.0	15.2	6.8	17.3
n	40		15		24		50	

	QB		RB		TE		WR	
% rank	in.	cm	in.	cm	in.	cm	in.	cm
90	118.5	301.0	126.3	320.8	122.8	311.9	127.0	322.6
80	116.0	294.6	122.2	310.4	121.2	307.8	122.2	310.4
70	114.0	289.6	120.0	304.8	115.2	292.6	120.3	305.6
60	110.0	279.4	119.0	302.3	111.2	282.4	118.0	299.7
50	106.5	270.5	116.0	294.6	111.0	281.9	117.0	297.2
40	104.0	264.2	114.8	291.6	109.0	276.9	113.6	288.5
30	103.5	262.9	111.1	282.2	108.2	274.8	112.0	284.5
20	102.0	259.1	110.0	279.4	106.4	270.3	111.0	281.9
10	98.5	250.2	108.7	276.1	96.4	244.9	110.0	279.4
$\bar{X}$	108.1	274.6	116.5	295.9	111.3	282.7	116.7	296.4
SD	7.1	18.0	6.5	16.5	8.3	21.1	5.9	15.0
n	14		36		11		38	

DB = defensive backs; DL = defensive linemen; LB = linebackers; OL = offensive linemen; QB = quarterbacks; RB = running backs; TE = tight ends; WR = wide receivers.

Data from 1999 NFL combine.

VERTICAL JUMP

The vertical jump is perhaps the most popular field test used to assess anaerobic power in athletic populations. It is relatively easy to perform and provides a measurement of power specific to sports that involve jumps (i.e., basketball and volleyball).

📱 For a description of how to perform the vertical jump, please see page 199 in the appendix.

The primary drawback of the vertical jump test is that it only measures jump height, so two athletes who jump the same height appear to have the same power output. Jump height alone, though, does not consider the mass of the athlete. In two athletes who have the same vertical jump height but different body masses, the athlete with the greater body mass has the greater power output. To assess power more accurately, the Lewis formula was developed to estimate power output from the vertical jump test (Fox and Mathews 1981). The formula is

$$power = \sqrt{4.9} \cdot weight \cdot \sqrt{jump\ height},$$

where power is in kg × m/s, weight is in kg, and jump height is in m.

Since power should be reported in standard units (W), the formula is adjusted as follows:

$$power = \sqrt{4.9} \cdot 9.807 \cdot weight \cdot \sqrt{jump\ height}.$$

The Lewis formula for converting vertical jump height to power output was popular among coaches, physical educators, and researchers (Harman et al. 1991). However, when compared to power outputs attained on a force plate, the Lewis formula underestimated peak and mean power by 70% and 12%, respectively (Harman et al. 1991). Harman and colleagues (1991) developed a more effective formula by using a multiple regression. The resulting equations were

$$peak\ power = 61.9\ (jump\ height) + 36\ (body\ mass) + 1,822,\ and$$

$$mean\ power = 21.2\ (jump\ height) + 23\ (body\ mass) - 1,393,$$

where power is in W, jump height is in cm, and body mass is in kg.

Percentile ranks for vertical jump heights in youth (ages 7-18) can be seen in table 5.8. The vertical jump heights in football and basketball players are shown in tables 5.9 and 5.10, respectively. The data for high school football and basketball athletes provide a year-by-year comparison to highlight the age-associated improvements. The data on collegiate and professional athletes combine all years of competition at each respective

TABLE 5.8 Percentile Ranks for Vertical Jump Heights in Youth

% rank	7-8 Y		9-10 Y		11-12 Y	
	in.	cm	in.	cm	in.	cm
90	9.6	24.4	11.5	29.2	16.5	41.9
80	9.3	23.6	11.0	27.9	14.3	36.3
70	8.7	22.1	10.4	26.4	12.3	31.2
60	8.1	20.6	9.9	25.1	11.8	30.0
50	8.0	20.3	9.5	24.1	10.5	26.7
40	7.7	19.6	9.0	22.9	10.0	25.4
30	7.5	19.1	8.6	21.8	9.6	24.4
20	7.1	18.0	7.8	19.8	8.8	22.4
10	6.9	17.5	7.0	17.8	6.8	17.3
$\bar{X}$	8.1	20.6	9.3	23.6	11.2	28.4
SD	1.0	2.5	1.7	4.3	3.5	8.9
n	26		67		74	

(continued)

TABLE 5.8 Percentile Ranks for Vertical Jump Heights in Youth *(continued)*

% rank	13-14 Y MALE in.	13-14 Y MALE cm	13-14 Y FEMALE in.	13-14 Y FEMALE cm	15-16 Y MALE in.	15-16 Y MALE cm	15-16 Y FEMALE in.	15-16 Y FEMALE cm	17-18 Y MALE in.	17-18 Y MALE cm
90	21.0	53.3	17.0	43.2	27.0	68.6	18.5	47.0	28.2	71.6
80	20.0	50.8	16.0	40.6	24.0	61.0	17.5	44.5	26.0	66.0
70	19.0	48.3	16.0	40.6	22.5	57.2	16.9	42.9	25.0	63.5
60	18.4	46.7	15.0	38.1	22.0	55.9	16.0	40.6	23.8	60.5
50	17.0	43.2	14.5	36.8	20.5	52.1	15.5	39.4	22.0	55.9
40	16.0	40.6	14.0	35.6	20.0	50.8	14.9	37.8	20.2	51.3
30	15.0	38.1	14.0	35.6	20.0	50.8	14.1	35.8	19.4	49.3
20	13.8	35.1	13.5	34.3	17.0	43.2	13.2	33.5	18.6	47.2
10	12.3	31.2	13.0	33.0	17.0	43.2	10.0	25.4	18.0	45.7
$\bar{X}$	16.8	42.7	14.6	37.1	20.9	53.1	15.2	38.6	22.6	57.4
SD	3.4	8.6	1.5	3.8	3.4	8.6	2.7	6.9	3.8	9.7
n	42		19		29		16		27	

TABLE 5.9 Percentile Ranks for Vertical Jump (No Step) in Football

% rank	HS 9TH GRADE in.	HS 9TH GRADE cm	HS 10TH GRADE in.	HS 10TH GRADE cm	HS 11TH GRADE in.	HS 11TH GRADE cm	HS 12TH GRADE in.	HS 12TH GRADE cm
90	27.6	70.1	27.4	69.6	28.5	72.4	30.0	76.2
80	25.5	64.8	26.0	66.0	26.9	68.3	28.0	71.1
70	24.0	61.0	24.6	62.5	25.5	64.8	26.5	67.3
60	23.5	59.7	23.9	60.7	25.0	63.5	26.0	66.0
50	22.3	56.6	23.0	58.4	24.0	61.0	25.0	63.5
40	21.9	55.6	22.0	55.9	23.5	59.7	23.5	59.7
30	21.2	53.8	21.0	53.3	22.0	55.9	22.5	57.2
20	19.3	49.0	19.0	48.3	20.5	52.1	21.5	54.6
10	17.7	45.0	18.0	45.7	18.8	47.8	19.5	49.5
$\bar{X}$	22.6	57.4	22.7	57.7	23.9	60.7	25.0	63.5
SD	3.6	9.1	4.1	10.4	3.5	8.9	4.1	10.4
n	30		102		95		114	

% rank	NCAA DIII in.	NCAA DIII cm	NCAA DI in.	NCAA DI cm
90	30.0	76.2	33.5	85.1
80	28.5	72.4	31.5	80.0
70	27.5	69.9	30.0	76.2
60	26.5	67.3	29.0	73.7
50	25.5	64.8	28.0	71.1
40	24.5	62.2	27.0	68.6
30	23.5	59.7	25.5	64.8
20	22.0	55.9	24.0	61.0
10	20.0	50.8	21.5	54.6
$\bar{X}$	25.3	64.3	27.6	70.1
SD	4	10.2	4.4	11.2
n	567		1,495	

level. Table 5.11 provides vertical jump heights for college football players (organized by position) invited to the NFL combine. (These results were collected from Web sites providing 2 y of data from the combine. NFL scouts present at the combine confirmed the accuracy of these Web sites.) Table 5.12 provides the percentile ranks for vertical jump heights of various NCAA Division I female athletes. Normative data for different sports are limited. To help rate vertical jump heights of various sports and levels of competition, table 5.13 shows descriptive data of vertical jump heights and jump power performance of various athletic populations reported in the literature or through personal communications.

HS = high school.

TABLE 5.10 Percentile Ranks for Vertical Jump (No Step) in Basketball Players

% rank	HS 14 Y in.	HS 14 Y cm	HS 15 Y in.	HS 15 Y cm	HS 16 Y in.	HS 16 Y cm	HS 17 Y in.	HS 17 Y cm
90	25.6	65.0	27.1	68.8	29.0	73.7	28.3	71.9
80	23.4	59.4	25.0	63.5	27.5	69.9	26.5	67.3
70	22.5	57.2	24.0	61.0	25.7	65.3	24.5	62.2
60	21.6	54.9	23.0	58.4	24.7	62.7	24.0	61.0
50	21.0	53.3	23.0	58.4	24.0	61.0	24.0	61.0
40	20.9	53.1	22.0	55.9	23.0	58.4	23.5	59.7
30	20.3	51.6	21.5	54.6	22.4	56.9	22.9	58.2
20	18.0	45.7	20.5	52.1	20.9	53.1	21.6	54.9
10	15.4	39.1	20.0	50.8	19.5	49.5	21.0	53.3
$\bar{X}$	21.0	53.3	23.1	58.7	24.0	61.0	24.0	61.0
SD	3.1	7.9	3.0	7.6	3.9	9.9	2.3	5.8
n	21		87		58		22	

% rank	NCAA DI in.	NCAA DI cm	NCAA DI FEMALE in.	NCAA DI FEMALE cm	NBA in.	NBA cm
90	30.5	77.5	21.6	54.9	31.2	79.2
80	30.0	76.2	20.1	51.1	29.5	74.9
70	28.5	72.4	19.7	50.0	28.4	72.1
60	28.0	71.1	18.5	47.0	27.5	69.9
50	27.5	69.9	18.0	45.7	27.0	68.6
40	26.8	68.1	17.5	44.5	26.2	66.5
30	26.0	66.0	16.5	41.9	24.6	62.5
20	25.5	64.8	15.9	40.4	23.6	59.9
10	24.5	62.2	14.5	36.8	22.4	56.9
$\bar{X}$	27.7	70.4	18.0	45.7	26.7	67.8
SD	2.4	6.1	2.5	6.4	3.3	8.4
n	138		118		40	

HS = high school.

TABLE 5.11 Vertical Jump Heights for College Football Players Participating in the NFL Combine

% rank	DB in.	DB cm	DL in.	DL cm	LB in.	LB cm	OL in.	OL cm
90	40.0	101.6	36.8	93.5	37.0	94.0	33.0	83.8
80	38.5	97.8	35.0	88.9	36.4	92.5	31.6	80.3
70	37.5	95.3	34.1	86.6	35.0	88.9	30.5	77.5
60	37.0	94.0	32.5	82.6	34.0	86.4	29.5	74.9
50	36.0	91.4	32.0	81.3	33.5	85.1	28.5	72.4
40	35.5	90.2	30.5	77.5	32.5	82.6	27.8	70.6
30	34.5	87.6	30.5	77.5	32.4	82.3	27.0	68.6
20	33.5	85.1	30.0	76.2	31.0	78.7	26.0	66.0
10	32.5	82.6	28.5	72.4	30.0	76.2	25.0	63.5
$\bar{X}$	36.2	91.9	32.0	81.3	33.5	85.1	28.8	73.2
SD	2.6	6.6	3.5	8.9	2.9	7.4	3.1	7.9
n	120		102		65		148	

(continued)

TABLE 5.11 Vertical Jump Heights for College Football Players Participating in the NFL Combine *(continued)*

	QB		RB		TE		WR	
% rank	in.	cm	in.	cm	in.	cm	in.	cm
90	35.5	90.2	38.5	97.8	37.9	96.3	39.5	100.3
80	35.5	90.2	36.6	93.0	36.2	91.9	38.5	97.8
70	34.5	87.6	35.0	88.9	35.6	90.4	36.5	92.7
60	33.2	84.3	34.5	87.6	34.9	88.6	36.0	91.4
50	31.8	80.8	33.5	85.1	34.0	86.4	35.5	90.2
40	31.0	78.7	32.5	82.6	33.5	85.1	34.5	87.6
30	30.0	76.2	32.0	81.3	31.0	78.7	34.0	86.4
20	29.0	73.7	31.0	78.7	30.5	77.5	32.5	82.6
10	26.5	67.3	29.7	75.4	28.5	72.4	31.5	80.0
$\bar{X}$	31.8	80.8	33.8	85.9	33.6	85.3	35.5	90.2
SD	3.6	9.1	3.1	7.9	3.3	8.4	3.4	8.6
n	38		73		42		100	

DB = defensive backs; DL = defensive linemen; LB = linebackers; OL = offensive linemen; QB = quarterbacks; RB = running backs; TE = tight ends; WR = wide receivers.

Data collected 1999 NFL combine and from ESPN.com, Redeyesports.com, and ffmastermind.com.

TABLE 5.12 Percentile Ranks for Vertical Jump (No Step) in NCAA Division I Female Athletes

	VOLLEYBALL		SOFTBALL		SWIMMING	
% rank	in.	cm	in.	cm	in.	cm
90	20.0	50.8	18.5	47.0	19.9	50.5
80	18.9	48.0	17.0	43.2	18.0	45.7
70	18.0	45.7	16.0	40.6	17.4	44.2
60	17.5	44.5	15.0	38.1	16.1	40.9
50	17.0	43.2	14.5	36.8	15.0	38.1
40	16.7	42.4	14.0	35.6	14.5	36.8
30	16.5	41.9	13.0	33.0	13.0	33.0
20	16.0	40.6	12.0	30.5	12.5	31.8
10	15.5	39.4	11.0	27.9	11.6	29.5
$\bar{X}$	17.3	43.9	14.6	37.1	15.3	38.9
SD	2.1	5.3	2.9	7.4	3.0	7.6
n	90		118		40	

TABLE 5.13 Descriptive Data for the Vertical Jump Test in Athletic Populations

Population	Gender	VERTICAL JUMP HEIGHT		VERTICAL JUMP POWER	Source
		(in.)	(cm)	(W)	
Baseball					
Elite youth	M				Unpublished data
13 y		16.0 ± 3.8	35.1 ± 8.4		
14 y		18.4 ± 3.4	40.4 ± 7.4		
15 y		20.5 ± 3.4	45.2 ± 7.4		
16 y		21.1 ± 3.5	46.5 ± 7.6		
17 y		23.0 ± 3.2	50.6 ± 7.1		
NAIA	M	23.7 ± 3.2	60.2 ± 8.2		Unpublished data
NCAA DIII	M	22.3 ± 2.5	56.6 ± 6.4		Unpublished data

Population	Gender	VERTICAL JUMP HEIGHT		VERTICAL JUMP POWER	Source
		(in.)	(cm)	(W)	
Basketball					
NCAA DI	M	28.1 ± 4.1	71.4 ± 10.4	1,671 ± 210	Latin, Berg, and Baechle 1994
G		28.9 ± 3.8	73.4 ± 9.6	1,551 ± 162	
F		28.1 ± 4.1	71.4 ± 10.4	1,751 ± 211	
C		26.3 ± 4.2	66.8 ± 10.7	1,786 ± 163	
NCAA DI	F	19.0 ± 3.3	48.2 ± 8.5		LaMonte et al. 1999
G		19.4 ± 2.4	49.4 ± 6.2		
F		19.4 ± 4.4	49.4 ± 11.1		
C		17.1 ± 1.8	43.5 ± 4.5		
Canadian national team	F	17.6 ± 2.1	44.7 ± 5.3		Smith and Thomas 1991
G		19.3 ± 1.9	48.9 ± 4.9		
F		17.5 ± 1.7	44.5 ± 4.4		
C		16.5 ± 1.2	42.0 ± 3.0		
Football					
NCAA DI	M	31.5 ± 4.0	80.1 ± 10.2	2,078 ± 307	Garstecki, Latin, and Cuppett 2004
DL		30.7 ± 3.2	77.9 ± 8.2	2,303 ± 178	
LB		34.0 ± 3.1	83.2 ± 7.8	2,050 ± 135	
DB		34.6 ± 3.1	87.8 ± 7.8	1,725 ± 139	
QB		31.8 ± 2.5	80.7 ± 6.4	1,804 ± 151	
RB		33.8 ± 3.0	85.9 ± 7.7	1,953 ± 185	
WR		34.4 ± 2.8	87.4 ± 7.0	1,736 ± 176	
OL		27.1 ± 2.4	68.8 ± 6.2	2,395 ± 166	
TE		31.3 ± 2.8	79.6 ± 7.2	2,202 ± 150	
NCAA DII	M	27.6 ± 4.8	70.1 ± 12.1	1,898 ± 371	Garstecki, Latin, and Cuppett 2004
DL		26.3 ± 4.4	66.9 ± 11.3	2,063 ± 231	
LB		28.5 ± 4.3	72.4 ± 10.8	1,849 ± 161	
DB		30.7 ± 4.1	78.0 ± 10.3	1,602 ± 185	
QB		27.7 ± 3.7	70.3 ± 9.3	1,715 ± 161	
RB		29.2 ± 4.3	74.2 ± 11.0	1,783 ± 157	
WR		30.6 ± 4.8	77.8 ± 12.1	1,593 ± 168	
OL		23.8 ± 3.4	60.4 ± 8.6	2,163 ± 229	
TE		27.6 ± 3.4	70.1 ± 8.7	1,903 ± 182	
NFL drafted rookies	M				McGee and Burkett 2003
Rounds 1 + 2		33.3 ± 3.3	84.3 ± 8.4		
Rounds 6 + 7		31.2 ± 4.2	79.2 ± 10.7		
Soccer					
Portuguese youth (13-15 y)	M	11.5 ± 1.8	29.3 ± 4.6		Malina et al. 2004
Defensemen		11.9 ± 2.0	30.3 ± 5.0		
Midfielders		11.1 ± 1.5	28.2 ± 3.9		
Forwards		11.9 ± 2.0	30.1 ± 5.2		
Elite Norwegian	M				Wisloff, Helgerud, and Hoff 1998
Defensemen		21.7 ± 2.6	55.1 ± 6.5		
Midfielders		19.9 ± 1.7	50.5 ± 4.4		
Forwards		22.7 ± 2.0	57.6 ± 5.1		
American elite youth and adult*	F				Kirkendall 2000
U12		15.9	40.3		
U13		16.1	40.8		
U14		16.9	42.8		
U15		17.7	44.9		
U16		18.0	45.6		
U17		19.5	49.6		
U18		17.0	43.1		

(continued)

TABLE 5.13 Descriptive Data for the Vertical Jump Test in Athletic Populations *(continued)*

Population	Gender	VERTICAL JUMP HEIGHT (in.)	VERTICAL JUMP HEIGHT (cm)	VERTICAL JUMP POWER (W)	Source
Soccer					
National	M	20.6	52.4		Kirkendall 2000
U13		18.6	47.2		
U14		21.2	53.8		
U15		24.0	61.0		
U16		25.7	65.2		
16 National		24.0	61.0		
17 National		25.7	65.3		
20 National		26.1	66.3		
23 National		27.7	70.4		
Volleyball					
NCAA DI	F	18.9 ± 1.7	48.0 ± 4.2		Fry et al. 1991
Weightlifting					
National	F	19.7 ± 3.1	50.0 ± 8.0	962 ± 232	Stoessel et al. 1991
	M	23.9 ± 1.5	60.8 ± 3.9	5,377 ± 395	Fry et al. 2003
Wrestling					
National	M	23.6 ± 3.9	60 ± 10		Callan et al. 2000
NCAA DI	M	23.6 ± 3.9		4,916 ± 395#	Kraemer et al. 2001

* = one step permitted; # = jump power assessed from a force plate. C = centers; F = forwards; G = guards; DB = defensive back; DL = defensive line; LB = linebacker; OL = offensive line; QB = quarterback; RB = running back; TE = tight end; WR = wide receiver.

SHUTTLE RUN

The 300 yd (274.3 m) shuttle run is a field test often used to assess anaerobic capacity (Gillam 1983). Normative data for this assessment are shown in table 5.14.

📄 For a description of how to perform the 300 yd (274.3 m) shuttle run, please see page 199 in the appendix.

TABLE 5.14 Percentile Ranks for Shuttle Run Times (s) in NCAA Division I Athletes

% rank	Baseball	Men's basketball	Women's basketball	Softball
90	56.7	54.1	58.4	63.3
80	58.9	55.1	61.8	65.1
70	59.9	55.6	63.6	66.5
60	61.3	56.3	64.7	67.9
50	62.0	56.7	65.2	69.2
40	63.2	57.2	65.9	71.3
30	63.9	58.1	66.8	72.4
20	65.3	58.9	68.1	74.6
10	67.7	60.2	68.9	78.0
$\bar{X}$	62.2	57.1	64.7	70.0
SD	4.2	2.7	4.1	6.3
n	107	125	82	114

Adapted from G.M. Gillam, 1983, "300 yard shuttle run," *National Strength and Conditioning Association Journal* 5:46.

LINE DRILL

The line drill is a field test that measures anaerobic capacity in athletes (Seminick 1994). Recent studies have demonstrated that the line drill is an acceptable measure for anaerobic power performance, and it may also indicate anaerobic fitness (Hoffman et al. 2000; Hoffman and Kaminsky 2000). Although descriptive data for the line drill are limited, table 5.15 provides percentile ranks in NCAA Division III football players and in elite high school basketball players. A major concern in many anaerobic sports is the lack of a valid assessment to indicate an athlete's preparedness to play an anaerobic sport. To address this concern, some coaches have their athletes perform repeated line drills. This assessment has been performed with the football team at The College of New Jersey. The line drill is slightly altered for football in that cones are placed at the goal line and the 10, 20, 30, and 40 yd (9.1, 18.3, 27.4, and 36.6 m) lines of the field. The athletes begin at the goal line and sprint to each cone and then back to the goal line. Three line drills are performed with 2 min rest between each. Table 5.15 also provides the percentile ranks for fatigue rates in college football players performing repeated (3) line drills.

📄 For a description of how to perform the line drill, please see page 200 in the appendix.

TABLE 5.15 Percentile Ranks for the Line Drill			
	NCAA DIII FOOTBALL		**MEN'S BASKET-BALL (ISRAELI NATIONAL HIGH SCHOOL)**
% rank	Time (s)	FI (%)	Time (s)
90	34.2	.93	27.4
80	34.8	.91	27.6
70	35.5	.89	28.0
60	36.3	.87	28.0
50	36.8	.86	28.1
40	37.5	.84	28.3
30	38.1	.83	28.6
20	39.5	.81	29.1
10	41.7	.78	30.6
$\bar{X}$	37.4	.85	28.5
SD	3.1	.08	1.2
n	335	335	59

FI = fatigue index (fastest time / slowest time of 3 sprints).

Summary

- ⊃ Numerous anaerobic tests varying in style and sophistication have been developed.
- ⊃ Laboratory assessments of anaerobic power may be highly sophisticated and sensitive.
- ⊃ Field tests are easier to perform and can assess both anaerobic power and capacity.
- ⊃ The test selected should be specific to the movement patterns of the athlete.

CHAPTER 6

Aerobic Power and Endurance

Aerobic power, also referred to as *aerobic capacity,* measures a person's capacity for aerobic synthesis of ATP (McArdle, Katch, and Katch 1996) and so indicates the ability to perform sustained, high-intensity exercise. During exercise of increasing intensity (whether by running faster or up a greater incline), oxygen consumption increases. As the workload continues to increase, oxygen uptake plateaus and the athlete begins to utilize other energy sources (e.g., glycolytic sources) to produce ATP. The point at which oxygen uptake plateaus with an increase in workload is called *maximal aerobic power, maximal oxygen uptake, maximal oxygen consumption,* or simply $\dot{V}O_2max$. Maximal aerobic power is a critical component in determining the success of endurance athletes. In addition, aerobic capacity may be used to assess the fitness and health status of recreational athletes and sedentary individuals. This chapter discusses both laboratory and field measurements of aerobic capacity and provides normative data for general and athletic populations.

Aerobic Power Assessment

Maximal aerobic power can be determined either by directly measuring oxygen consumption ($\dot{V}O_2$) while the athlete exercises to exhaustion or by administering submaximal exercise tests. Directly measuring $\dot{V}O_2$ while the athlete performs a graded exercise is considered the gold standard of maximal aerobic power assessment. However, $\dot{V}O_2max$ can also be determined on a cycle ergometer or through tethered swimming. The choice of exercise depends on the sport that the athlete plays or the exercise that the individual is most accustomed to performing. However, if specificity is not an issue, the treadmill produces the best results. In a study of triathletes, the results for $\dot{V}O_2max$ from tethered swimming and cycle ergometry were 13% to 18% and 3% to 6% lower, respectively, than values obtained from treadmill running (O'Toole, Douglas, and Hiller 1989).

LABORATORY TESTS

Figures 6.1, 6.2, and 6.3 describe popular treadmill and cycle ergometer protocols for assessing maximal aerobic capacity. Many protocols have been developed, some of which are population specific. For instance, some are designed for cardiac subjects whereas others are designed for athletes. The primary differences between the two are the starting points (beginning elevation and speed of the treadmill) and the increments between stages of exercise (increases in elevation and speed).

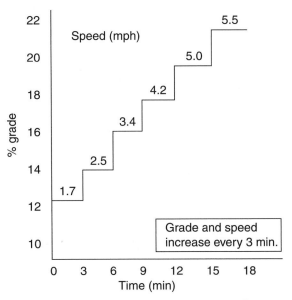

FIGURE 6.1 The Bruce treadmill protocol for assessing maximal oxygen consumption.

Reprinted from *American Heart Journal*, 85, R.A. Bruce, F. Kusumi and D. Hosmer, "Maximal oxygen uptake and nomographic assessment of functional aerobic impairment in cardiovascular disease," 546-562, Copyright 1973, with permission of Elsevier.

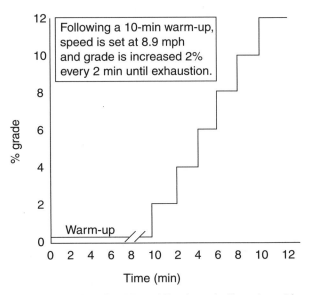

FIGURE 6.2 The Costill and Fox treadmill protocol for assessing maximal oxygen consumption.

Adapted, by permission, from D.L. Costill and E.L. Fox, 1969, "Energetics of marathon running," *Med Sci Sports Exerc* 1: 81-86.

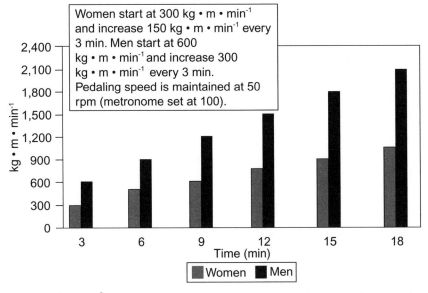

Figure 6.3 The Åstrand cycle ergometer protocol for assessing maximal oxygen consumption.

Adapted, by permission, from P.O. Åstrand, 1960, "Aerobic capacity in men & women with special reference to age," *Acta Physiologica Scandinavica* 49 (Suppl. 169): 45-60.

Before beginning a maximal exercise test, the subject should warm up for a minimum of 5 min or until she feels ready to proceed. Generally the warm-up is performed at a 0% grade and at a speed that the subject considers comfortable. Following the warm-up, the subject is attached to the breathing apparatus, and the test begins. The test ends when the subject indicates that she has reached exhaustion or when the subject has met at least two of the first three criteria listed here:

1. An increase in oxygen uptake no greater than $150 \ ml \cdot min^{-1}$, despite an increase in exercise intensity (plateau criterion)

2. The attainment of the age-predicted maximal heart rate

3. A respiratory exchange ratio $(\dot{V}CO_2/\dot{V}O_2)$ greater than 1.10

4. A plasma lactate concentration of at least 8 $mmol \cdot L^{-1}$ 4 min after exercise

The fourth criterion can only be assessed once the test has been completed and is used to confirm that $\dot{V}O_2$max has been attained.

In general, the testing protocols used for adults are also suitable for children (>8 y of age) (Bar-Or 1993). However, a treadmill test is recommended for children as they often experience early fatigue in the knee extensors during the cycle ergometer exercise. Still, due to safety, space, and cost considerations cycle ergometers are used to aerobically test children. Tables 6.1 and 6.2 detail examples of treadmill and cycle ergometer testing protocols for children of different heights. These protocols can be used for both maximal and submaximal tests.

Tethered swimming is not a common method of assessing aerobic capacity, but it is the most specific method for swimming and other water sports (e.g., water polo). The subject swims in a stationary position, using the freestyle stroke. He is attached to a harness connected to a rope or series of pulleys and to a pan containing weights (Costill 1966). The swimmer swims to maintain a constant body position in the pool. Initial resistance may be 50% of the subject's maximum (determined in a familiarization session) and is increased during each stage of exercise. Expired air collected in a meteorological balloon during the last minute of each stage is analyzed. A swimming flume, which

uses propeller pumps to vary the resistance that the swimmer must swim against, eliminates the need for any attachment to the swimmer. This allows the swimmer to swim more naturally.

Considering the costs that are associated with the equipment, space, and personnel needed to directly measure oxygen consumption, this methodology is generally reserved for research or clinical settings. When directly measuring $\dot{V}O_2$max is not possible, there are a variety of submaximal and maximal tests for predicting $\dot{V}O_2$max. These tests are generally performed in a controlled environment and are administered on an individual basis by the exercise technician. The validity of these tests has been well established and is based on several assumptions:

- A steady-state heart rate is obtained for each stage of exercise.
- The relationship between heart rate and exercise intensity is linear.
- The maximal heart rate for a given age is consistent.
- The efficiency of exercise (i.e., $\dot{V}O_2$ for the intensity of exercise) is the same for everyone (ACSM 2000).

If these assumptions are not met, the test may be less valid.

Submaximal testing can be performed on either a cycle ergometer or a treadmill. Generally a submaximal test uses an end point that equals 85% of the age-predicted maximal heart rate. With a treadmill, the speed and grade of the final exercise stage can be used to estimate $\dot{V}O_2$max (see figure 6.4). The benefit of using a treadmill is that most individuals are more familiar with walking or running than with riding a cycle ergometer. However, cycle ergometers may still be more popular because of the ease in performing other measurements (i.e., blood pressure and electrocardiogram (ECG) readings) during the test and the non-weight-bearing nature of the test. That cycle ergometers are less expensive but safer than treadmills (e.g., subject is less likely to trip or fall while cycling as compared to running on a treadmill) may contribute to a greater use of submaximal cycle ergometer testing. Normative data for the Åstrand-Rhyming cycle ergometer test can be found in tables 6.3 to 6.6.

📄 For descriptions of the YMCA submaximal cycle ergometer test and the Åstrand-Rhyming cycle ergometer test, please see page 201 in the appendix.

TABLE 6.1 Treadmill Walking Protocol for the Child

Body height (cm)	Speed (km · h⁻¹)	Initial slope (%)	Slope increment (%)	Stage duration (min)
<110	4	10	2.5	2
110-129.9	5	10	2.5	2
130-149.9	6	10	2.5	2
>150	6	10 (females) 12.5 (males)	2.5	2

Adapted from Bar-Or O. 1993. Importance of differences between children and adults for exercise testing and prescription. In Skinner J.S. (ed) *Exercise Testing and Exercise Prescription for Special Cases.* 2nd Edition Williams and Wilkins: Baltimore, MD. 57-74.

TABLE 6.2 Cycle Ergometer Protocol for the Child

Body height (cm)	Initial load (W)	Increments (W)	Stage duration (min)
<120	12.5	12.5	2
120-139.9	12.5	25	2
140-159.9	25	25	2
>160	25	25 (females) 50 (males)	2

Adapted, by permission, from O. Bar-Or, 1993, Importance of differences between children and adults for exercise testing and prescription. In *Exercise testing and exercise prescription for special cases,* 2nd ed., edited by J.S. Skinner (Baltimore, MD: Lippincott, Williams & Wilkins), 57-74.

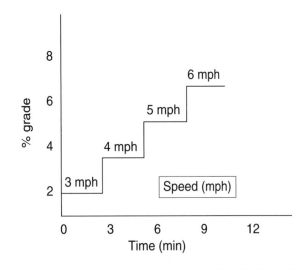

FIGURE 6.4 Submaximal treadmill protocol for estimating aerobic fitness. Each stage should last for 3 min to allow a steady-state heart rate to be achieved. To estimate $\dot{V}O_2$max the following formula is used (from Ebbeling et al. 1991):

$\dot{V}O_2$max (ml · kg^{-1} · min^{-1}) = 15.1 + (21.8 × speed in mph)
    − (0.327 × heart rate)
    − (0.263 × speed in mph × age)
    + (0.00504 × heart rate × age)
    + (5.98 × gender),

For gender 0 = females and 1 = males. This formula is reported to predict $\dot{V}O_2$max within 4.85 ml · kg^{-1} · min^{-1} of actual $\dot{V}O_2$max.

Adapted, by permission, from C.B. Ebeling et al. 1991, "Development of a single-stage submaximal treadmill walking test," Med Sci Sports Exerc 23: 966-973.

TABLE 6.3 Prediction of Maximal Oxygen Consumption from Heart Rate and Cycling Power in Men

Maximal oxygen consumption (L · min⁻¹)					Maximal oxygen consumption (L · min⁻¹)				
	POWER (KG · M · MIN⁻¹; W)					POWER (KG · M · MIN⁻¹; W)			
HR (beats/ min)	300; 50	600; 100	900; 150	1,200; 200	1,500; 250	HR (beats/ min)	600; 100	900; 150	1,200; 200	1,500; 250
120	2.2	3.5	4.8			146	2.4	3.3	4.4	5.5
121	2.2	3.4	4.7			147	2.4	3.3	4.4	5.5
122	2.2	3.4	4.6			148	2.4	3.2	4.3	5.4
123	2.1	3.4	4.6			149	2.3	3.2	4.3	5.4
124	2.1	3.3	4.5	6.0		150	2.3	3.2	4.2	5.3
125	2.0	3.2	4.4	5.9		151	2.3	3.1	4.2	5.2
126	2.0	3.2	4.4	5.8		152	2.3	3.1	4.1	5.2
127	2.0	3.1	4.3	5.7		153	2.2	3.0	4.1	5.1
128	2.0	3.1	4.2	5.6		154	2.2	3.0	4.0	5.1
129	1.9	3.0	4.2	5.6		155	2.2	3.0	4.0	5.0
130	1.9	3.0	4.1	5.5		156	2.2	2.9	4.0	5.0
131	1.9	2.9	4.0	5.4		157	2.1	2.9	3.9	4.9
132	1.8	2.9	4.0	5.3		158	2.1	2.9	3.9	4.9
133	1.8	2.8	3.9	5.3		159	2.1	2.8	3.8	4.8
134	1.8	2.8	3.9	5.2		160	2.1	2.8	3.8	4.8
135	1.7	2.8	3.8	5.1		161	2.0	2.8	3.7	4.7
136	1.7	2.7	3.8	5.0		162	2.0	2.8	3.7	4.6
137	1.7	2.7	3.7	5.0		163	2.0	2.8	3.7	4.6
138	1.6	2.7	3.7	4.9		164	2.0	2.7	3.6	4.5
139	1.6	2.6	3.6	4.8		165	2.0	2.7	3.6	4.5
140	1.6	2.6	3.6	4.8	6.0	166	1.9	2.7	3.6	4.4
141		2.6	3.5	4.7	5.9	167	1.9	2.6	3.5	4.4
142		2.5	3.5	4.6	5.8	168	1.9	2.6	3.5	4.3
143		2.5	3.4	4.6	5.7	169	1.9	2.6	3.5	4.3
144		2.5	3.4	4.5	5.7	170	1.8	2.6	3.4	4.3
145		2.4	3.4	4.5	5.6					

Reprinted from G.M. Adams, 2002, Exercise physiology laboratory manual, 4th ed. (New York, NY: McGraw-Hill), with permission of The McGraw-Hill Companies; adapted, by permission, from P.O. Åstrand and I. Rhyming, 1954, "A nomogram for calculation of aerobic capacity (physical fitness) from pulse rate during submaximal work," Journal of Applied Physiology 7: 218-221.

TABLE 6.4 Prediction of Maximal Oxygen Consumption from Heart Rate and Cycling Power in Women

Maximal oxygen consumption (L · min⁻¹)						Maximal oxygen consumption (L · min⁻¹)					
	POWER (KG · M · MIN⁻¹; W)						POWER (KG · M · MIN⁻¹; W)				
HR (beats/min)	300; 50	450; 75	600; 100	750; 125	900; 150	HR (beats/min)	300; 50	450; 75	600; 100	750; 125	900; 150
120	2.6	3.4	4.1	4.8		146	1.6	2.2	2.6	3.2	3.7
121	2.5	3.3	2.0	4.8		147	1.6	2.1	2.6	3.1	3.6
122	2.5	3.2	3.9	4.7		148	1.6	2.1	2.6	3.1	3.6
123	2.4	3.1	3.9	4.6		149		2.1	2.6	3.0	3.5
124	2.4	3.1	3.8	4.5		150		2.0	2.5	3.0	3.5
125	2.3	3.0	3.7	4.4		151		2.0	2.5	3.0	3.4
126	2.3	3.0	3.7	4.4		152		2.0	2.5	2.9	3.4
127	2.2	2.9	3.5	4.2		153		2.0	2.4	2.9	3.3
128	2.2	2.8	3.5	4.2		154		2.0	2.4	2.8	3.3
129	2.2	2.8	3.4	4.1		155		1.9	2.4	2.8	3.2
130	2.1	2.7	3.4	4.0	4.7	156		1.9	2.3	2.8	3.2
131	2.1	2.7	3.4	4.0	4.6	157		1.9	2.3	2.7	3.2
132	2.0	2.7	3.3	4.0	4.5	158		1.8	2.3	2.7	3.1
133	2.0	2.6	3.2	3.8	4.4	159		1.8	2.2	2.7	3.1
134	2.0	2.6	3.2	3.8	4.4	160		1.8	2.2	2.6	3.0
135	2.0	2.6	3.1	3.7	4.3	161		1.8	2.2	2.6	3.0
136	1.9	2.5	3.1	3.6	4.2	162		1.8	2.2	2.6	3.0
137	1.9	2.5	3.0	3.6	4.2	163		1.7	2.2	2.6	2.9
138	1.8	2.4	2.9	3.5	4.1	164		1.7	2.1	2.5	2.9
139	1.8	2.4	2.8	3.5	4.0	165		1.7	2.1	2.5	2.9
140	1.8	2.4	2.8	3.4	4.0	166		1.7	2.1	2.5	2.8
141	1.8	2.3	2.8	3.4	3.9	167		1.6	2.1	2.4	2.8
142	1.7	2.3	2.8	3.3	3.9	168		1.6	2.0	2.4	2.8
143	1.7	2.2	2.7	3.3	3.8	169		1.6	2.0	2.4	2.8
144	1.7	2.2	2.7	3.2	3.8	170		1.6	2.0	2.4	2.7
145	1.6	2.2	2.7	3.2	3.7						

Reprinted from G.M. Adams, 2002, *Exercise physiology laboratory manual*, 4th ed. (New York, NY: McGraw-Hill), with permission of The McGraw-Hill Companies; adapted, by permission, from P.O. Åstrand and I. Rhyming, 1954, "A nomogram for calculation of aerobic capacity (physical fitness) from pulse rate during submaximal work," *Journal of Applied Physiology* 7: 218-221.

TABLE 6.5 Age Correction Factors (CF) for Age-Adjusted Maximal Oxygen Consumption

Age	CF	Age	CF	Age	CF	Age	CF	Age	CF
15	1.10	20	1.05	25	1.00	30	0.93	35	0.87
16	1.10	21	1.04	26	0.99	31	0.93	36	0.86
17	1.09	22	1.03	27	0.98	32	0.91	37	0.85
18	1.07	23	1.02	28	0.96	33	0.90	38	0.85
19	1.06	24	1.01	29	0.95	34	0.88	39	0.84

(continued)

Age	CF	Age	CF	Age	CF	Age	CF	Age	CF
40	0.83	45	0.78	50	0.75	55	0.71	60	0.68
41	0.82	46	0.77	51	0.74	56	0.70	61	0.67
42	0.81	47	0.77	52	0.73	57	0.70	62	0.67
43	0.80	48	0.76	53	0.73	58	0.69	63	0.66
44	0.79	49	0.76	54	0.72	59	0.69	64	0.66

Reprinted, by permission, from J.T. Cramer and J.W. Coburn, 2004, Fitness testing protocols and norms. In *NSCA's Essentials of Personal Training*, edited by R.W. Earle and T.R. Baechle (Champaign, IL: Human Kinetics), 252; adapted, by permission, from P.O. Åstrand, 1960, "Aerobic capacity in men & women with special reference to age," *Acta Physiologica Scandinavica* 49(Suppl. 169): 45-60.

TABLE 6.6 Norms for Evaluating Åstrand-Ryhming Cycle Test Performance

Age (y)	AEROBIC FITNESS CATEGORIES					
	VERY HIGH	HIGH	GOOD	AVERAGE	FAIR	LOW
	Maximal oxygen consumption (ml · kg · min⁻¹)					
Men						
20-29	>61	53-61	43-52	34-42	25-33	<25
30-39	>57	49-57	39-48	31-38	23-30	<23
40-49	>53	45-53	36-44	27-35	20-26	<20
50-59	>49	43-49	34-42	25-33	18-24	<18
60-69	>45	41-45	31-40	23-30	16-22	<16
Women						
20-29	>57	49-57	38-48	31-37	24-30	<24
30-39	>53	45-53	34-44	28-33	20-27	<20
40-49	>50	42-50	31-41	24-30	17-23	<17
50-59	>42	38-42	28-37	21-27	15-20	<15
60-69	>39	35-39	24-34	18-23	13-17	<13

Reprinted from G.M. Adams, 2002, *Exercise physiology laboratory manual*, 4th ed. (New York, NY: McGraw-Hill), with permission of The McGraw-Hill Companies.

All of the indirect protocols discussed in this chapter have been shown to be both reliable and accurate in directly measuring aerobic capacity. However, recent research has shown that the Bruce treadmill protocol and the Åstrand-Rhyming cycle ergometer test produce the least amount of error with the highest validity coefficient (Grant, Joseph, and Campagna 1999).

FIELD TESTS

In situations where large groups are being tested, it may be more timely to administer a field test. Field tests measuring the time required to run 1 to 2 mi (1.6-3.2 km) or the distance that can be run in 12 min have been used to estimate aerobic fitness. The most popular tests are the Cooper 12 min run and the 1.5 mi (2.41 km) test for time (ACSM 2000). In the Cooper test the individual runs as great a distance as possible in the allotted time (12 min). Percentile ranks of distance run in the 12 min test and of time required for the 1.5 mi (2.41 km) test can be seen in tables 6.7 and 6.8, respectively.

To estimate an individual's $\dot{V}O_2$max for the 12 min run, the following formula is used:

$\dot{V}O_2$max = 0.0268 (distance covered) – 11.3,

where $\dot{V}O_2$max is in ml·kg⁻¹·min⁻¹ and distance covered is in m.

The distance of a single lap around most oval tracks is 400 m. An individual who runs 5.5 laps runs 2,200 m. The estimated $\dot{V}O_2$max for that individual is

0.0268 (2,200) – 11.3 = 47.7 ml · kg⁻¹ · min⁻¹.

For the 1.5 mi (2.41 km) run, $\dot{V}O_2$max can be estimated by

$\dot{V}O_2$max = 3.5 + 483 / (time to run 1.5 mi or 2.41 km),

where $\dot{V}O_2$max is in ml·kg⁻¹·min⁻¹ and time is in min.

The Rockport walking test was developed specifically for individuals who are not comfortable running (Kline et al. 1987). It requires an individual to walk at a fast pace for 1.0 mi (1.6 km). Walk times can be compared to the normative values in table 6.9.

TABLE 6.7 Percentile Ranks for Distance Run During 12 Min Run

Percentile	AGE (Y)									
	20-29		30-39		40-49		50-59		60+	
Men	n = 1,675		n = 7,095		n = 6,837		n = 3,808		n = 1,005	
	mi	km	mi	km	mi	km	mi	km	mi	km
90	1.74	2.78	1.71	2.74	1.65	2.64	1.57	2.51	1.49	2.38
80	1.65	2.64	1.61	2.58	1.54	2.46	1.45	2.32	1.37	2.19
70	1.61	2.58	1.55	2.48	1.47	2.35	1.38	2.21	1.29	2.06
60	1.54	2.46	1.49	2.38	1.42	2.27	1.33	2.13	1.24	1.98
50	1.50	2.40	1.45	2.32	1.37	2.19	1.29	2.06	1.19	1.90
40	1.45	2.32	1.39	2.22	1.33	2.13	1.25	2.00	1.15	1.84
30	1.41	2.26	1.35	2.16	1.29	2.06	1.21	1.94	1.11	1.78
20	1.34	2.14	1.29	2.06	1.23	1.97	1.15	1.84	1.05	1.68
10	1.27	2.03	1.21	1.94	1.17	1.87	1.09	1.74	0.95	1.52
Women	n = 764		n = 2,049		n = 1,630		n = 878		n = 202	
90	1.54	2.46	1.45	2.32	1.41	2.26	1.29	2.06	1.29	2.06
80	1.45	2.32	1.38	2.21	1.32	2.11	1.21	1.94	1.18	1.89
70	1.37	2.19	1.33	2.13	1.25	2.00	1.17	1.87	1.13	1.81
60	1.33	2.13	1.27	2.03	1.21	1.94	1.13	1.81	1.07	1.71
50	1.29	2.06	1.25	2.00	1.17	1.87	1.10	1.76	1.03	1.65
40	1.25	2.00	1.21	1.94	1.13	1.81	1.06	1.70	0.99	1.58
30	1.21	1.94	1.16	1.86	1.10	1.76	1.02	1.63	0.97	1.55
20	1.16	1.86	1.11	1.78	1.05	1.68	0.98	1.57	0.94	1.50
10	1.10	1.76	1.05	1.68	1.01	1.62	0.93	1.49	0.89	1.42

Adapted, by permission, from American College of Sports Medicine, 1995, *Guidelines for exercise testing and prescription* (Philadelphia, PA: Lippincott, Williams & Wilkins), 113-115.

TABLE 6.8 Percentile Ranks for 1.5 Mi (2.41 km) Run Time (min:s)

Percentile	AGE (Y)				
	20-29	30-39	40-49	50-59	60+
Men	n = 1,675	n = 7,095	n = 6,837	n = 3,808	n = 1,005
90	9:09	9:30	10:16	11:18	12:20
80	10:16	10:47	11:44	12:51	13:53
70	10:47	11:34	12:34	13:45	14:53
60	11:41	12:20	13:14	14:24	15:29
50	12:18	12:51	13:53	14:55	16:07
40	12:51	13:36	14:29	15:26	16:43
30	13:22	14:08	14:56	15:57	17:14
20	14:13	14:52	15:41	16:43	18:00
10	15:10	15:52	16:28	17:29	19:15
Women	n = 764	n = 2,049	n = 1,630	n = 878	n = 202
90	11:43	12:51	13:22	14:55	14:55
80	12:51	13:43	14:31	15:57	16:20
70	13:53	14:24	15:16	16:27	16:58
60	14:24	15:08	15:57	16:58	17:46
50	14:55	15:26	16:27	17:24	18:16
40	15:26	15:57	16:58	17:55	18:44
30	15:57	16:35	17:24	18:23	18:59
20	16:33	17:14	18:00	18:49	19:21
10	17:21	18:00	18:31	19:30	20:04

Adapted, by permission, from American College of Sports Medicine, 1995, *Guidelines for exercise testing and prescription* (Philadelphia, PA: Lippincott, Williams & Wilkins), 113-115.

Maximal aerobic capacity can also be estimated from the Rockport walking test. To estimate $\dot{V}O_2$max, the individual's time for walking 1 mi (1.6 km) and the ending heart rate are entered into the following formula:

$\dot{V}O_2$max (ml · kg^{-1} · min^{-1}) = 132.853 – (0.0769 × BW)
– (0.3877 × age)
+ (6.315 × gender (1 for males, 0 for females))
– 3.2649 × time in minutes to walk 1.0 miles
– (0.1565 × heart rate),

TABLE 6.9 Normative Values for the Rockport Walking Test

Rating	Males	Females
Ages 30-69 y (min:s)		
Excellent	<10:12	<11:40
Good	10:13-11:42	11:41-13:08
High average	11:43-13:13	13:09-14:36
Low average	13:14-14:44	14:37-16:04
Fair	14:45-16:23	16:05-17:31
Poor	>16:24	>17:32
18-30 y (min:s)		
90%	11:08	11:45
75%	11:42	12:49
50%	12:38	13:15
25%	13:38	14:12
10%	14:37	15:03

Reprinted, by permission, from J.R. Morrow, A. Jackson, J. Disch and D. Mood, 2005, *Measurement and evaluation in human performance*, 3rd ed. (Champaign, IL: Human Kinetics), 235.

In addition to the run and walk tests, $\dot{V}O_2$max can be estimated for large groups with a step test. There are a variety of step tests with both acceptable reliability and validity. The Queens College step test was developed by McArdle and colleagues (1996) for predicting aerobic capacity in college-aged individuals. Slightly different protocols were established for males and females. Males step to a bench 16.25 in. (41.28 cm) in height (approximate height of a gymnasium bench) at a rate of 24 steps per minute. Females step at a rate of 22 steps per minute. The duration of the test is 3 min. At the conclusion of the test the subject remains standing and takes a 15 s heart rate. The heart rate is then entered into the appropriate equation:

Males: predicted $\dot{V}O_2$max = 111.33 – (0.42 × heart rate),

Females: predicted $\dot{V}O_2$max = 65.81 – (0.1847 × heart rate),

where $\dot{V}O_2$max is in ml · kg^{-1} · min^{-1} and heart rate is in beats/min.

The error associated with this prediction is approximately 16%. However, this large error may be acceptable when testing large populations (McArdle, Katch, and Katch 1996).

Another cardiovascular endurance test is the YMCA step test. It uses the same protocol as the Queens College step test, but in the YMCA test heart rate is taken 1 min postexercise. The recovery heart rate is then compared to the normative values in table 6.10.

TABLE 6.10 Normative Values for Males and Females for Recovery Heart Rate Following the 3 Min Step Test (beats/min)

Heart rate rating	AGE (Y)					
	18-25	26-35	36-45	46-55	56-65	66+
Males						
Excellent	70-78	73-79	72-81	78-84	72-82	72-86
Good	82-88	83-88	86-94	89-96	89-97	89-95
Above average	91-97	91-97	98-102	99-103	98-101	97-102
Average	101-104	101-106	105-111	109-115	105-111	104-113
Below average	107-114	109-116	113-118	118-121	113-118	114-119
Poor	118-126	119-126	120-128	124-130	122-128	122-128
Very poor	131-164	130-164	132-168	135-158	131-150	133-152
Females						
Excellent	72-83	72-86	74-87	76-93	74-92	73-86
Good	88-97	91-97	93-101	96-102	97-103	93-100

Heart rate rating	AGE (Y)					
	18-25	26-35	36-45	46-55	56-65	66+
Females						
Above average	100-106	103-110	104-109	106-113	106-111	104-114
Average	110-116	112-118	111-117	117-120	113-117	117-121
Below average	118-124	121-127	120-127	121-126	119-127	123-127
Poor	128-137	129-135	130-138	127-133	129-136	129-134
Very poor	142-155	141-154	143-152	138-152	142-151	135-151

Reprinted, by permission, from J.R. Morrow, A. Jackson, J. Disch and D. Mood, 2005, *Measurement and evaluation in human performance*, 3rd ed. (Champaign, IL: Human Kinetics), 234; adapted from *Y's Way to Physical Fitness*, 3rd edition, 1989, with permission of YMCA of the USA, 101 N. Wacker Drive, Chicago, IL 60606.

Normative Values for Aerobic Power and Endurance

Normative values for maximal aerobic power in male and female adult populations can be seen in table 6.11. Whether $\dot{V}O_2$max is directly measured or is predicted from the various equations discussed throughout the chapter, the values obtained can be compared to the normative values established for the general population. Youth are generally evaluated in school settings that utilize field tests to assess cardiovascular endurance. The President's Council of Physical Fitness, through the President's Challenge, has developed normative values for 1 mi (1.6 km) run and walk times for youth. These can be seen in table 6.12.

TABLE 6.11 Percentile Values for Maximal Aerobic Power (ml · kg · min^{-1})

Percentile	AGE (Y)				
	20-29	30-39	40-49	50-59	60+
Men					
90	51.4	50.4	48.2	45.3	42.5
80	48.2	46.8	44.1	41.0	38.1
70	46.8	44.6	41.8	38.5	35.3
60	44.2	42.4	39.9	36.7	33.6
50	42.5	41.0	38.1	35.2	31.8
40	41.0	38.9	36.7	33.8	30.2
30	39.5	37.4	35.1	32.3	28.7
20	37.1	35.4	33.0	30.2	26.5
10	34.5	32.5	30.9	28.0	23.1
Women					
90	44.2	41.0	39.5	35.2	35.2
80	41.0	38.6	36.3	32.3	31.2
70	38.1	36.7	33.8	30.9	29.4
60	36.7	34.6	32.3	29.4	27.2
50	35.2	33.8	30.9	28.2	25.8
40	33.8	32.3	29.5	26.9	24.5
30	32.3	30.5	28.3	25.5	23.8
20	30.6	28.7	26.5	24.3	22.8
10	28.4	26.5	25.1	22.3	20.8

Reprinted, by permission, from American College of Sports Medicine, 2000, *ACSM's Guidelines for Exercise Testing and Prescription*, 6th ed. (Philadelphia, PA: Lippincott, Williams & Wilkins), 77.

AEROBIC POWER AND ENDURANCE TESTING FOR CIVIL SERVICE AND MILITARY PERSONNEL

Testing for aerobic fitness is a common tool in the selection and fitness assessment of police, fire, and military personnel. As with other tests utilized by these agencies, aerobic fitness tests measure physical fitness to indicate whether individuals are ready and able to perform their tasks. As mentioned in other chapters, information concerning police and firefighters is limited. Tables 6.13 and 6.14 provide the percentile scores of law enforcement personnel and the standard passing scores for police depart-

TABLE 6.12 One Mile (1.6 km) Run and Walk Times (min:s) for Youth

% rank	AGE (Y)											
	6	7	8	9	10	11	12	13	14	15	16	17+
Boys												
90	9:41	5:56	8:28	8:14	7:39	7:17	6:57	6:39	6:13	6:07	5:56	5:57
80	10:32	9:43	9:00	8:47	8:08	7:45	7:25	7:00	6:33	6:29	6:18	6:14
70	11:17	10:20	9:38	9:12	8:37	8:14	7:56	7:20	6:59	6:48	6:33	6:32
60	12:00	10:55	10:15	9:47	9:11	8:45	8:14	7:41	7:19	7:06	6:50	6:50
50	12:36	11:40	11:05	10:30	9:48	9:20	8:40	8:06	7:44	7:30	7:10	7:04
40	13:39	12:17	11:55	11:03	10:32	10:07	9:11	8:35	8:13	7:52	7:35	7:24
30	14:48	13:23	12:30	11:44	11:14	10:54	10:00	9:10	8:48	8:29	8:09	7:52
20	15:34	14:16	13:23	12:33	12:15	12:00	10:52	10:02	9:35	9:05	8:56	8:25
10	17:25	16:12	14:57	13:52	13:50	13:08	12:11	11:43	11:22	10:10	10:17	9:23
Girls												
90	10:29	10:05	9:45	9:07	8:49	8:40	8:00	7:49	7:43	7:52	7:55	7:58
80	11:37	10:55	10:20	10:03	9:38	9:22	8:52	8:29	8:20	8:24	8:39	8:34
70	12:12	11:25	11:20	10:45	10:19	10:04	9:36	9:09	8:50	8:55	9:11	9:15
60	12:31	12:20	11:53	11:13	10:52	10:42	10:26	9:50	9:27	9:23	9:48	9:51
50	13:12	12:56	12:30	11:52	11:22	11:17	11:05	10:23	10:06	9:58	10:31	10:22
40	14:14	13:44	13:07	12:24	11:58	12:00	11:47	11:20	10:51	10:40	11:15	11:05
30	15:09	14:32	13:56	13:19	12:30	12:42	12:24	12:00	11:36	11:20	12:08	12:00
20	16:10	15:12	14:53	14:07	13:29	13:44	13:35	13:01	12:18	12:19	13:23	12:40
10	17:36	16:35	15:45	15:40	14:30	14:44	14:39	14:49	14:10	14:13	16:03	14:01

Reprinted, by permission, from Presidents Council for Physical Fitness, *Presidents Challenge Normative Data Spreadsheet* (Online). Available: www.presidentschallenge.org.

TABLE 6.13 Percentile Scores of Police Recruits

Category	PERCENTILE								
	90	80	70	60	50	40	30	20	10
1.5 mi (2.41 km) run time (min:s)	11:31	12:32	13:14	13:58	14:40	15:20	15:55	16:55	17:00

Data from Hoffman R.J.and T.R. Collingwood, Fit for Duty-2nd Edition; Champaign, Ill: Human Kinetics, 2005.

TABLE 6.14 Standard Passing Scores (min:s) for 1.5 Mi (2.41 km) Run in Police Department Personnel

Gender	AGE (Y)			
	20-29	30-39	40-49	50-59
Females	15:26	15:57	16:58	17:54
Males	12:51	13:36	14:29	15:26

Consistent with data from various police forces around the United States.

ment personnel, respectively. The standard passing scores across age groups and gender for the 1.5 mi (2.41 km) run (see table 6.14) appear to be consistent with physical fitness requirements reported by various police departments around the United States. Minimum standards in aerobic endurance for U.S. Army, Navy, Air Force, and Marines personnel can be seen in table 6.15. These measurements are reported across age groups and gender. Table 6.16 classifies endurance performance

TABLE 6.15 Minimum Standards for Cardiovascular Endurance Assessments in American Military Personnel, Adjusted for Age and Gender

	2 MI (3.2 KM) RUN (MIN:S)	
Age	M	F
Army		
17-21	15:54	15:54
22-26	16:36	19:36
27-31	17:00	20:30
32-36	17:42	21:42
37-41	18:18	22:42
42-46	18:42	23:42
47-51	19:30	24:00
52-56	19:48	24:24
57-61	19:54	24:48
62+	20:00	25:00
Army basic training		
17-21	16:36	19:42
22-26	17:30	20:36
27-31	17:54	21:42
32-36	18:48	23:06

	1.5 MI (2.41 KM) RUN (MIN:S)	
Age	M	F
Navy		
17-19	12:30	15:00
20-29	13:30	15:30
30-39	14:30	16:45

Age	M	F
Navy		
40-49	15:30	17:15
50+	16:45	17:30
Navy basic training		
17-19	11:00	13:30
20-29	12:00	14:15
30-39	13:45	15:30

	2 MI (3.2 KM) RUN (MIN:S)	
Age	M	F
Air Force basic training		
<30	18:00	21:00
>30	20:00	23:00

	3 MI (4.8 KM) RUN (MIN)	
Age	M	F
Marines		
17-26	28	31
27-39	29	32
40-45	30	33
46+	33	36
Marines basic training		
Same as active force		

Adapted from B. Singer, B. Palmer, B. Rogers and J. Smith, 2002, Military services physical fitness and weight management database: A review and analysis. *U.S. Army Medical Research*, Document No. HSIAC-RA-2002-001.

TABLE 6.16 Physical Readiness Classification for Cardiovascular Endurance in U.S. Naval Personnel

	1.5 MI (2.41 KM) RUN TIME (MIN:S)							
	OUTSTANDING		EXCELLENT		GOOD		SATISFACTORY	
Age	M	F	M	F	M	F	M	F
17-19	9:00	11:30	9:45	13:30	11:00	15:00	12:45	16:15
20-29	9:15	11:30	10:30	13:15	12:00	15:00	13:45	16:45
30-39	10:00	12:00	11:45	13:45	13:45	15:30	15:30	17:15
40-49	10:15	12:15	12:15	14:15	14:30	16:15	15:15	16:45
50+	10:45	12:45	12:30	14:45	15:15	16:45	17:00	19:00

Adapted from J.A. Hodgdon, 1999, "A history of the U.S. Navy physical readiness program from 1976 to 1999," *Technical Document Number 99-6F* (Washington, DC: Office of Naval Research).

measurements for the physical readiness of U.S. Navy personnel.

AEROBIC POWER AND ENDURANCE TESTING IN COMPETITIVE ATHLETES

The means and standard deviations of maximal aerobic power and of endurance in collegiate, professional, and national athletes are provided in tables 6.17 and 6.18, respectively (values are those reported in the literature). These normative values can be used for comparative purposes, but they should not be interpreted as levels required for success. The importance of aerobic power and endurance depends on the sport. For some sports, maximal aerobic capacity has little to no relation to success (Hoffman et al., 1996), while in others aerobic capacity directly influences performance success.

TABLE 6.17 Maximal Aerobic Power ($ml \cdot kg^{-1} \cdot min^{-1}$) in Collegiate, Professional, and National Athletes

Population	Gender	Treadmill	Cycle ergometer	Tethered swimming	Source
Alpine skiing					
Austrian national	M		60 ± 4.7		Neumayr et al. 2003
	F		55 ± 3.5		
Baseball					
MLB	M		40.4 ± 0.52		Hagerman, Starr, and Murray 1989
NAIA college	M	52.6 ± 5.9			Potteiger et al. 1992
Basketball					
Canadian national team	F	51.3 ± 4.9			Smith and Thomas 1991
Finnish professional	F	48.0 ± 6.6			Hakkinen 1993
Israeli national	M	50.2 ± 3.8			Hoffman et al. 1999
Collegiate team	M	50.0 ± 7.7			Hunter, Hilyer, and Forster 1993
NCAA DI	M	53.0 ± 4.7			Caterisano et al. 1997
Biathlon					
U.S. national team	F	59.0 ± 2.7			Unpublished data
	M	70.9 ± 3.0			
Cross-country skiing					
Canadian collegiate	M	70.4 ± 7.2			Boulay et al. 1994
Cycling					
Puerto Rican national road	M		68.3 ± 6.5		Rivera, Rivera-Brown, and Frontera 1998
	F		51.7 ± 10.2		
Ice hockey					
U.S. national	F	49.4			Unpublished data
Judo					
U.S. national	M	53.2 ± 1.4			Callister et al. 1990
	F	51.9 ± 0.8			
Kickboxing					
Professional	M		62.7		Zabukovec and Tiidus 1995

Population	Gender	Treadmill	Cycle ergometer	Tethered swimming	Source
Soccer					
French professional	M	60.5 ± 0.3			Filaire et al. 2001
German national team	M	63			Nowacki et al. 1988
German professional	M	69.2			Nowacki et al. 1988
Elite youth	M	68.8			Nowacki et al. 1988
2nd division	M	52.1			Nowacki et al. 1988
Regional amateur	M	50			Nowacki et al. 1988
Youth	M	48.4			Nowacki et al. 1988
Speed skating					
Canadian national	M F		62.0 ± 5.3 53.9 ± 2.8		Smith and Roberts 1991
U.S. national	M F		61.3 ± 4.7 49.1 ± 3.1		Unpublished data
Swimming					
NCAA DI	M	52.4 ± 6.7			Delistraty, Noble, and Wilkinson 1990
NCAA DI	M F			58.6 ± 1.9 51.3 ± 6.9	Flynn et al. 1994 Raglin et al. 1996
Team handball					
French national team	M F	48.1 ± 4.2 46.7 ± 6.4			Filaire and Lac 1999 Filaire et al. 1999
Tennis					
Collegiate	F	51.0 ± 3.2			Kraemer et al. 2003
NCAA DI	M	58.5 ± 9.4			Bergeron et al. 1991
Track and field—distance					
NCAA DI	M	69 ± 4.4 65.2 ± 1.3			Armstrong et al. 1994
Puerto Rican national team	M F	79.7 ± 3.1 62.4 ± 2.5			Flynn et al. 1994 Rivera, Rivera-Brown, and Frontera 1998
Track and field—sprint					
Puerto Rican national team	M F	59.1 ± 7.5 53.4 ± 9.8			Rivera, Rivera-Brown, and Frontera 1998
Triathlon					
Amateur	M	67.0 ± 3.8	62.9 ± 3.5	59.4 ± 4.1	Millard-Stafford et al. 1991
Volleyball					
French national team	F	46.2 ± 8.1			Filaire et al. 1999
Wrestling					
U.S. national	M	54.6 ± 2.0	41.2 ± 6.1		Callan et al. 2000
Canadian national	M	61.8	57.8		Sharratt, Taylor, and Song 1986

TABLE 6.18 Endurance in Collegiate, Professional, and National Athletes

Population	Gender	1 mi (1.61 km) run (min:s)	1.5 mi (2.41 km) run (min:s)	2 mi (3.2 km) run (min:s)	Source
Baseball					
NAIA	M		12:52 ± 1:48		Unpublished data
Basketball					
NCAA DI	M	5:40 ± 0:32	9:43 ± 1:06		Latin, Berg, and Baechle 1994
Football					
NCAA DIAA	M	6:37 ± 0:45			Unpublished data
	M			13:59 ± 1:12	Hoffman et al. 1990
Soccer					
Elite youth (16.2 ± 0.5 y)	M			14:15 ± 1:36	Unpublished data
Volleyball					
NCAA DI	F			15:46 ± 0:58	Fry et al. 1991

Summary

⊃ Aerobic power indicates the ability of an individual to perform sustained, high-intensity exercise.

⊃ Aerobic capacity may be used to assess the fitness and health status of both recreational athletes and sedentary individuals.

⊃ Aerobic capacity can be assessed with running, cycling, or swimming protocols.

⊃ In the laboratory, oxygen consumption can be directly measured with a metabolic cart during a maximal effort test or predicted with an individual's heart rate or workload obtained from a submaximal test.

⊃ A variety of field tests can also be used to predict maximal oxygen consumption.

CHAPTER 7

Anthropometry and Body Composition

Anthropometry and body composition are staples in the descriptive statistics used in human performance. These measurements are important assessments in both research and nonresearch settings. Height and weight, girth ratio, and body composition not only serve as important descriptions but also contribute to health and fitness assessments. This chapter briefly discusses common anthropometric and body composition measurements and provides, where appropriate, normative values for general and athletic populations.

Anthropometry

Anthropometry refers to the measurement of the human body. Such assessments usually include height, weight, and various body and limb girths.

HEIGHT

Height is easy to measure. The individual removes her shoes and stands against a wall, next to a tape measure (attached or unattached). A rectangular object is placed flat on top of her head and the corresponding height is read. Commercial stadiometers or other measuring devices can also be purchased for measuring height. Typically, individuals remove their shoes before assessment.

Height is measured to the nearest quarter of an inch or half a centimeter (Harman et al. 2000). To validate the accuracy of commercial devices such as a physician's scale or a stadiometer, height can be calibrated to a commercially available tape measure.

WEIGHT

Body mass is typically measured on a certified balance scale or calibrated electronic scale, with the individual wearing gym shorts, a T-shirt, and no shoes. The most reliable measurements are performed in the morning following voiding and elimination (going to the bathroom). When individuals are weighed several times (i.e., for a research study), all measurements should be performed at the same time of day. Body mass is reported to the nearest 0.1 lb or kg.

HEIGHT AND WEIGHT NORMS

Tables 7.1 and 7.2 provide the average heights of children and adults in the United States, stratified by gender and race or ethnicity, respectively. Tables 7.3 and 7.4 provide average weights for children and adults in the United States, stratified by gender and race or ethnicity, respectively. Tables 7.5, 7.6, and 7.7 provide height and weight norms for elite athletes who play professional football, baseball, and basketball, respectively.

TABLE 7.1 Average Height for American Children and Adults, Based on Gender and Age

Age (y)	MALES		FEMALES	
	in.	cm	in.	cm
Children				
2	35.9	91.2	35.5	90.1
3	38.8	98.6	38.4	97.6
4	41.9	106.5	41.7	105.9
5	44.5	113.0	44.3	112.4
6	46.9	119.2	46.1	117.1
7	49.7	126.2	49.0	124.4
8	52.2	132.5	51.5	130.9
9	54.4	138.1	53.9	136.9
10	55.7	141.4	56.4	143.3
11	58.5	148.7	59.6	151.4
12	60.9	154.8	61.4	156.0
13	63.1	160.1	62.6	159.1
14	66.3	168.5	63.7	161.8
15	68.4	173.8	63.8	162.0
16	69.0	175.3	63.8	161.9
17	69.0	175.3	64.2	163.2
18	69.5	176.4	64.2	163.0
19	69.6	176.7	64.2	163.1
Adults				
20-29	69.6	176.7	64.1	162.8
30-39	69.5	176.4	64.2	163.0
40-49	69.7	177.2	64.3	163.4
50-59	69.2	175.8	63.9	162.3
60-74	68.6	174.4	63.0	160.0
75+	67.4	171.3	62.0	157.4

Adapted from C.L. Ogden, C.D. Fryar, M.D. Carroll and K.M. Flegal, 2004, "Mean body weight, height, and body mass index, United States 1960-2002," *Advance data from vital and health statistics,* no. 347. (Hyattsville, MD: National Center for Health Statistics).

TABLE 7.2 Average Height for Adults, Based on Gender and Race or Ethnicity

Age (y)	MALES		FEMALES	
	in.	cm	in.	cm
Non-Hispanic White				
20-39	70.2	178.2	64.6	164.1
40-59	70.0	177.8	64.6	164.0
60+	68.6	174.3	62.8	159.6
Non-Hispanic Black				
20-39	70.0	177.8	64.6	164.0
40-59	69.6	176.8	64.3	163.4
60+	68.5	174.1	63.2	160.6
Mexican American				
20-39	66.8	169.7	62.3	158.1
40-59	66.9	169.0	61.9	157.3
60+	66.5	168.5	60.9	154.8

Data from the United States.

Adapted from C.L. Ogden, C.D. Fryar, M.D. Carroll and K.M. Flegal, 2004, "Mean body weight, height, and body mass index, United States 1960-2002," *Advance data from vital and health statistics,* no. 347. (Hyattsville, MD: National Center for Health Statistics).

TABLE 7.3 Average Weight for Children and Adults, Based on Gender and Age

Age (y)	MALES		FEMALES	
	lb	kg	lb	kg
Children				
2	30.2	13.7	29.2	13.3
3	35.0	15.9	33.4	15.2
4	40.8	18.5	39.5	17.9
5	46.9	21.3	45.3	20.6
6	51.7	23.5	49.2	22.4
7	59.8	27.2	56.9	25.9
8	72.0	32.7	70.1	31.9
9	79.2	36.0	78.0	35.4
10	84.9	38.6	87.9	40.0
11	96.2	43.7	105.4	47.9
12	110.9	50.4	114.3	52.0
13	118.6	53.9	127.0	57.7
14	140.5	63.9	131.7	59.9
15	150.3	68.3	134.4	61.1
16	163.7	74.4	138.5	63.0
17	166.3	75.6	135.8	61.7
18	166.4	75.6	143.5	65.2
19	172.1	78.2	149.3	67.9
Adults				
20-29	183.4	83.4	156.5	71.1
30-39	189.1	86.0	163.0	74.1
40-49	196.0	89.1	168.2	76.5
50-59	195.4	88.8	169.2	76.9
60-74	191.5	87.1	164.7	74.9
75+	172.7	78.5	146.6	66.6

Data from the United States.

Adapted from C.L. Ogden, C.D. Fryar, M.D. Carroll and K.M. Flegal, 2004, "Mean body weight, height, and body mass index, United States 1960-2002," *Advance data from vital and health statistics*, no. 347. (Hyattsville, MD: National Center for Health Statistics).

TABLE 7.4 Average Weight for Adults, Based on Gender and Race or Ethnicity

Age (y)	MALES		FEMALES	
	lb	kg	lb	kg
Non-Hispanic White				
20-39	189.7	86.2	158.4	72.0
40-59	199.5	90.7	167.6	76.2
60+	188.8	85.8	158.0	71.8
Non-Hispanic Black				
20-39	189.1	85.9	179.2	81.5
40-59	191.1	86.8	189.3	86.0
60+	186.5	84.8	176.6	80.3
Mexican American				
20-39	172.5	78.4	152.9	69.5
40-59	183.6	83.4	165.5	75.2
60+	180.3	82.0	155.0	70.5

Data from the United States.

Adapted from C.L. Ogden, C.D. Fryar, M.D. Carroll and K.M. Flegal, 2004, "Mean body weight, height, and body mass index, United States 1960-2002," *Advance data from vital and health statistics*, no. 347. (Hyattsville, MD: National Center for Health Statistics).

TABLE 7.5 Percentile Ranks for Height and Weight in Players Participating in the NFL Combine

HEIGHT

% rank	DB in.	DB cm	DL in.	DL cm	LB in.	LB cm	OL in.	OL cm
90	73.5	186.7	76.9	195.3	75.6	192.0	78.8	200.2
80	72.8	184.9	76.6	194.6	74.9	190.2	78.0	198.1
70	72.3	183.6	76.4	194.1	74.2	188.5	77.3	196.3
60	71.8	182.4	76.0	193.0	73.9	187.7	76.7	194.8
50	71.0	180.3	75.6	192.0	73.5	186.7	76.6	194.6
40	70.6	179.3	75.5	191.8	73.4	186.4	76.3	193.8
30	70.1	178.1	75.0	190.5	72.9	185.2	75.6	192.0
20	69.9	177.5	74.4	189.0	72.4	183.9	75.3	191.3
10	69.4	176.3	73.8	187.5	72.0	182.9	74.8	190.0
$\bar{X}$	71.3	181.1	75.6	192.0	73.7	187.2	76.6	194.6
SD	1.6	4.1	1.2	3.0	1.3	3.3	1.5	3.8
n	49		47		35		59	

WEIGHT

% rank	DB lb	DB kg	DL lb	DL kg	LB lb	LB kg	OL lb	OL kg
90	211	95.9	306	139.1	252	114.5	337	153.2
80	206	93.6	297	135.0	250	113.6	325	147.7
70	198	90.0	290	131.8	246	111.8	318	144.5
60	195	88.6	285	129.5	244	110.9	314	142.7
50	192	87.3	281	127.7	239	108.6	309	140.5
40	191	86.8	278	126.4	237	107.7	302	137.3
30	186	84.5	272	123.6	233	105.9	300	136.4
20	182	82.7	268	121.8	228	103.6	296	134.5
10	176	80.0	252	114.5	224	101.8	292	132.7
$\bar{X}$	193	87.7	281	127.7	239	108.6	311	141.4
SD	12.8	5.8	19	8.6	11.1	5.0	17	7.7
n	49		47		35		59	

HEIGHT

% rank	QB in.	QB cm	RB in.	RB cm	TE in.	TE cm	WR in.	WR cm
90	77.4	196.6	73.3	186.2	78.4	199.1	75.7	192.3
80	77.1	195.8	72.3	183.6	76.9	195.3	74.4	189.0
70	76.2	193.5	72.0	182.9	76.8	195.1	73.7	187.2
60	75.4	191.5	71.7	182.1	76.4	194.1	73.1	185.7
50	74.6	189.5	71.5	181.6	76.3	193.8	72.5	184.2
40	74.0	188.0	70.8	179.8	76.1	193.3	72.0	182.9
30	73.8	187.5	70.2	178.3	75.9	192.8	71.6	181.9
20	73.6	186.9	69.6	176.8	75.5	191.8	70.8	179.8
10	73.0	185.4	68.8	174.8	75.2	191.0	68.9	175.0
$\bar{X}$	75.0	190.5	71.0	180.3	76.4	194.1	72.5	184.2
SD	1.6	4.1	1.6	4.1	1.0	2.5	2.3	5.8
n	15		45		14		47	

	WEIGHT							
	QB		RB		TE		WR	
% rank	lb	kg	lb	kg	lb	kg	lb	kg
90	248	112.7	243	110.5	278	126.4	213	96.8
80	228	103.6	235	106.8	272	123.6	207	94.1
70	223	101.4	230	104.5	271	123.2	201	91.4
60	220	100.0	224	101.8	263	119.5	195	88.6
50	219	99.5	218	99.1	256	116.4	192	87.3
40	218	99.1	215	97.7	253	115.0	187	85.0
30	216	98.2	208	94.5	251	114.1	186	84.5
20	212	96.4	204	92.7	249	113.2	184	83.6
10	209	95.0	195	88.6	241	109.5	180	81.8
$\bar{X}$	221	100.5	219	99.5	259	117.7	195	88.6
SD	13.7	6.2	17.6	8.0	13.1	6.0	14.8	6.7
n	15		45		14		47	

DB = defensive backs; DL = defensive linemen; LB = linebackers; OL = offensive linemen; QB = quarterbacks; RB = running backs; TE = tight ends; WR = wide receivers.

TABLE 7.6   Average Height and Weight of Major League Baseball Players

	HEIGHT							
	P		C		IF		OF	
% rank	in.	cm	in.	cm	in.	cm	in.	cm
90	77.0	195.6	75.0	190.5	75.0	190.5	75.0	190.5
80	76.0	193.0	75.0	190.5	74.0	188.0	74.0	188.0
70	75.0	190.5	74.0	188.0	73.0	185.4	74.0	188.0
60	75.0	190.5	74.0	188.0	73.0	185.4	73.0	185.4
50	74.0	188.0	73.0	185.4	72.0	182.9	73.0	185.4
40	74.0	188.0	72.6	184.4	72.0	182.9	72.0	182.9
30	73.0	185.4	71.2	180.8	71.0	180.3	72.0	182.9
20	73.0	185.4	71.0	180.3	71.0	180.3	71.0	180.3
10	72.0	182.9	70.0	177.8	70.0	177.8	70.0	177.8
$\bar{X}$	74.4	189.0	72.9	185.2	72.5	184.2	72.8	184.9
SD	2.2	5.6	1.9	4.8	2.3	5.8	2.0	5.1
n	356		63		206		141	

	WEIGHT							
	P		C		IF		OF	
% rank	lb	kg	lb	kg	lb	kg	lb	kg
90	240.0	109.1	230.0	104.5	225.0	102.3	225.0	102.3
80	230.0	104.5	225.0	102.3	218.0	99.1	220.0	100.0
70	220.0	100.0	220.0	100.0	210.0	95.5	215.0	97.7
60	215.0	97.7	216.0	98.2	200.0	90.9	209.0	95.0
50	210.0	95.5	210.0	95.5	198.0	90.0	205.0	93.2
40	205.0	93.2	210.0	95.5	190.0	86.4	200.0	90.9
30	200.0	90.9	200.0	90.9	186.0	84.5	195.0	88.6
20	190.0	86.4	195.0	88.6	180.0	81.8	190.0	86.4

(continued)

TABLE 7.6 Average Height and Weight of Major League Baseball Players *(continued)*

	WEIGHT							
	P		**C**		**IF**		**OF**	
% rank	**lb**	**kg**	**lb**	**kg**	**lb**	**kg**	**lb**	**kg**
10	180.0	81.8	190.0	86.4	175.0	79.5	180.0	81.8
$\bar{X}$	210.0	95.5	212.0	96.4	199.0	90.5	204.0	92.7
SD	22.6	10.3	14.3	6.5	19.5	8.9	18.4	8.4
n	356		63		206		141	

P = pitchers; C = catchers; IF = infielders; OF = outfielders.

Data collected from MLB team Web sites

TABLE 7.7 Average Height and Weight of National Basketball Association Players

	HEIGHT					
	G		**F**		**C**	
% rank	**in.**	**cm**	**in.**	**cm**	**in.**	**cm**
90	79.0	200.7	83.0	210.8	86.0	218.4
80	78.0	198.1	82.0	208.3	85.0	215.9
70	78.0	198.1	82.0	208.3	84.0	213.4
60	77.0	195.6	81.0	205.7	84.0	213.4
50	76.0	193.0	81.0	205.7	84.0	213.4
40	75.0	190.5	81.0	205.7	83.0	210.8
30	75.0	190.5	80.0	203.2	83.0	210.8
20	74.0	188.0	80.0	203.2	83.0	210.8
10	73.0	185.4	79.0	200.7	82.0	208.3
$\bar{X}$	76.0	193.0	80.9	205.5	84.0	213.4
SD	2.6	6.6	1.3	3.3	1.8	4.6
n	184		157		73	

	WEIGHT					
	G		**F**		**C**	
% rank	**lb**	**kg**	**lb**	**kg**	**lb**	**kg**
90	220.0	100.0	260.0	118.2	280.0	127.3
80	215.0	97.7	248.0	112.7	275.0	125.0
70	210.0	95.5	245.0	111.4	265.0	120.5
60	208.0	94.5	240.0	109.1	260.0	118.2
50	202.0	91.8	235.0	106.8	260.0	118.2
40	195.0	88.6	234.0	106.4	255.0	115.9
30	190.0	86.4	229.0	104.1	250.0	113.6
20	185.0	84.1	222.0	100.9	242.0	110.0
10	179.0	81.4	215.0	97.7	240.0	109.1
$\bar{X}$	201.0	91.4	236.0	107.3	260.0	118.2
SD	17.1	7.8	16.1	7.3	18.6	8.5
n	184		157		73	

G = guards; F = forwards; C = centers.

Data from NBA team Web sites.

BODY GIRTH

Body girths are typically assessed with a flexible measuring tape equipped with a spring-loaded attachment. The tape should be lightly applied to the skin to avoid compression that would artificially lower scores. Girth measurements have been used to compare muscular size differences in individuals in various sporting endeavors and to determine fat distribution on the body. Although specific equations can predict body fat composition from girth measurements, ratios of various girths, such as the waist-to-hip ratio, have been used to assess risks of morbidity and mortality. A larger ratio represents a greater distribution of fat in the abdomen and upper body. Such a distribution is associated with a greater risk for cardiovascular disease (Shimokata et al. 1989). Waist circumference is measured at the narrowest portion of the torso (about 2-3 in.

or 5.1-7.6 cm above the umbilicus), while hip circumference is measured at the level of the greater trochanters. Table 7.8 provides waist-to-hip ratios and disease risks for men and women.

BODY MASS INDEX

The body mass index (BMI) is calculated (in kg/m^2) by dividing body weight (in kg) by the square of height (in m). BMI standards are used to classify obesity and to assess disease risk. As BMI increases, mortality rate from cardiovascular disease and diabetes increases as well (Bray and Gray 1988). A problem with the BMI is that it does not differentiate between lean body mass and fat mass. As a result it is not appropriate to use with an athletic population. Table 7.9 classifies weight by BMI, waist circumference, and associated disease risks.

TABLE 7.8 Waist-to-Hip Ratio Norms for Men and Women

| | RISK FOR HEART DISEASE | | | | | | | |
| | LOW | | MODERATE | | HIGH | | VERY HIGH | |
Age (y)	Men	Women	Men	Women	Men	Women	Men	Women
20-29	<0.83	<0.71	0.83-0.88	0.71-0.77	0.89-0.94	0.78-0.82	>0.94	>0.82
30-39	<0.84	<0.72	0.84-0.91	0.72-0.78	0.92-0.96	0.79-0.84	>0 .96	>0.84
40-49	<0 .88	<0.73	0.88-0.95	0.73-0.79	0.96-1.00	0.80-0.87	>1.00	>0.87
50-59	<0.90	<0.74	0.90-0.96	0.74-0.81	0.97-1.02	0.82-0.88	>1.02	>0.88
60-69	<0.91	<0.76	0.91-0.98	0.76-0.83	0.99-1.03	0.84-0.90	>1.03	>0.90

Adapted from G.A. Bray and D.S. Gray, 1988, "Obesity part I—Pathogenesis," *Western Journal of Medicine* 149:432, with permission of the BMJ Publishing group.

TABLE 7.9 Classification of Weight by Body Mass Index (BMI), Waist Circumference, and Associated Disease Risks

| Category | BMI (kg/m^2) | Obesity class | DISEASE RISK* RELATIVE TO NORMAL WEIGHT AND WAIST CIRCUMFERENCE | |
			Men ≤102 cm (40 in.) Women ≤88 cm (35 in.)	Men >102 cm (40 in.) Women >88 cm (35 in.)
Underweight	<18.5		—	—
Normal	18.5-24.9		—	—
Overweight	25.0-29.9		Increased	High
Obese	30.0-34.9	I	High	Very high
	35.0-39.9	II	Very high	Very high
Extremely obese	≥40.0	III	Extremely high	Extremely high

* Disease risk for type 2 diabetes, hypertension, and coronary heart disease.

From the National Institute of Health (NIH), and the National Heart, Lung, and Blood Institute, 1998, *Clinical Guidelines on the Identification, Evaluation, and Treatment of Overweight and Obesity in Adults (Executive Summary)*, NIH Publication 98-4083.

Body Composition

Body composition refers to the proportion of body weight that is from fat relative to the amount of weight that is from lean tissue. High body fat is a known risk factor for heart disease, diabetes, cancer, and other health problems (Blair and Brodney 1999). Measuring body composition differentiates being overweight from being overfat. For many years, height and weight tables set the acceptable body weights. Individuals who were heavier than the weight suggested for their height were classified as being overweight and at high risk for disease. Unfortunately, these tables are still used by insurance companies in setting insurance premiums for individuals. The major drawback to using height and weight scales is that it does not differentiate between lean mass and fat mass. Heaviness does not relate to disease risk. If it did, many elite athletes would be considered to be at high risk for diseases of obesity. Yet these individuals are healthy and are often quite lean. To accurately assess an individual's disease risk with anthropometric measurements, body composition should be used. Numerous methods can be used to assess body composition. These methods, which vary in complexity, cost, and accuracy, are briefly described.

HYDROSTATIC WEIGHING

For many years hydrostatic weighing was considered the gold standard of body composition analysis. However, the relatively new dual X-ray absorptiometry and plethysmography have gained large acceptance in sport science as primary methods of body composition analysis. Hydrostatic weighing measures the amount of water that is displaced when an individual is submerged in a tank. As a body sinks under water, it is buoyed by a counterforce equal to the weight of the water displaced. The loss of weight in water, corrected by the density of water, can be used to calculate body density in the following formula:

$$\text{Body density} = \frac{\text{weight in air}}{\left[\frac{(\text{weight in air} - \text{weight in water})}{\text{density of water}} - \text{residual volume}\right]}.$$

Once body density is known, percent body fat can be calculated through various equations. Since body density varies and is affected by age, growth and maturation, gender, and ethnicity, equations are often specific to a population. In addition, a lung residual volume is needed to accurately assess body density. This volume can be measured directly or predicted through various formulas. A common equation for deriving percent body fat from body density is

$$\% \text{ body fat} = \frac{495}{\text{body density}} - 450.$$

This method of calculating body composition is highly reproducible, but several factors may reduce its accuracy. For instance, an accurate measurement of residual volume is important to reduce error, and residual volume does not account for possible air in the intestines. In addition, several assumptions in the calculation of body density may increase error in atypical populations. It is generally assumed that the hydrostatic method estimates body fat to within 2.5% of the "true" value (Gettman 1993). Table 7.10 provides population-specific formulas for converting body density to percent body fat.

DUAL X RAY ABSORPTIOMETRY

Dual energy X-ray absorptiometry (DEXA) is becoming a popular method of body composition assessment. It is a noninvasive procedure that measures regional and total-body lean and fat tissue as well as bone density and bone mineral content. The reliability and validity of DEXA for assessing body composition have been established at low, moderate, and high levels of body fat and with athletic and nonathletic populations (Fornetti et al. 1999; Visser et al. 1999). Although older DEXA models relied on a pencil-beam scanner that required 20 min for an assessment, newer fan-beam models scan at a much faster speed (requiring 5-10 min). One of the major advantages of DEXA measurements is that they use a three-compartment model (fat mass, lean-tissue mass, and bone density) to determine body composition. Such a method is superior to the more common two-compartment model (fat and lean-tissue mass) and measures body composition more accurately, eliminating sources of error (e.g., from residual volume) seen when estimating body density. Figure 7.1 on page 90 shows a full-body DEXA scan. The major drawback to DEXA is the cost for purchasing and operating the machine. The cost makes assessing body composition via DEXA unrealistic for most assessment facilities.

TABLE 7.10 Population-Specific Formulas for Converting Body Density to % Body Fat

Population	Age (y)	Gender	% body fat (%BF) formula*	FFBd (g/cc)**
African American	9-17	Female	(5.24 / Db) – 4.82	1.088
	19-45	Male	(4.86 / Db) – 4.39	1.106
	24-79	Female	(4.86 / Db) – 4.39	1.106
American Indian	18-62	Male	(4.97 / Db) – 4.52	1.099
	18-60	Female	(4.81 / Db) – 4.34	1.108
Asian Japanese native	18-48	Male	(4.97 / Db) – 4.52	1.099
		Female	(4.76 / Db) – 4.28	1.111
	61-78	Male	(4.87 / Db) – 4.41	1.105
		Female	(4.95 / Db) – 4.50	1.100
Singaporean (Chinese, Indian, Malay)	61-78	Male	(4.94 / Db) – 4.48	1.102
		Female	(4.84 / Db) – 4.37	1.107
Caucasian	8-12	Male	(5.27 / Db) – 4.85	1.086
		Female	(5.27 / Db) – 4.85	1.086
	13-17	Male	(5.12 / Db) – 4.69	1.092
		Female	(5.19 / Db) – 4.76	1.090
	18-59	Male	(4.95 / Db) – 4.50	1.100
		Female	(4.96 / Db) – 4.51	1.101
	60-90	Male	(4.97 / Db) – 4.52	1.099
		Female	(5.02 / Db) – 4.57	1.098
Hispanic	20-40	Male	NA	NA
		Female	(4.87 / Db) – 4.41	1.105

* Multiply by 100 for percentage value.

** FFBd = fat-free body density based on average values reported in selected research articles.

Adapted, by permission, from V.H. Heyward and L.M. Stolarczyk, 2004, *Applied body composition*, 2nd ed. (Champaign, IL: Human Kinetics), 9.

PLETHYSMOGRAPHY

Recent technological advances have led to air displacement plethysmography (ADP), a system that measures air displacement rather than water displacement. Air displacement is an attractive method of assessing body composition, especially for individuals who are uncomfortable being fully immersed in the hydrostatic tank. The plethysmograph (a closed chamber that assesses body volume by measuring changes in pressure) has been found to be highly reliable, yet its validity for lean individuals has not been established (Vescovi et al. 2001, 2002). In studies comparing ADP to hydrostatic weighing and to skinfold measurement, ADP tended to overestimate body composition in female college athletes. However, when ADP was compared to DEXA, it was shown to be a valid measurement of body composition in female athletes (Ballard, Fafara, and Vukovich 2004). Apparently the three-compartment method

of DEXA, which considers the density of bone minerals, reduces the errors seen in the two-compartment method of hydrostatic weighing (Fornetti et al. 1999). Thus, if DEXA is better than hydrostatic weighing for body composition analysis, then ADP appears to be a reliable and valid measurement of body composition.

SKINFOLD MEASUREMENT

Skinfold measurement is a popular assessment of body composition. It takes significantly less time to complete than hydrostatic weighing, DEXA, or ADP. The principle behind skinfold measurement is that subcutaneous fat is proportional to total-body fat. By measuring the skinfold thickness at various sites on the body, percent body fat can be calculated through a regression equation. Because the proportion of subcutaneous fat to total-body fat varies according to age, gender, and ethnicity (Lohman 1981), the appropriate regression

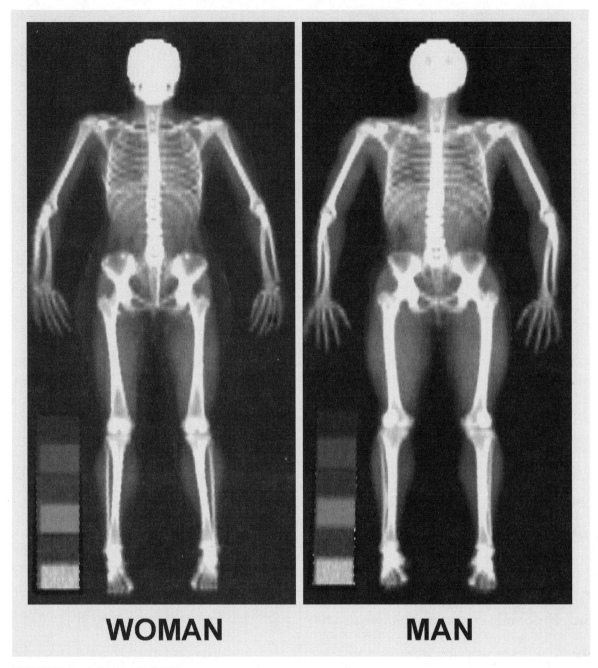

WOMAN **MAN**

FIGURE 7.1   A full-body DEXA scan.

Courtesy of Henry C. Lukaski.

equation must be selected. Regression equations also vary in the number of skinfold sites needed. Even when the appropriate regression equation is used, there may be a 3% to 4% error in the calculated percent body fat (Lohman 1981). Thus, the correct regression equation must be carefully selected. Table 7.11 provides several commonly used regression equations, and table 7.12 describes skinfold sites.

BIOELECTRICAL IMPEDANCE

Bioelectrical impedance (BI) is gaining popularity because of its ease in administration and its similarity to skinfold measurements regarding

TABLE 7.11 Commonly Used Regression Equations for Computing % Body Fat From Skinfold Measurements

Population subgroups	Sites	Formula	Source
Males 17-19 y 20-29 y 30-39 y Females 17-19 y 20-29 y 30-39 y	Biceps, triceps, subscapular, and suprailiac	D = body density $D = 1.1620 - 0.0630 \times (\log \Sigma \text{ skinfolds})$ $D = 1.1631 - 0.0632 \times (\log \Sigma \text{ skinfolds})$ $D = 1.1422 - 0.0544 \times (\log \Sigma \text{ skinfolds})$ $D = 1.1549 - 0.0678 \times (\log \Sigma \text{ skinfolds})$ $D = 1.1599 - 0.0717 \times (\log \Sigma \text{ skinfolds})$ $D = 1.1423 - 0.0632 \times (\log \Sigma \text{ skinfolds})$	Durnin and Womersley 1974
Males Females	Chest, midaxillary, triceps, subscapular, abdomen, suprailiac, and thigh	$D = 1.112 - 0.00043499 (\Sigma 7 \text{ skinfolds})$ $+ 0.00000055 (\Sigma \text{skinfolds})^2 - 0.00028826 \text{ (age)}$ $D = 1.097 - 0.00046971 (\Sigma 7 \text{ skinfolds})$ $+ 0.00000056 (\Sigma \text{skinfolds})^2 - 0.00012828 \text{ (age)}$	Jackson, Pollock, and Ward 1980 (7 site)
Female athletes (18-29 y)	Triceps, suprailiac, abdomen, and thigh	$D = 1.096095 - 0.0006952 (\Sigma 4 \text{ skinfolds})$ $+ 0.0000011 (\Sigma 4 \text{ skinfolds})^2 - 0.0000714 \text{ (age)}$	Jackson and Pollock 1980 (4 site)
Males (18-61 y)	Chest, abdomen, and thigh	$D = 1.10938 - 0.0008267 (\Sigma 3 \text{ skinfolds})$ $+ 0.0000016 (\Sigma \text{skinfolds})^2 - 0.0002574 \text{ (age)}$	Jackson and Pollock 1978 (3 site)
Females (18-55 y)	Triceps, suprailiac, and thigh	$D = 1.1099421 - 0.0009929 (\Sigma 3 \text{ skinfolds})$ $+ 0.0000023 (\Sigma \text{skinfolds})^2 - 0.0001392 \text{ (age)}$	
Black and White boys (6-17 y)	Triceps and calf	$\% BF = 0.735 (\Sigma \text{skinfolds}) + 1$	Slaughter et al. 1988
Black and White girls (6-17 y)	Triceps and calf	$\% BF = 0.610 (\Sigma \text{skinfolds}) + 5.1 (\Sigma \text{ skinfolds})$	

D = body density. Use population-specific conversion formulas to calculate % body fat (% BF).

TABLE 7.12 Skinfold Sites

Site	Description
Abdominal	Horizontal fold 2 cm to the right of the umbilicus
Biceps	Vertical fold on the anterior aspect of the arm over the belly of the biceps muscle
Chest	Diagonal fold 1/2 the distance between the anterior axillary line and the nipple (men) or 1/3 the distance between the anterior axillary line and the nipple (women)
Midaxillary	Horizontal fold on the midaxillary line at the level of the xiphoid process of the sternum
Subscapular	Diagonal fold at a 45° angle 1-2 cm below the inferior angle of the scapula
Suprailiac	Diagonal fold in line with the natural angle of the iliac crest taken in the anterior axillary line
Thigh	Vertical fold on the anterior midline of the thigh midway between the proximal border of the patella and the inguinal crease
Triceps	Vertical fold on the posterior midline of the upper arm midway between the acromion process of the scapula and the inferior part of the olecranon process of the elbow

Reprinted, by permission, from J. Hoffman, 2002, *Physiological aspects of sport training and performance* (Champaign, IL: Human Kinetics), 183.

accuracy. BI is based on the relationship between total body water and lean body mass. Since water is an excellent conductor of electricity, a greater resistance to an electrical current passing through the body indicates a higher percentage of body fat. Likewise, resistance decreases when there is a higher percentage of lean tissue. Since BI is sensitive to changes in body water, subjects should refrain from drinking or eating within 4 h of the measurement, void completely before the measurement, and refrain from consuming any alcohol, caffeine, or diuretic agent before assessment (Hoffman 2002). Failure to do so increases measurement error.

Standards of body composition for men and women can be seen in table 7.13.

TABLE 7.13 Body Composition Standards

Percentile	20–29 y	30–39 y	40–49 y	50–59 y	60+ y
Men					
90	7.1	11.3	13.6	15.3	15.3
80	9.4	13.9	16.3	17.9	18.4
70	11.8	15.9	18.1	19.8	20.3
60	14.1	17.5	19.6	21.3	22.0
50	15.9	19.0	21.1	22.7	23.5
40	17.4	20.5	22.5	24.1	25.0
30	19.5	22.3	24.1	25.7	26.7
20	22.4	24.2	26.1	27.5	28.5
10	25.9	27.3	28.9	30.3	31.2
Women					
90	14.5	15.5	18.5	21.6	21.1
80	17.1	18.0	21.3	25.0	25.1
70	19.0	20.0	23.5	26.6	27.5
60	20.6	21.6	24.9	28.5	29.3
50	22.1	23.1	26.4	30.1	30.9
40	23.7	24.9	28.1	31.6	32.5
30	25.4	27.0	30.1	33.5	34.3
20	27.7	29.3	32.1	35.6	36.6
10	32.1	32.8	35.0	37.7	39.3

Adapted, by permission, from American College of Sports Medicine (ACSM), 2000, *Guidelines for exercise testing and prescription* (Philadelphia, PA: Lippincott, Williams & Wilkins), 67-68.

BODY COMPOSITION IN ATHLETES

The range in percent body fat varies among athletes (see table 7.14), primarily because of the specific demands of each sport. While some athletes are very lean, others such as football players (primarily linemen) may be borderline obese. Despite possessing superior athletic skills, some football players may be in the lower 20th percentile of body composition standards. Recent studies have reported that the body fat of both National Football League (NFL) and National Collegiate Athletic Association (NCAA) linemen may exceed 25% (Noel et al. 2003; Snow, Millard-Stafford, and Rosskopf 1998). Though these body fat percentages are categorized as borderline obesity, the needs of the lineman position (extreme physical contact) require a higher percentage of fat. However, the athlete's long-term health should be considered once the playing career is over. The examples in table 7.14 focus on studies published in the last decade or on recently collected but as of yet unpublished data from various training centers.

As previously suggested, body fat percentages may vary within a sport due to the different positional demands. Tables 7.15 and 7.16 provide a positional analysis of body composition in collegiate football and basketball players, respectively. The positional differences, especially those in football, are quite obvious. Interestingly, body fat percentages in Division I football players have

TABLE 7.14 Body Composition Characteristics of Athletes ($\bar{X} \pm SD$)

Population	G	n	Age (y)	% BF	Method	Source
Baseball						
High school	M	76	13	21.7 ± 9.6	SF	Unpublished data
		91	14	20.2 ± 7.6		
		140	15	19.7 ± 7.7		
		153	16	19.5 ± 7.1		
		124	17	18.5 ± 8.8		
NCAA DIII	M	44		16.2 ± 3.8	SF	Unpublished data
NAIA	M	109	19.7 ± 1.4	14.2 ± 5.3		Unpublished data
Professional	M				SF	Coleman and Lasky 1992
MLB		27	27.6 ± 4.2	14.9 ± 6.4		
AAA		29	26.5 ± 2.8	11.3 ± 4.3		
AA		22	23.4 ± 1.8	10.5 ± 3.8		
A		132	22.6 ± 2.0	8.2 ± 7.9		
Basketball						
NBA	M	41		10.1 ± 3.0	SF	Unpublished data
NCAA DI	M	255		9.4 ± 3.8	—	Latin, Berg, and Baechle 1994

Population	G	n	Age (y)	% BF	Method	Source
Crew						
NCAA DI	F	22	20.4 ± 1.9	21.9 ± 2.3	DEXA	Fornetti et al. 1999
Distance running						
NCAA DI	F	24	20.3 ± 1.1	18.3 ± 2.7	DEXA	Fornetti et al. 1999
Field hockey						
NCAA DI	F	10	19.8 ± 1.2	20.9 ± 4.1	DEXA	Fornetti et al. 1999
Football						
NCAA DI	M	41		15.6 ± 6.5	HW	Prior et al. 2001
	M	69	19.5 ± 1.1	17.0 ± 6.6	HW	Collins et al. 1999
	M	632		12.3 ± 4.8	—	Berg, Latin, and Baechle 1990
NCAA DII	M	53	20.3 ± 1.1	11.9 ± 3.4	SF	Mayhew et al. 1989
NCAA DIII	M	225	19.6 ± 1.3	17.2 ± 5.4	HW	Unpublished data
				16.9 ± 5.2	SF	
Gymnastics						
NCAA DI	F	11		16.4 ± 3.4	HW	Prior et al. 2001
	F	15	19.8 ± 1.0	19.1 ± 2.2	DEXA	Fornetti et al. 1999
Hockey						
NHL	M	86		12.6 ± 2.0	SF	Unpublished data
U.S. national team	F	26	23.8	16.0	SF	Unpublished data
Rowing						
NCAA DI	F	10	21.5 ± 2.8	22.2 ± 7.3	HW	Vescovi et al. 2002
Skating						
U.S. national team	F	7	16.7 ± 2.1	16.9 ± 1.9	SF	Unpublished data
	M	11	18.2 ± 2.6	5.6 ± 1.0	SF	Unpublished data
Soccer						
NCAA DI	F	10	19.8 ± 0.9	21.8 ± 2.7	DEXA	Fornetti et al. 1999
NCAA DI	M	44		8.5 ± 1.2	SF	Unpublished data
Softball						
NCAA DI	F	17	20.4 ± 1.4	20.9 ± 3.9	DEXA	Fornetti et al. 1999
	F	17	21.5 ± 2.8	21.7 ± 5.7	HW	Vescovi et al. 2002
Masters players	F	9	40.6 ± 7.0	24.1 ± 7.4	HW	Terbizan et al. 1996
Swimming						
NCAA DI	M	10		15.1 ± 3.8	HW	Prior et al. 2001
	F	14		23.5 ± 5.8	HW	Prior et al. 2001
Track and field						
NCAA DI	F	32	20.0 ± 1.2	15.7 ± 4.5	HW	Vescovi et al. 2002
Volleyball						
NCAA DI	F	17	20.4 ± 1.1	22.1 ± 6.2	HW	Vescovi et al. 2002
	F	10	19.6 ± 0.6	19.1 ± 2.7	SF	Fry et al. 1991
Weightlifting						
Elite (U.S. national)	M	6	27.0 ± 2.1	20.4 ± 1.9	SF	Fry et al. 2003
Wrestling						
NCAA DI	M	33	19.5 ± 1.3	11.0 ± 2.9	4C	Clark et al. 2003
	M	12	19.3 ± 1.2	7.3 ± 0.7	SF	Kraemer et al. 2001
Elite (U.S. national)	M	8		7.6 ± 3.4	SF	Callan et al. 2000

4C = 4 compartment method; DEXA = dual energy X-ray absorbtiometry; HW = hydrostatic weighing; SF = skinfolds.

increased in the past decade. Some of these differences may be due to methodology of measurement, but demands on the athletes to get bigger also may have contributed to the elevated body fat. Table 7.17 provides a composition profile in a percentile format for college football players. The data presented in this table are from Division III football players. Table 7.18 provides body fat percentiles of football players invited to the NFL combine (the top college football players in the United States).

TABLE 7.15 Body Composition in NFL and College Football Players

| Position | NFL COMBINE 1999 DATA | | NCAA DIVISION I | | | | NCAA DIVISION III 2000-2004 | |
| | | | 1990 | | 2003 | | | |
	n	$\bar{X} \pm SD$	n	$\bar{X} \pm SD$	n	$\bar{X} \pm SD$	n	$\bar{X} \pm SD$
DB	45	6.3 ± 1.9	116	8.6 ± 2.6	12	13.4 ± 4.1	43	13.1 ± 3.1
DL	47	14.7 ± 4.0	114	14.6 ± 4.0	14	23.6 ± 7.3	32	20.9 ± 5.0
LB	34	10.1 ± 2.8	85	11.6 ± 3.4	6	18.5 ± 4.3	33	16.9 ± 4.2
OL	59	19.3 ± 2.8	145	17.1 ± 4.0	16	25.8 ± 8.2*	37	21.2 ± 4.8
QB	16	11.4 ± 2.5	29	9.9 ± 3.0	6	15.5 ± 4.0**	12	15.4 ± 3.8
RB	46	8.6 ± 3.2	86	8.8 ± 2.7	15	13.8 ± 4.9#	28	15.9 ± 4.6
TE	14	12.6 ± 4.0	28	12.0 ± 2.8			8	18.6 ± 3.4
WR	48	6.6 ± 1.6	29	8.0 ± 2.6			31	13.1 ± 4.6
Source	Unpublished data		Berg, Latin, and Baechle 1990		Noel et al. 2003		Unpublished data	

DB = defensive backs; DL = defensive linemen; LB = linebackers; OL = offensive linemen; QB = quarterbacks; RB = running backs; TE = tight ends; WR = wide receivers. * includes offensive linemen and tight ends; ** includes quarterbacks and kickers; # includes running backs and wide receivers.

TABLE 7.16 Anthropometric and Body Composition Measurements in NCAA Division I College Basketball Players

| Position | Height | | Weight | | Body fat % |
	in.	cm	lb	kg	
Guards	73.8 ± 2.3	187.4 ± 5.8	182.4 ± 15.0	82.9 ± 6.8	8.4 ± 3.0
Forwards	78.1 ± 1.5	198.4 ± 3.8	209.2 ± 18.3	95.1 ± 8.3	9.7 ± 3.9
Centers	80.9 ± 2.4	205.5 ± 6.1	224.2 ± 21.3	101.9 ± 9.7	11.2 ± 4.5

Data from R.W. Latin, K. Berg and T. Baechle, 1994, "Physical and performance characteristics of NCAA Division I male basketball players," *Journal of Strength and Conditioning Research* 8:214-218.

TABLE 7.17 Percentile Ranks of % Body Fat in NCAA Division III College Football Players

Percentage	Body fat %
90	10.6
80	12.3
70	13.6
60	14.9
50	16.1
40	17.4
30	19.6
20	22.0
10	24.9

n = 224.

TABLE 7.18 Percentile Ranks of % Body Fat in Players Participating in the NFL Combine

% rank	BODY FAT %							
	DB	DL	LB	OL	QB	RB	TE	WR
90	4.1	7.7	6.3	15.0	8.5	5.0	7.3	4.6
80	4.4	11.8	7.8	17.3	8.9	5.7	9.8	5.0
70	5.5	12.9	8.6	18.3	9.2	6.3	10.2	5.3
60	5.8	14.1	9.5	19.1	10.1	7.3	11.1	5.8
50	6.1	15.0	10.1	19.6	11.1	7.9	12.1	6.6
40	6.5	16.1	10.8	20.4	12.0	9.0	13.4	7.1
30	6.8	17.1	11.2	20.7	12.5	10.5	14.0	7.8
20	7.4	18.0	12.9	21.4	13.8	11.4	16.1	8.2
10	9.2	19.7	13.9	22.0	15.5	13.4	19.8	8.9
n	45	47	34	59	16	46	14	48

DB = defensive backs; DL = defensive linemen; LB = linebackers; OL = offensive linemen; QB = quarterbacks; RB = running backs; TE = tight ends; WR = wide receivers.

Unpublished data using Jackson-Pollock 3-site equation.

CALCULATING DESIRED BODY WEIGHT

Once a person's body fat is calculated and compared to standards for individuals of similar gender and age, the individual may desire to reduce body fat. An ideal body weight can be computed for the desired percent body fat. Although the ideal weight may correspond to the values in table 7.13, for athletes it may be lower or higher depending on the sport and sport position. Regardless, the formula for calculating desired body weight is as follows:

$$\text{Desired body weight} = \frac{\text{Lean body mass (LBM)}}{1 - \text{desired body fat \%}}.$$

For example, the ideal body weight for a 25-year-old recreational athlete weighing 200 lb (90.7 kg) with 22% body fat can be computed as follows (assume the desired body fat is 15%):

1. *Compute fat mass and lean body mass (LBM):*

200 lb (90.7 kg) × 0.22 body fat = 44 lb (20.0 kg) of fat mass,

200 lb (90.7 kg) − 44 lb (20.0 kg) of fat mass
= 156 lb (70.8 kg) of lean mass.

2. *Calculate ideal body weight:*

Ideal body weight = LBM / (1 − desired % body fat)
= 156 / (1 − 0.15) = 156 / 0.85
= 184 lb (83.5 kg).

Summary

⊃ Anthropometry and body composition analysis are often used as descriptive measurements in both research and nonresearch settings.

⊃ The various methods for assessing body composition range in complexity and ease of administration.

⊃ Equations used should be specific to the population being assessed.

CHAPTER 8

Flexibility

Flexibility is the ability to move a muscle, or a group of muscles, through its complete range of motion (ROM). The role of flexibility in sport performance is not clearly understood. In some sports the range of motion for a given joint may have important implications for performance. For instance, flexibility is important in gymnastics and weightlifting, yet its ability to predict performance has not been established. Baseball pitchers also benefit from increased flexibility of specific joints, as an increase in the external rotation of the dominant shoulder joint (throwing arm) increases the distance through which force is applied during a pitch and results in a higher throw velocity. Lack of flexibility may predispose athletes to muscle and tendon injuries, while high flexibility may enhance the risk for joint dislocations and ligament strains (Maud and Cortez-Cooper 2002). Still, a direct relationship between flexibility and injury risk has not been established. In this chapter various flexibility assessments are reviewed and population norms and specific sport measurements are given when possible.

Flexibility Assessment

Numerous tests can be used to measure the flexibility of a joint or a group of muscles. Flexibility can be assessed either directly by measuring the range of joint rotation in degrees or indirectly by measuring static flexibility in linear units. Flexibility testing identifies joints or muscles that have a poor range of motion and are at a greater risk for injury.

DIRECT MEASURES

Direct measurements of flexibility use a goniometer, a flexometer, or an inclinometer. All measure the range of motion of a joint in degrees. The goniometer is a device like a protractor that measures the angle of the joint at both extremes of the range of motion (see figure 8.1). The center of the goniometer is placed at the axis of rotation (of the joint). The arms of the goniometer are aligned with the longitudinal axis of each moving body segment. The initial joint angle is recorded and the proximal

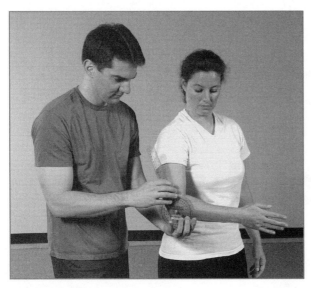

FIGURE 8.1 Using a goniometer to examine the range of motion for elbow flexion.

limb is then moved through its complete range of motion until it reaches its other extreme. At that point the angle is recorded again. The difference between the angles indicates the range of motion of that joint. Table 8.1 presents the average ranges of motion for healthy adults.

The flexometer and inclinometer also directly measure the range of motion of a joint or body segment. Both of these devices can be placed on the subject (either strapped on or held by hand), and the range of motion for a particular joint or body segment is easily recorded. Although both the validity and reliability of these tests have been established, the reliability may depend on the skill of the technician and on the joint being measured. Measurements of the upper extremities appear more reliable than measurements of the lower extremities (Norkin and White 1995).

The flexometer was invented by Jack Leighton and consists of a weighted 360° dial and a weighted pointer. The dial and pointer are controlled by gravity and act independently of each other. The instrument records movement in a position that is ≥20° from horizontal. The flexometer is strapped to the body segment being tested, the dial is locked in one extreme position (full flexion or extension), the movement is performed, and the pointer is locked at the other extreme position (full extension or flexion). The reading of the pointer on the dial is the range of motion (in degrees). Norms from the Leighton flexometer can be seen in table 8.2.

TABLE 8.1 Average Range of Motion (ROM) for Healthy Adults

Joint and movement	ROM (°)
Shoulder	
Flexion	150-180
Extension	50-60
Abduction	180
Medial rotation	70-90
Lateral rotation	90
Elbow	
Flexion	140-150
Extension	0
Radioulnar	
Pronation	80
Supination	80
Wrist	
Flexion	60-80
Extension	60-70
Radial deviation	20
Ulnar deviation	30
Cervical spine	
Flexion	45-60
Extension	45-75
Lateral flexion	45
Rotation	60-80
Thoracic-lumbar spine	
Flexion	60-80
Extension	20-30
Lateral flexion	25-35
Rotation	30-45
Hip	
Flexion	100-120
Extension	30
Abduction	40-45
Adduction	20-30
Medial rotation	40-45
Lateral rotation	45-50
Knee	
Flexion	135-150
Extension	0-10
Ankle	
Dorsiflexion	20
Plantar flexion	40-50
Subtalar	
Inversion	30-35
Eversion	15-20

Adapted, by permission, from V.H. Heyward, 2002, *Advanced fitness assessment & exercise prescription*, 4th ed. (Champaign, IL: Human Kinetics), 234. Data from the American Academy of Orthopedic Surgeons (Greene and Heckman, 1994) and the American Medical Association (1988).

TABLE 8.2 Norms for Joint Range of Motion (°) Using Leighton Flexometer

Joint movement	MALES					FEMALES				
	Low	Mod. low	Avg.	Mod. high	High	Low	Mod. low	Avg.	Mod. high	High
Neck										
Flexion/extension	<107	107-128	129-142	143-160	>160	<125	125-141	142-160	161-177	>177
Lateral flexion	<74	74-89	90-106	107-122	>122	<84	84-99	100-116	117-132	>132
Rotation	<141	141-160	161-181	182-201	>201	<158	158-177	178-198	199-218	>218
Shoulder										
Flexion/extension	<207	207-223	224-242	243-259	>259	<226	226-242	243-261	262-278	>278
Adduction/abduction	<158	158-171	172-186	187-200	>200	<167	167-180	181-195	196-209	>209
Rotation	<154	154-171	172-192	193-210	>210	<189	189-206	207-227	228-245	>245
Elbow										
Flexion/extension	<133	133-143	144-156	157-167	>167	<133	133-143	144-156	157-167	>167
Forearm										
Supination/pronation	<151	151-170	171-191	192-211	>211	<160	160-179	180-200	201-220	>220
Wrist										
Flexion/ extension	<112	112-131	132-152	153-172	>172	<136	136-155	156-176	177-196	>196
Ulnar/radial deviation	<64	64-77	78-92	93-105	>105	<75	75-88	89-101	102-117	>117
Hip										
Flexion/extension	<50	50-67	68-88	89-106	>106	<82	82-99	100-120	121-138	>138
Adduction/abduction	<41	41-50	51-61	62-71	>71	<45	45-54	55-65	66-75	>75
Rotation	<59	59-78	79-99	100-119	>119	<90	90-109	110-130	131-150	>150
Knee										
Flexion/extension	<122	122-133	134-146	147-157	>157	<134	134-144	145-157	158-168	>168
Ankle										
Plantar flexion/ dorsiflexion	<48	48-58	59-71	72-82	>82	<56	56-66	67-79	80-90	>90
Inversion/ eversion	<30	30-41	42-56	57-68	>68	<39	39-50	51-65	66-77	>77
Trunk										
Flexion/extension	<45	45-62	63-83	84-101	>101	<30	30-47	48-68	69-86	>86
Lateral flexion	<74	74-89	90-106	107-122	>122	<104	104-119	120-136	137-152	>152
Rotation	<108	108-126	127-147	148-166	>166	<134	134-152	153-173	174-192	>192

Adapted, by permission, from J.R. Leighton, 1987, *Manual of Instruction for Leighton Flexometer*.

An inclinometer is similar to the flexometer in that it operates through gravity, but it is held in the hand instead of being strapped into position. In addition, for measurements of the vertebral column the inclinometer differentiates between the thoracic and lumbosacral regions. To achieve this differentiation, two inclinometers are generally used. Table 8.3 provides methods for selected spinal measurements that use the flexometer or inclinometer. The ranges of motion in which impairment exists in these measurements can be seen in table 8.4.

TABLE 8.3 Methods for Selected Spinal Measurements Using the Flexometer or Inclinometer

Movement	Starting position	Method	Stabilization
Flexometer			
Cervical			
Flexion/ extension	• Subject is in supine position with arms at side of body. • Shoulders are on edge of bench, with head and neck projecting beyond bench. • Flexometer is attached over ears on either side of head.	• Subject raises head toward chest as far as possible. • Dial is locked in position. • Subject lowers head as far back as possible and pointer is locked. • Reading is taken.	• Buttocks and shoulders remain in contact with bench during movement. • Lumbar region is not allowed to arch.
Lateral flexion	• Subject is seated in armchair, with back straight. • Upper arm is hooked over back of chair. • Hands grasp the arms of the chair. • Flexometer is attached to the back of the head.	• Subject moves head sideways to extreme left and the dial is locked. • Subject moves head in an arc to the extreme right and the pointer is locked. • A reading is taken.	• Body position in chair remains steady throughout measurement. • No raising or lowering of shoulders during movement.
Rotation	• Subject is in similar position as for flexion and extension. • Flexometer is placed on top of head.	• Subject rotates head to extreme left and dial is locked. • Subject rotates head to extreme right and pointer is locked. • A reading is taken.	• Shoulders must remain in contact with bench.

Movement	Starting position	Method
Inclinometer		
Cervical		
Flexion/ extension	• Subject is seated in a chair with thoracic and lumbar spine in contact with back of chair. • Inclinometers are placed on spinous process of T1 and over the occiput of the head.	• Subject flexes the neck maximally and the reading from T1 is subtracted from the occiput. The difference is recorded as cervical flexion. • Subject returns to neutral position. • Subject extends head maximally and the reading of T1 is again subtracted from the reading at the occiput. The difference is recorded as cervical extension.
Lateral flexion	• Same starting position as flexion and extension. • Inclinometers are positioned in the coronal plane.	• Subject maximally flexes the neck laterally. • The difference between the reading at T1 and at the occiput is maximal lateral flexion for that side. • The subject returns to neutral position and repeats to opposite side.
Rotation	• Subject lies supine on bench, with shoulders off the bench. • One inclinometer is placed near the back of the head, approximately in line with the cervico–occipital junction.	• Subject rotates head maximally to one side and inclinometer reading is recorded as maximal cervical rotation to that side. • Subject returns to starting position and repeats movement to the opposite side.

Movement	Starting position	Method
Thoracic		
Flexion/extension	• Subject is seated upright with shoulders back and hands resting on hips. • Inclinometers are placed on spinous processes of T1 and T12.	• Subject maximally flexes the thoracic spine. • Some hip flexion is permitted. • T12 reading is subtracted from T1 and the difference is recorded as maximal thoracic flexion.
Rotation	• Subject stands and flexes at hip so that thoracic spine is horizontal to floor. • Inclinometers are placed at the spinous processes of T1 and T12.	• Subject rotates trunk maximally to one side. • T12 reading is subtracted from the T1 reading and the difference is recorded as maximal thoracic rotation. • Subject returns to neutral position and repeats to the opposite side.
Lumbosacral		
Flexion/extension	• Subject stands with knees straight, with weight evenly distributed and hands on hips. • Inclinometers are placed on the spinous process of T12 and on the midpoint of the sacrum. • Trunk is in neutral position.	• Subject flexes at hip and the reading of the inclinometer at the sacrum is subtracted from the reading from T12. The difference is recorded as lumbar flexion. • Subject returns to starting position. • Subject extends backward as far as possible. The reading from the sacrum is again subtracted from the reading of T12 to obtain maximal lumbar extension.
Lateral flexion	• Same as for flexion and extension.	• Subject laterally flexes to one side. The sacral reading is subtracted from the T12 reading. • Subject returns to neutral position. • Subject repeats lateral flexion to the opposite side.

Adapted from P.J. Maud and M.Y. Cortez-Cooper, 1995, Static techniques for the evaluation of joint range of motion. In *Physiological assessment of human fitness,* edited by P.J. Maud and C. Foster (Champaign, IL: Human Kinetics), 230-242.

TABLE 8.4   Range of Motion at Which Impairment Exists for Selected Measurements of Spine Motion

Movement	Range at which impairment may exist (°)
Neck	
Flexion	<40
Extension	<50
Right lateral flexion	<30
Left lateral flexion	<30
Right rotation	<60
Left rotation	<60
Thoracic region	
Flexion/extension	<30
Right rotation	<20
Left rotation	<20
Lumbosacral region	
Right lateral flexion	<20
Left lateral flexion	<20

Adapted, by permission, from P.J. Maud and M.Y. Cortez-Cooper, 2006, Static techniques for the evaluation of joint range of motion. In *Physiological assessment of human fitness,* 2nd ed., edited by P.J. Maud and C. Foster (Champaign, IL: Human Kinetics), 232.

INDIRECT MEASURES

Indirect measurements of the range of motion about a joint are also easily assessed. Indirect measures are reported as inches or centimeters rather than as degrees. A commonly used indirect measurement is the sit-and-reach test (see figure 8.2). Although this test is used to evaluate lower back and hip flexibility, it appears to be more valid for hamstring flexibility than for lower back flexibility (Minkler and Patterson 1994). This test can be performed with or without a sit-and-reach box. When a sit-and-reach box is used, the subject sits

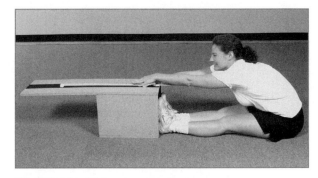

FIGURE 8.2   Sit-and-reach test.

on the ground with the soles of her feet against the edge of the box and with her knees extended but not locked. Keeping her back straight, the subject reaches as far forward as possible, with one hand on top of the other, and slides her fingers along the measuring device. The most distant point that she reaches is recorded (in either inches or centimeters). The percentile ranks for the sit-and-reach test for both men and women can be seen in table 8.5. This table, however, does not indicate the flexibility requirements for athletes or predict performance capabilities. It is primarily for evaluating a normal adult population.

One of the potential limitations of the sit-and-reach test is that it does not allow for differences in limb length or proportional differences between the arms and legs (Hopkins and Hoeger 1992). The starting position for a sit-and-reach test (the subject's feet against the box) places the subject's

hands at a zero point of 23 or 26 cm. The subject's ability to reach depends on limb length. Subjects with long legs or short arms are at a disadvantage for this test and do not score well. Hopkins and Hoeger (1992) suggested that the starting point for subjects be measured while the subject's back is at 90° and his feet are against the box. The subject places one hand over the other, and the only movement allowed is scapular adduction. The point that the subject is able to reach while in this position is the zero point. The subject then completes the reach test and the total distance reached is recorded. This test, the *modified sit-and-reach test*, appears to negate the bias in limb length. Differences in testing methodologies for the modified and regular sit-and-reach tests are likely responsible for the varying results in the sport science literature. Percentile scores for the modified sit-and-reach test can be seen in table 8.6

TABLE 8.5 Percentile Ranks for the Sit-and-Reach Test (cm)

| | AGE (Y) | | | | | | | | | |
| | 20-29 | | 30-39 | | 40-49 | | 50-59 | | 60-69 | |
% rank	M	F	M	F	M	F	M	F	M	F
90	39	40	37	39	34	37	35	37	32	34
80	35	37	34	36	31	33	29	34	27	31
70	33	35	31	34	27	32	26	32	23	28
60	30	33	29	32	25	30	24	29	21	27
50	28	31	26	30	22	28	22	27	19	25
40	26	29	24	28	20	26	19	26	15	23
30	23	26	21	25	17	23	15	23	13	21
20	20	23	18	22	13	21	12	20	11	20
10	15	19	14	18	9	16	9	16	8	15

Reprinted, by permission, from V.H. Heyward, 2002, *Advanced fitness assessment & exercise prescription*, 4th ed. (Champaign, IL: Human Kinetics), 236; from the *Canadian Standardized Test of Fitness (CSTF) Operations Manual*, 3rd ed., Public Health Agency of Canada, 1986. Adapted and reproduced with permission of the Minister of Public Works and Government Services, Canada, 2006.

TABLE 8.6 Percentile Ranks for the Modified Sit-and-Reach Test

| | FEMALES | | | | | | | |
| | <18 Y | | 19-35 Y | | 36-49 Y | | >50 Y | |
% rank	in.	cm	in.	cm	in.	cm	in.	cm
99	22.6	57.4	21.0	53.3	19.8	50.3	17.2	43.7
95	19.5	49.5	19.3	49.0	19.2	48.8	15.7	39.9
90	18.7	47.5	17.9	45.5	17.4	44.2	15.0	38.1
80	17.8	45.2	16.7	42.4	16.2	41.1	14.2	36.1
70	16.5	41.9	16.2	41.1	15.2	38.6	13.6	34.5
60	16.0	40.6	15.8	40.1	14.5	36.8	12.3	31.2

	FEMALES							
	<18 Y		19-35 Y		36-49 Y		>50 Y	
% rank	in.	cm	in.	cm	in.	cm	in.	cm
50	15.2	38.6	14.8	37.6	13.5	34.3	11.1	28.2
40	14.5	36.8	14.5	36.8	12.8	32.5	10.1	25.7
30	13.7	34.8	13.7	34.8	12.2	31.0	9.2	23.4
20	12.6	32.0	12.6	32.0	11.0	27.9	8.3	21.1
10	11.4	29.0	10.1	25.7	9.7	24.6	7.5	19.1

	MALES							
	<18 Y		19-35 Y		36-49 Y		>50 Y	
% rank	in.	cm	in.	cm	in.	cm	in.	cm
99	20.1	51.1	24.7	62.7	18.9	48.0	16.2	41.1
95	19.6	49.8	18.9	48.0	18.2	46.2	15.8	40.1
90	18.2	46.2	17.2	43.7	16.1	40.9	15.0	38.1
80	17.8	45.2	17.0	43.2	14.6	37.1	13.3	33.8
70	16.0	40.6	15.8	40.1	13.9	35.3	12.3	31.2
60	15.2	38.6	15.0	38.1	13.4	34.0	11.5	29.2
50	14.5	36.8	14.4	36.6	12.6	32.0	10.2	25.9
40	14.0	35.6	13.5	34.3	11.6	29.5	9.7	24.6
30	13.4	34.0	13.0	33.0	10.8	27.4	9.3	23.6
20	11.8	30.0	11.6	29.5	9.9	25.1	8.8	22.4
10	9.5	24.1	9.2	23.4	8.3	21.1	7.8	19.8

Flexibility Measures in Athletic Populations

Flexibility is important in preparing for sport participation and recovering from exercise; however, as mentioned previously, its role in sport performance is not well understood. Although it may not directly affect athletic achievement, it may indirectly influence performance by helping athletes stay clear of musculotendon injuries. Unfortunately, whether an athlete is too flexible or not flexible enough too often relies on empirical evidence. Table 8.7 provides percentile ranks of male and female high school athletes participating in various scholastic sports. Table 8.8 shows the mean and standard deviation of the sit-and-reach test in high school athletes playing specific sports. These results were compiled from assessments of scholastic athletes shared by various strength and conditioning coaches. Table 8.9 provides the mean and standard deviation of sit-and-reach measurements of athletes participating in various sports and athletic events. When applicable, sit-and-reach performance measurements of the various positions within a sport are provided as well. These values were taken from the scientific literature. Table 8.10 reports the shoulder range of motion in collegiate and professional baseball pitchers. Both collegiate and professional pitchers appear to have greater external rotation and lower internal rotation in their dominant arm as compared to their nondominant arm. These differences are not seen in control subjects.

TABLE 8.7 Percentile Ranks in the Sit and Reach (cm) for High School Athletes

% rank	MALES (BASEBALL, BASKETBALL, SOCCER, SWIMMING)		FEMALES (BASKETBALL, FIELD HOCKEY, SWIMMING)	
	13-15 y $n = 194$	16-18 y $n = 157$	13-15 y $n = 73$	16-18 y $n = 37$
90	39.3	42.0	46.5	47.1
80	36.0	38.5	43.5	44.3
70	33.0	37.0	41.0	41.5
60	31.0	35.0	38.7	40.9
50	29.0	33.5	37.0	40.0
40	27.0	31.6	33.8	37.4
30	25.5	28.7	32.1	35.4
20	23.5	27.8	29.5	32.4
10	19.5	23.0	24.8	30.4

TABLE 8.8 Mean and Standard Deviation of the Sit-and-Reach Test in High School Athletes

	Baseball ($n = 76$)	Basketball ($n = 206$)	Soccer ($n = 43$)	Swimming ($n = 20$)	Swimming ($n = 42$)	Field hockey ($n = 43$)
Gender	M	M	M	M	F	F
Age (y)	16.1 ± 1.0	15.5 ± 0.8	15.2 ± 1.0	15.6 ± 1.5	15.8 ± 1.7	14.6 ± 1.1
Sit and reach (cm)	30.5 ± 7.7	31.8 ± 6.7	30.1 ± 7	31.9 ± 9.7	40.2 ± 7.6	36.9 ± 7

Data reported as $\bar{X} \pm SD$.

TABLE 8.9 Mean and Standard Deviation of the Sit-and-Reach Test in Competitive Athletes

Sport	League	Gender	Age	Sit and reach (cm)	Reference
Volleyball	NCAA DI	F	19.6 ± 0.6	17.3 ± 4.9	Fry et al. 1991
Basketball	Professional—NBA	M			Parr et al. 1978
C			27.7 ± 5.2	14.8 ± 0.00	
F			25.3 ± 3.8	16.2 ± 2.7	
G			25.2 ±3.6	15.9 ± 3.1	
Football	NCAA DIII	M			Schmidt 1999
DB			19.9 ± 1.4	11.4 ± 3.8	
L			19.9 ± 1.6	14.2 ± 5.2	
TE/LB			19.9 ± 1.2	10.5 ± 6.5	
Football	NCAA DIII	M			Stuempfle, Katch, and Petrie 2003
Team			19.6 ± 1.3	12.1 ± 5.9	
OL			19.0 ± 1.1	10.7 ± 3.9	
DL			19.5 ± 1.2	14.3 ± 6.1	
OB			19.9 ± 1.4	11.4 ± 6.4	
DB			19.8 ± 1.2	12.1 ± 5.9	

C = centers; F = forwards; G = guards; DB = defensive backs; L = linemen; TE/LB = tight ends and linebackers; OL = offensive linemen; DL = defensive linemen; OB = offensive backs.

TABLE 8.10 Shoulder Range of Motion (°) in Baseball Pitchers		
Measurement	**Pitchers**	**Controls**
Comparison between collegiate pitchers and controls		
Flexion, dominant arm	169	164
Flexion, nondominant arm	172	169
Extension, dominant arm	60	58
Extension, nondominant arm	63	60
Internal rotation, dominant arm	66	64
Internal rotation, nondominant arm	72	64
External rotation, dominant arm	99	105
External rotation, nondominant arm	95	106
Comparison of external and internal rotation in professional pitchers and controls		
Internal rotation, dominant arm at 90° abduction	61	61
Internal rotation, nondominant arm at 90° abduction	73	67
External rotation, dominant arm at 90° abduction	134	106
External rotation, nondominant arm at 90° abduction	129	102
Measurement	**Dominant arm ($\bar{X} \pm SD$)**	**Nondominant arm ($\bar{X} \pm SD$)**
Examination of external and internal rotation at varying degrees of abduction		
External rotation at 0° of abduction	90.1 ± 10.8	81.0 ± 10.7
External rotation at 90° of abduction	126.8 ± 12.0	114.5 ± 9.1
Internal rotation at 90° of abduction	79.3 ± 13.3	91.4 ± 13.6

Comparison between Collegiate Pitchers and Controls data adapted from Cook et al., 1987. Comparison of External and Internal Rotation in Professional Pitchers and Controls data adapted from Magnusson et al., 1994. Examination of External and Internal Rotation at Varying Degrees of Abduction Data adapted from Osbahr et al., 2002.

Summary

⊃ Direct and indirect flexibility measurements are used to assess both general and athletic populations.

⊃ Direct measurements of flexibility use a goniometer, a flexometer, or an inclinometer to provide the range of motion of specific joints.

⊃ The sit-and-reach test indirectly assesses flexibility and is one of the most common flexibility measurements used by coaches, trainers, and educators.

CHAPTER 9

Speed and Agility

The importance of speed and agility for success in a variety of sports (i.e., baseball, basketball, football, hockey, soccer) has been well acknowledged (Hoffman 2002; Hoffman et al. 1996; Kraemer and Gotshalk 2000; Kirkendall 2000). As a result, these variables are often part of the testing battery for these athletes. Surprisingly, there are very little normative data that can be used for comparisons in the various athletic populations.

Coaches are reluctant to share their results with peers or researchers for a variety of reasons. As a result, it is often difficult for many coaches, exercise scientists, physical educators, and trainers to evaluate their athletes, subjects, students, and clients in respect to their sport activity. In addition, the specific tests used to evaluate speed and agility often differ among sports and within sports as well. Many coaches develop their own tests, while others change test methodologies, which limits their ability to compare their results to those of similar testing populations. Other factors that may limit the ability to share data among teams or groups are the technique (e.g., athlete performing the test in a 2-point or 3-point stance) and timing method (e.g., handheld stopwatch or electronic timer) used. This chapter describes common speed and agility tests used in athletic and student populations. When possible, norma-tive data for various sports are provided. For sports in which normative data are not available, descriptive data are presented.

Speed

Speed is the ability to perform a movement in as short a time as possible. It is relatively easy to measure and requires only a timer and a court, field, or running track. The 40 yd (36.6 m) sprint is the most popular speed assessment for many athletes, probably because most coaches are familiar with the sprint times associated with this distance. The 40 yd (36.6 m) sprint has achieved tremendous popularity among football coaches and is a staple of most football testing programs. The justification for using 40 yd (36.6 m) for football, though, is not entirely clear. The distance may have arbitrarily originated and become well accepted over time. Since the backgrounds of many strength and conditioning coaches in North America evolved from football, the 40 yd (36.6 m) sprint is often used in other sports. However, as strength and conditioning professionals have begun to work with other sports, more specific sprinting distances have become more commonplace.

Some strength and conditioning coaches for basketball use a 30 yd (27.4 m) sprint to assess speed in their athletes since 30 yd (27.4 m) is the approximate length of a basketball court. Baseball has used the 60 yd (54.9 m) sprint, most likely because 60 yd (54.9 m) is the distance between three bases (i.e., distance from home to second or from first to third). For many other sports, the sprint distance is quite arbitrary; however, most strength and conditioning coaches can easily interpret the 40 yd (36.6 m) sprint.

📄 For a description of how to perform the 40 yd (36.6 m) sprint, please see page 201 in the appendix.

ASSESSMENT METHOD

In programs with large training budgets, electronic timers are becoming more popular. Using a stopwatch has the potential for measurement error. Even under ideal conditions and with an experienced tester, stopwatch times may be 0.24 s faster than electronically measured times because of the tester's reaction time in pressing the start and stop buttons as the athlete begins and ends the sprint (Harman, Garhammer, and Pandorf 2000). Figure 9.1 compares 40 yd (36.6 m) sprint times measured by these two timing methods. Electronic timers and handheld stopwatches were simultaneously used to time 70 male American football players. As can be seen by the scatter diagram in figure 9.1, the correlation between the two methods was very high ($r = 0.98$). Although these two methods are valid, electronic timers result in slower sprint times. Thus, knowing the method of assessment

is important when comparing sprint times from different programs. In addition, when choosing a timing method some coaches may be concerned with the confidence and motivation issues of their athletes. Coaches may not want to risk having their athletes think they are slow due to the slower than expected sprint times when speed is assessed from electronic timing compared to handheld stopwatches.

NORMATIVE AND DESCRIPTIVE SPRINT DATA

As discussed previously, normative data of sprint times for various athletic populations are quite limited. Through the cooperation of numerous coaches around the United States, percentile ranks for several athletic populations have been developed. Table 9.1 provides 40 yd (36.6 m) sprint times for high school and National Collegiate Athletic Association (NCAA) Division I and III football players. Table 9.2 provides 40 yd (36.6 m) sprint times for college football players that were invited to the National Football League (NFL) combine. Table 9.3 provides percentile ranks for 30 and 60 yd (27.4 and 54.9 m) sprint times of high school baseball and basketball players. These times were collected with a handheld stopwatch. Percentile ranks for the 40 yd (36.6 m) sprint in active male youth are shown in table 9.4. Descriptive data for the 30, 40, and 60 yd (27.4, 36.6, and 54.9 m) sprints, which were in the literature or provided by various coaches around the country, can be seen in table 9.5. Sprint times assessed by electronic timers are followed by an *E*.

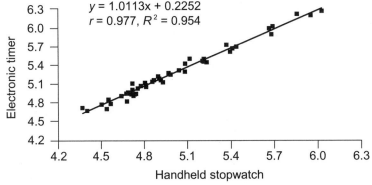

FIGURE 9.1 Comparison of 40 yd (36.6 m) sprint times measured with an electronic timer and a handheld stopwatch.

TABLE 9.1 Percentile Ranks for 40 Yd (36.6 m) Sprint Times (sec) in American Football Players

% rank	High school (14-15 y)	High school (16-18 y)	High school (14-15 y) E	High school (16-18 y) E	NCAA DIII	NCAA DI	NCAA DI E
90	4.86	4.70	5.08	4.98	4.59	4.58	4.75
80	5.00	4.80	5.17	5.10	4.70	4.67	4.84
70	5.10	4.89	5.28	5.21	4.77	4.73	4.92
60	5.20	4.96	5.31	5.30	4.85	4.80	5.01
50	5.28	5.08	5.43	5.40	4.95	4.87	5.10
40	5.38	5.17	5.52	5.46	5.02	4.93	5.18
30	5.50	5.30	5.63	5.63	5.12	5.02	5.32
20	5.84	5.45	5.84	5.73	5.26	5.18	5.48
10	6.16	5.73	6.22	5.84	5.47	5.33	5.70
$\bar{X}$	5.40	5.15	5.54	5.41	4.99	4.92	5.17
SD	0.53	0.45	0.52	0.35	0.35	0.32	0.37
n	113	205	94	151	538	757	608

E = electronic timing device; other measurements were from handheld stopwatches.

TABLE 9.2 40 Yd (36.6 m) Sprint Times (sec) for College Football Players Participating in the NFL Combine

% rank	DB	DL	LB	OL	QB	RB	TE	WR
90	4.41	4.72	4.57	5.07	4.60	4.44	4.66	4.42
80	4.45	4.80	4.62	5.15	4.70	4.50	4.78	4.46
70	4.48	4.87	4.66	5.21	4.75	4.55	4.80	4.50
60	4.51	4.90	4.72	5.25	4.79	4.58	4.83	4.52
50	4.54	4.90	4.76	5.30	4.81	4.62	4.90	4.55
40	4.57	4.96	4.78	5.33	4.86	4.65	4.96	4.57
30	4.59	5.03	4.81	5.40	4.91	4.69	4.99	4.61
20	4.62	5.09	4.86	5.47	4.99	4.74	5.02	4.65
10	4.67	5.15	4.92	5.56	5.10	4.82	5.07	4.68
$\bar{X}$	4.54	4.97	4.75	5.31	4.84	4.62	4.89	4.55
SD	0.11	0.19	0.13	0.20	0.17	0.16	0.15	0.10
n	111	100	62	155	41	67	42	98

DB = defensive backs; DL = defensive linemen; LB = linebackers; OL = offensive linemen; QB = quarterbacks; RB = running backs; TE = tight ends; WR = wide receivers.

Data collected from 1999 NFL combine.

TABLE 9.3 Percentile Ranks for 30 Yd (27.4 m) and 60 Yd (54.9 m) Sprint Times (sec) in Male High School Baseball and Basketball Players

% rank	Baseball (14-15 y) 30 yd	Baseball (16-18 y) 30 yd	Baseball (elite 15-18 y)* 60 yd	Basketball (14-15 y) 30 yd	Basketball (16-18 y) 30 yd
90	3.86	3.78	6.8	4.07	3.91
80	3.90	3.85	6.9	4.17	3.96
70	3.99	3.89	7.0	4.23	4.00
60	4.00	3.90	7.1	4.28	4.11
50	4.11	3.91	7.2	4.31	4.19
40	4.20	3.99	7.3	4.38	4.26
30	4.25	4.00	7.4	4.44	4.31
20	4.30	4.09	7.5	4.53	4.34
10	4.45	4.20	7.6	4.75	4.47
$\bar{X}$	4.12	3.95	7.21	4.35	4.19
SD	0.21	0.16	0.29	0.25	0.22
n	45	27	118	150	109

* Subjects were selected to participate in a national high school baseball showcase held at the Cleveland Indians training complex (in October of 2003).

TABLE 9.4 Percentile Ranks for 40 yd (36.6 m) Sprint Times (sec) in Male Youth

% rank	12-13 y	14-15 y	16-18 y
90	5.41	5.02	4.76
80	5.63	5.15	4.85
70	5.77	5.24	4.90
60	5.84	5.32	4.98
50	5.97	5.46	5.10
40	6.08	5.54	5.13
30	6.25	5.78	5.21
20	6.32	6.02	5.30
10	6.64	6.08	5.46
$\bar{X}$	5.99	5.54	5.09
SD	0.39	0.43	0.28
n	28	92	94

TABLE 9.5 Descriptive Data for Sprint Tests in Athletic Populations

Population	Gender	SPRINT TIMES (SEC) 30 yd (27.4 m)	40 yd (36.6 m)	60 yd (54.9 m)	Source
Baseball					
Youth	M				Unpublished data
13 y				8.7 ± 0.5 E	
14 y				8.4 ± 0.7 E	
15 y				7.9 ± 0.5 E	
16 y				7.8 ± 0.5 E	
17 y				7.5 ± 0.5 E	

		SPRINT TIMES (SEC)			
Population	Gender	30 yd (27.4 m)	40 yd (36.6 m)	60 yd (54.9 m)	Source
Baseball					
Elite high school	M	4.34 ± 0.94 E		7.21 ± 0.29 E	Unpublished data
NAIA	M			7.61 ± 0.36 E	Unpublished data
NCAA DIII	M			7.42 ± 0.31	Unpublished data
NCAA DI	M			7.05 ± 0.28	Unpublished data
Professional MLB AAA AA A	M	 3.75 ± 0.11 3.66 ± 0.15 3.64 ± 0.12 3.77 ± 0.18		 6.96 ± 0.16 6.86 ± 0.29 6.79 ± 0.23 7.05 ± 0.31	Coleman and Lasky 1992
Basketball					
NCAA DI G F C	M	3.79 ± 0.19 3.68 ± 0.14 3.83 ± 0.16 3.97 ± 0.21	4.81 ± 0.26 4.68 ± 0.20 4.84 ± 0.29 4.97 ± 0.21		Latin, Berg, and Baechle 1994
Bobsled					
U.S. national	M	30 m E 3.81 ± 0.12		60 m E 6.95 ± 0.28	Osbeck, Maiorca, and Rundell 1996
Field hockey					
South African college-aged players	F		40 m E 6.37 ± 0.27		Boddington, Lambert, and Waldeck 2004
Football					
NCAA DI DL LB DB QB RB WR OL TE	M		4.74 ± 0.3 4.85 ± 0.2 4.64 ± 0.2 4.52 ± 0.2 4.70 ± 0.1 4.53 ± 0.2 4.48 ± 0.1 5.12 ± 0.2 4.78 ± 0.2		Garstecki, Latin, and Cuppett 2004
NCAA DII DL LB DB QB RB WR OL TE			4.88 ± 0.3 5.03 ± 0.3 4.76 ± 0.2 4.61 ± 0.1 4.81 ± 0.1 4.69 ± 0.2 4.59 ± 0.2 5.25 ± 0.2 4.84 ± 0.1		Garstecki, Latin, and Cuppett 2004
NFL drafted rookies Rounds 1 + 2 Rounds 6 + 7	M		 4.81 ± 0.31 4.93 ± 0.34		McGee and Burkett 2003
Ice hockey					
Youth (8-16 y, $\bar{X} \pm SD$ = 12.2 ± 2.1 y)	F		7.19 ± 0.70		Bracko and George 2001

(continued)

TABLE 9.5 Descriptive Data for Sprint Tests in Athletic Populations *(continued)*

Population	Gender	SPRINT TIMES (SEC)			Source
		30 yd (27.4 m)	40 yd (36.6 m)	60 yd (54.9 m)	
Rugby					
Australian professional	M		40 m E 5.32 ± 0.26		Baker and Nance 1999
Australian/English professional Forwards Backs	M		40 m E 5.27 ± 0.19 5.08 ± 0.20		Meir et al. 2001
Soccer					
Youth (13-15 y) Defense Midfield Forward	M	30 m 4.88 ± 0.30 4.83 ± 0.28 4.94 ± 0.33 4.81 ± 0.26			Malina et al. 2004
NCAA DIII	F M		5.34 ± 0.17 4.73 ± 0.18		Unpublished data
Sprinting and hurdling					
Irish national	F	30 m E 4.58 ± 0.17			Hennessy and Kilty 2001
Tennis					
NCAA	F	20 m E 3.66 ± 0.19			Kraemer et al. 2003
Volleyball					
NCAA DI	F		5.62 ± 0.24		Fry et al. 1991

E = Electronic timing; C = centers; F = forwards; G = guards; DB = defensive backs; DL = defensive linemen; LB = linebackers; OL = offensive linemen; QB = quarterbacks; RB = running backs; TE = tight ends; WR = wide receivers.

Agility

Agility is the ability to change direction rapidly. It is a common variable measured during most athletic performance testing. Like speed, it is relatively easy to measure. Times can be assessed with handheld stopwatches or electronic timers. The only additional equipment needed are cones or tape marks and a tape measure to mark the appropriate distances.

Agility testing provides more relevant information if the selected test incorporates movements that are similar to those the athlete performs during competition and if the selected test is part of the athlete's training program. Normative data for agility performance are scarce, primarily due to a lack of consensus on which agility measure to use for a specific athlete. Numerous agility tests are available to coaches, educators, exercise scientists, and trainers. Some of the more popular tests are the T-test, Edgren side step test, hexagon agility test, 3-cone drill, and pro agility test.

📖 For descriptions of how to perform the T-test, Edgren side step test, hexagon agility test, 3-cone drill, and pro agility test, please see pages 202-204 in the appendix.

Through the cooperation of a number of coaches around the country, percentile ranks for several athletic populations have been developed. Table 9.6 provides the percentile ranks for the T-test in NCAA Division III college football players. The data for this table were collected with a handheld stopwatch. Table 9.7 provides T-test percentile ranks for elite high school (16.2 ± 0.5 y) soccer players. This data pool was comprised of Olympic development and All-American players. Percentile ranks for the pro agility test, collected using electronic timers with various NCAA Division I athletes, are shown in table 9.8. Table 9.9 provides percentile ranks for the pro agility test and the 3-cone drill in college football players who were invited to the NFL combine. Descriptive data for agility tests in athletes, found in the sport science literature or provided by various coaches around the country, can be seen in table 9.10. This table

TABLE 9.6 Percentile Ranks for the T-Test (sec) in NCAA Division III College Football Players

% rank	Team	DB	DL	LB	OL	RB	WR	QB/TE
90	8.39	8.17	8.44	8.36	9.24	8.33	8.33	8.51
80	8.57	8.39	8.77	8.78	9.50	8.62	8.49	8.62
70	8.72	8.57	8.98	8.95	9.65	8.73	8.54	8.75
60	8.90	8.68	9.48	9.00	9.69	8.89	8.64	8.85
50	9.01	8.87	9.59	9.07	9.88	8.95	8.80	9.10
40	9.15	8.94	9.69	9.16	10.03	9.05	8.89	9.20
30	9.38	9.05	9.91	9.24	10.28	9.13	9.09	9.23
20	9.60	9.12	10.05	9.35	10.49	9.23	9.26	9.33
10	10.01	9.41	10.30	9.58	10.81	9.69	9.49	9.43
$\bar{X}$	9.11	8.81	9.45	9.05	9.96	8.95	8.85	8.99
SD	0.64	0.46	0.72	0.49	0.63	0.46	0.41	0.35
n	458	63	50	57	48	37	45	31

DB = defensive backs; DL = defensive linemen; LB = linebackers;OL = offensive linemen; RB = running backs; WR = wide receivers; QB = quarterbacks; TE = tight ends.

Data collected using handheld stopwatches.

TABLE 9.7 Percentile Ranks for the T-Test (sec) in Elite High School Soccer Players

% rank	Team
90	9.90
80	10.01
70	10.08
60	10.13
50	10.18
40	10.37
30	10.53
20	10.67
10	10.90
$\bar{X}$	10.30
SD	0.42
n	40

TABLE 9.8 Percentile Ranks for the Pro Agility Test (sec) in NCAA Division I College Athletes

% rank	Women's volleyball	Women's basketball	Women's softball	Men's basketball	Men's baseball	Men's football
90	4.75	4.65	4.88	4.22	4.25	4.21
80	4.84	4.82	4.96	4.29	4.36	4.31
70	4.91	4.86	5.03	4.35	4.41	4.38
60	4.98	4.94	5.10	4.39	4.46	4.44
50	5.01	5.06	5.17	4.41	4.50	4.52
40	5.08	5.10	5.24	4.44	4.55	4.59
30	5.17	5.14	5.33	4.48	4.61	4.66
20	5.23	5.23	5.40	4.51	4.69	4.76
10	5.32	5.36	5.55	4.61	4.76	4.89
$\bar{X}$	5.03	5.02	5.19	4.41	4.53	4.54
SD	0.20	0.26	0.26	0.18	0.23	0.27
n	81	128	118	97	165	869

Data collected using electronic timing devices.

TABLE 9.9 Pro Agility and 3-Cone Drill Times for College Football Players Participating in the NFL Combine

% rank	PRO AGILITY (SEC)								3-CONE (SEC)							
	DL	LB	DB	OL	QB	RB	TE	WR	DL	LB	DB	OL	QB	RB	TE	WR
90	4.22	4.07	3.89	4.45	4.07	4.02	4.18	3.97	7.22	7.05	6.87	7.66	7.06	7.17	7.12	6.85
80	4.32	4.13	3.96	4.53	4.12	4.14	4.21	4.03	7.45	7.16	6.97	7.82	7.13	7.29	7.16	7.01
70	4.38	4.16	4.05	4.57	4.16	4.18	4.26	4.07	7.52	7.30	7.07	7.98	7.19	7.32	7.27	7.10
60	4.41	4.21	4.07	4.61	4.20	4.22	4.31	4.10	7.64	7.38	7.09	8.07	7.31	7.36	7.38	7.19
50	4.46	4.24	4.12	4.69	4.25	4.25	4.35	4.15	7.71	7.49	7.14	8.15	7.36	7.47	7.42	7.28
40	4.52	4.28	4.18	4.77	4.33	4.31	4.39	4.20	7.78	7.54	7.22	8.28	7.40	7.53	7.48	7.35
30	4.58	4.31	4.19	4.83	4.36	4.34	4.42	4.24	7.89	7.61	7.29	8.38	7.54	7.60	7.57	7.41
20	4.68	4.41	4.21	4.93	4.38	4.38	4.46	4.26	8.07	7.70	7.39	8.51	7.59	7.71	7.71	7.49
10	4.75	4.53	4.27	5.06	4.41	4.49	4.56	4.33	8.47	7.84	7.47	8.66	7.70	7.82	8.04	7.58
$\bar{X}$	4.48	4.26	4.11	4.74	4.26	4.26	4.35	4.15	7.75	7.46	7.17	8.18	7.29	7.48	7.47	7.26
SD	0.22	0.17	0.15	0.39	0.15	0.16	0.13	0.15	0.43	0.30	0.22	0.43	0.57	0.27	0.34	0.30
n	89	38	76	125	38	58	39	85	88	57	102	139	38	58	41	86

DL = defensive linemen; DB = defensive backs; LB = linebackers; OL = offensive linemen; QB = quarterbacks; RB = running backs; TE = tight ends; WR = wide receivers.

Data collected from 1999 NFL combine.

TABLE 9.10 Descriptive Data for Agility Tests in Athletic Populations

Population	Gender	AGILITY TESTS (SEC)				Source
		3-cone	T-test	Hexagon test	Pro agility	
Baseball						
NAIA	M		10.11 ± 0.64			Unpublished data
Basketball						
NCAA DI	M		8.95 ± 0.53			Latin, Berg, and Baechle 1994
G			8.74 ± 0.41			
F			8.94 ± 0.38			
C			9.28 ± 0.81			
Football						
High school	M				5.02 ± 0.24	Wroble and Moxley 2001
NCAA DI	M				4.53 ± 0.22	Sawyer et al. 2002
OL, DL					4.35 ± 0.11	
WR, DB					4.35 ± 0.12	
RB, TE, LB					4.6 ± 0.2	
NCAA DIII	M				4.6 ± 0.2	Stuempfle, Katch, and Petrie 2003
OL					4.8 ± 0.2	
DL					4.8 ± 0.2	
OB					4.5 ± 0.2	
DB					4.6 ± 0.2	
NFL drafted rookies	M					McGee and Burkett 2003
Rounds 1 + 2		7.23 ± 0.41			4.38 ± 0.29	
Rounds 6 + 7		7.46 ± 0.46			4.45 ± 0.29	

Sport	Gender	AGILITY TESTS (SEC)				Source
		3-cone	T-test	Hexagon test	Pro agility	
Recreational						
College-aged	F		12.52 ± 0.90	13.21 ± 1.68		Pauole et al. 2000
	M		10.49 ± 0.89	12.33 ± 1.47		
Soccer						
Elite youth	M					Vanderford et al. 2004
U14			11.6 ± 0.1			
U15			11.0 ± 0.2			
U16			11.7 ± 0.1			
NCAA DIII	F				4.88 ± 0.18	Unpublished data
	M				4.43 ± 0.17	
Tennis						
Elite youth (11.62 ± 0.62 y)	M			15.93 ± 2.66		Roetart et al. 1992
Volleyball						
NCAA DI	F		11.16 ± 0.38			Fry et al. 1991
NCAA DIII	F				4.75 ± 0.19	Unpublished data

C = centers; F = forwards; G = guards; DB = defensive backs; DL = defensive linemen; LB = linebackers; OB = offensive backs; OL = offensive linemen; RB = running backs; TE = tight ends; WR = wide receivers.

clearly shows the diversity of the tests used within various sports as well as the limited data available.

Summary

⊃ Various speed and agility tests are utilized by coaches.

⊃ Using handheld stopwatches presents issues of intertester reliability. All testers must have sufficient experience in administering speed and agility tests.

⊃ Electronic timers provide a high degree of reliability but yield higher performance times.

⊃ The tests selected should simulate movements common to the respective sport.

PART III

Health Norms

CHAPTER 10

Cardiovascular Profiles

The cardiovascular system specifically adapts to the stresses placed upon it. These stresses may relate to a sedentary lifestyle or to exercise training. Depending on the stress experienced, the heart either makes a positive physiological adaptation or unfortunately changes to a more pathological condition. This chapter provides normative blood pressure and resting heart values (relative to age and gender) and shows the influence of exercise on these values. In addition, it explores the morphological changes to the heart associated with exercise.

Blood Pressure

The percentile norms for resting systolic and diastolic pressures can be seen in table 10.1. Systolic blood pressure represents the strain placed against the arterial walls during ventricular contraction. Diastolic blood pressure indicates the peripheral resistance, or the ease at which blood flows into the capillaries. Since the pumping action, or contraction, of the left ventricle of the heart is pulsatile, the arterial pressure fluctuates between its highest level during systole (the heart's contraction phase) to a lower level during diastole (the heart's relaxation phase). Recognizing elevated blood pressure,

or hypertension, is critical in assessing the risk for cardiovascular disease.

HYPERTENSION

Hypertension affects approximately 50 million people in the United States and nearly 1 billion people worldwide (USDHHS 2003). The well-acknowledged relationship between blood pressure and cardiovascular disease is independent of any of the other risk factors for heart disease (USDHHS 2003). Table 10.2 provides the latest classification of blood pressure for adults as published in the *Seventh Report of the Joint National Committee on Prevention, Detection, Evaluation and Treatment of High Blood Pressure* (USDHHS 2003). In individuals 50 y or older, a systolic blood pressure >140 mmHg is a more important risk factor for cardiovascular disease than is diastolic blood pressure. The risk of cardiovascular disease doubles with every 20/10 mmHg increase in systolic and diastolic blood pressure, respectively, from an initial level of 115/75 mmHg (Lewington et al. 2002).

ASSESSMENT

Considering the importance of blood pressure, accurate assessment is critical in achieving a valid and reliable reading. Two common methods of measuring blood pressure are auscultatory and ambulatory. The auscultatory method requires a

TABLE 10.1 Percentile Norms for Resting Blood Pressure in Men and Women

	SYSTOLIC (MMHG)					DIASTOLIC (MMHG)				
%	20-29 y	30-39 y	40-49 y	50-59 y	60+ y	20-29 y	30-39 y	40-49 y	50-59 y	60+ y
Blood pressure: men										
90	110	108	110	110	112	70	70	70	72	70
80	112	110	111	116	120	72	74	76	78	76
70	118	116	118	120	124	78	78	80	80	80
60	120	120	120	122	130	80	80	80	80	80
50	121	120	121	128	131	80	80	80	82	81
40	128	124	126	130	140	80	81	84	86	84
30	130	130	130	138	140	84	85	88	90	88
20	136	132	138	140	150	88	90	90	90	90
10	140	140	142	150	160	90	92	98	100	98
n	367	1,615	1,880	1,073	275	367	1,615	1,880	1,073	275
$\bar{X}$	124	123	124	129	135	80	81	85	84	83
SD	13.4	13.6	14.5	17.2	18.3	9.6	9.6	10.0	10.4	11.0
Blood pressure: women										
90	100	100	100	108	120	63	65	65	69	70
80	101	104	105	110	120	68	70	70	70	75
70	106	110	110	118	125	70	70	70	75	76
60	110	110	112	120	128	72	74	75	79	80
50	112	114	118	122	130	75	76	80	80	80
40	118	118	120	130	136	78	80	80	82	80
30	120	120	120	134	140	80	80	80	85	84
20	120	122	130	140	142	80	82	82	90	88
10	130	130	138	148	160	82	90	90	92	98
n	118	301	282	167	46	118	301	282	167	46
$\bar{X}$	114	115	118	126	135	74	77	78	80	81
SD	12.0	13.3	15.7	16.8	16.2	7.8	9.9	10.2	10.6	8.8

From *Health and Fitness Through Physical Activity* by Michael L. Pollock, Jack H. Wilmore and Samuel M. Fox III. Copyright © 1978 by John Wiley & Sons, Inc. Adapted by permission of Pearson Education, Inc.

TABLE 10.2 Classification of Blood Pressure for Adults

Blood pressure classification	Systolic blood pressure (mmHg)	Diastolic blood pressure (mmHg)
Normal	<120	And <80
Prehypertension	120-139	Or 80-89
Stage 1 hypertension	140-159	Or 90-99
Stage 2 hypertension	≥160	≥100

From the National Institutes of Health (NIH), and the National Heart, Lung, and Blood Institute (NHLBI), 2003, *The Seventh Report of the Joint National Committee on Prevention, Detection, Evaluation, and Treatment of High Blood Pressure* (JNC 7) (Washington, DC: U.S. Government Printing Office).

properly calibrated and validated instrument. In addition,

- the individual should be seated quietly in a chair with his feet flat on the floor and his arm at heart level for at least 5 min before his blood pressure is measured,

- an appropriately sized cuff bladder should be used,
- two measurements should be performed,
- systolic blood pressure should be determined by the point at which the first of two or more sounds are heard, and

- diastolic blood pressure should be determined by the point right before those sounds disappear.

Ambulatory methods are sometimes used to measure changes in blood pressure during activity and rest throughout the day. Ambulatory measurements are generally lower than those attained via auscultatory methods, and they may more accurately assess individuals who suffer white-coat hypertension (elevated blood pressure that occurs when a physician takes the measurement). As a result of the lower measurements attained using this method, an individual with an average blood pressure >135/85 mmHg during the day and >120/75 mmHg during sleep is considered hypertensive (USDHHS 2003).

Maximal Heart Rate

The percentile norms for resting and maximal heart rates are shown in table 10.3. The equation widely used in both fitness and clinical settings for computing maximal heart rate is 220 – age. The error in this equation is $\pm$ 10 to 12 beats/min (ACSM 1995), and table 10.3 clearly shows a wide range in maximal heart rates for a given age group. However, individuals older than 50 y may have maximal heart rates 20 beats/min greater than those predicted by the formula, and heavier, deconditioned individuals may have maximal heart rates that are 20 beats/min lower than the predicted levels (Whaley et al. 1992). This variability has important implications for exercise

TABLE 10.3 Resting and Maximal Heart Rates in Men and Women

	MEN					WOMEN				
%	20-29 y	30-39 y	40-49 y	50-59 y	60+ y	20-29 y	30-39 y	40-49 y	50-59 y	60+ y
Resting heart rates (beats/min)										
90	50	50	50	50	52	55	55	55	55	52
80	54	55	54	55	55	59	58	60	60	57
70	58	58	58	58	58	60	62	62	61	60
60	60	60	60	60	60	63	65	64	64	62
50	63	63	62	63	62	65	68	66	67	64
40	66	65	65	65	65	70	70	70	69	66
30	70	68	69	68	68	72	74	72	72	72
20	72	72	72	72	72	75	76	76	75	74
10	80	77	78	77	77	84	82	80	83	79
n	358	1,538	1,826	1,046	267	115	280	260	162	43
$\bar{X}$	64	63	64	63	63	67	68	68	68	65
SD	12.5	11.0	11.5	11.0	10.4	11.2	11.5	10.7	11.7	9.6
Maximal heart rates (beats/min)										
90	205	200	196	188	184	203	196	192	185	176
80	200	198	191	183	175	198	192	186	180	165
70	199	194	188	180	170	194	189	183	176	160
60	197	191	185	176	165	190	185	180	173	155
50	194	189	182	173	162	188	184	177	170	153
40	192	186	180	170	159	186	182	173	167	150
30	188	183	176	166	152	182	180	170	162	145
20	183	180	171	160	145	180	176	166	160	140
10	179	174	164	150	131	172	170	158	152	126
n	371	1,632	1,898	1,087	249	119	309	286	169	46
$\bar{X}$	192	188	181	171	159	188	183	175	169	151
SD	12.2	11.7	13.3	15.9	19.5	11.8	14.8	14.8	14.5	17.5

Data from the US Department of Health and Human Services.

testing considering that maximal heart rate may be overestimated in deconditioned individuals and underestimated in older individuals.

Training Effects

The effects of training on resting heart rate and blood pressure are shown in table 10.4, which includes compilations of several studies examining a variety of training regimens. In both endurance and strength and power athletes, resting heart rates tend to decrease following prolonged exercise training as a result of changes in the balance of sympathetic and parasympathetic activities (Hoffman 2002). Blood pressure that is initially elevated tends to decrease with training, but blood pressure levels in the normotensive range tend to remain steady following training (Hoffman 2002).

MORPHOLOGICAL CHANGES TO THE HEART

Long-term exercise training is associated with morphological changes to the heart, including an increased internal diameter of the left ventricle, an increased wall thickness, and a greater mass. Collectively these changes are referred to as *athlete's heart* (Pelliccia et al. 1999; Spirito et al. 1994), and

they are specific to the type of training. Concerning the volume and pressure stresses placed on the heart during exercise, endurance training and resistance training are at either ends of the spectrum. During *pressure overload,* common in resistance exercise programs, the septum and posterior wall of the left ventricle increase in size to normalize myocardial wall stress. However, the internal diameter of the left ventricle does not change. This adaptation is known as *concentric hypertrophy.* During prolonged endurance training the morphological changes of the heart are consistent with greater end-diastolic volumes, resulting in *volume overload.* Changes predominantly occur in the internal diameter of the left ventricle (increasing the size of the cavity), with both the septum and posterior wall of the ventricle proportionally increasing. This adaptation is termed *eccentric hypertrophy* (Morganroth et al. 1975; Pelliccia et al. 1991; Spirito et al. 1994).

CARDIAC DIMENSIONS IN ATHLETES

Most sports have a parallel effect on cavity dimension and wall thickness (Spirito et al. 1994). In these sports, the athletes perform some combination of aerobic and anaerobic training, which results in both an enlarged diastolic cavity dimension and a greater wall thickness. In sports that emphasize a single form of training the morphological changes of

Athletes by Sport	n	Age (y)	Body mass (kg)	SBP (mmHg)	DBP (mmHg)	RHR (beats/min)	Source
Bodybuilders	15	23.5 ± 7.6	84.7 ± 3.8	127 ± 11.8	79 ± 5.2	71 ± 11.7	Deligiannis, Zahopoulou, and Mandroukas 1988
Cyclists	13	17 ± 4.4	57 ± 8.7	123 ± 3.7	74 ± 5.5	63 ± 5.7	Lusiani et al. 1986
Cyclists	21	42 ± 8	77 ± 8	122 ± 13	71 ± 9	52 ± 6	Pluim et al. 1998
Cyclists and triathletes	30	26.1 ± 4.7	71.9 ± 6.3	119 ± 11.9	76 ± 8.0	51 ± 8.7	Schmidt-Trucksass et al. 2001
Runners	29	25 ± 6	77 ± 6	123 ± 9	80 ± 5	48 ± 6	Fisman et al. 1997
Runners	12	28.5 ± 1.6	67.7 ± 2.1	120 ± 2.5	78 ± 2.7	53 ± 2.9	Longhurst et al. 1980
Sprinters	6	19.3 ± 3.7	69 ± 8.0	124 ± 5.3	72 ± 4.8	59.3 ± 2.2	Lusiani et al. 1986
Weightlifters	15	22.6 ± 8.4	81.0 ± 3.2	130 ± 10.7	80 ± 6.1	71 ± 12	Deligiannis, Zahopoulou, and Mandroukas 1988
Weightlifters	16	23 ± 4	80 ± 7	122 ± 10	82 ± 7	52 ± 6	Fisman et al. 1997
Weightlifters	6	21.8 ± 3.9	72 ± 7.2	130 ± 5.7	75 ± 2.8	71 ± 4.2	Lusiani et al. 1986
Weightlifters (amateur)	7	28.1 ± 2.7	82.6 ± 4.7	122 ± 3.6	78 ± 2.0	63 ± 2.7	Longhurst et al. 1980
Weightlifters (competitive)	17	26.9 ± 1.2	89.8 ± 3.4	126 ± 3.3	82 ± 2.7	71 ± 2.5	Longhurst et al. 1980

SBP = systolic blood pressure; DBP = diastolic blood pressure; RHR = resting heart rate.

the heart may be more extreme. Table 10.5 provides the cardiac dimensions of athletes from various sports, using data from a number of studies.

Numerous variables relating to left ventricle function are reported in table 10.5. The data are separated into three categories representing endurance athletes, team athletes, and strength and power athletes. In addition, a range in the same type of athlete is reported for comparison purposes. The variables reported by each investigation varied and so some information on specific variables is not provided. In addition, some of the

TABLE 10.5 Cardiovascular Dimensions

Athletes by Sport	GENDER NUMBER		LEFT VENTRICLE									
	M	F	ID (ml)	EDV (ml)	ESV (ml)	Mass (g)	Mass index (g/m²)	LV wall (mm)	IVS (mm)	SV (ml)	LA (mm)	Source
Endurance athletes												
Canoeists	52	8	54.5 ± 3.4				110 ± 21	10.5 ± 1.6				Pelliccia, et al. 1991
Cross-country skiers	24	7	54.6 ± 4.1				107 ± 19	9.6 ± 0.9				Pelliccia, et al. 1991
Cyclists	13		51 ± 2.9					10.9 ± 1.4	8.0 ± 0.9	100 ± 12		Lusiani et al. 1986
Cyclists	21			222 ± 32		200 ± 23	102 ± 10			109 ± 11		Pluim et al. 1998
Cyclists	37	13	55.0 ± 5.3				115 ± 23	10.5 ± 1.2				Spirito et al. 1994
Cyclists and triathletes	18		58.8 ± 3.3				159.4 ± 18	10.5 ± 0.8	11.3 ± 0.7		39.4 ± 4.5	Schmidt-Trucksass et al. 2001
Orienteers		42	48.5 ± 2.6					9.2 ± 0.3	10.0 ± 0.4		35.1 ± 2.8	Henriksen et al. 1999
Rowers	92	3	56 ± 3.8				121 ± 22	11.3 ± 1.3				Pelliccia, et al. 1991
Runners	29			116 ± 11	42 ± 5	214 ± 18		10.8 ± 0.5	10.3 ± 0.4	74 ± 8		Fisman, et al. 1997
Runners	41	8	53.3 ± 3.6					10.3 ± 1.1				Spirito et al. 1994
Runners (collegiate)	15			160 ± 8.6		302 ± 9.0		11.3 ± 0.1	10.9 ± 0.2	117 ± 13		Morganroth et al. 1975
Runners (collegiate)	10		55.8 ± 3.3			312 ± 59		11.4 ± 1.6	10.5 ± 1.8			Cohen and Segal, 1985
Runners (world class)	10			155 ± 8.3		283 ± 10.6		10.8 ± 0.2	10.9 ± 0.2	113 ± 11.2		Morganroth et al. 1975
Swimmers	11		54 ± 5				136 ± 35					Colan et al. 1985
Swimmers	26	28	53 ± 4.8				98 ± 23	9.4 ± 1.3				Pelliccia, et al. 1991
Team sport athletes												
Soccer players	13		50.3 ± 3.0					11.0 ± 1.6	8.4 ± 0.5	94.4 ± 14		Lusiani et al. 1986
Soccer players	62		55 ± 4.3				105 ± 17	10 ± 0.8				Pelliccia, et al. 1991
Team handball players	9	17	51.9 ± 4.5				80 ± 13	8.5 ± 0.9				Pelliccia, et al. 1991

(continued)

TABLE 10.5 Cardiovascular Dimensions (*continued*)

Sport	GENDER NUMBER M	F	LEFT VENTRICLE ID (ml)	EDV (ml)	ESV (ml)	Mass (g)	Mass index (g/m²)	LV wall (mm)	IVS (mm)	SV (ml)	LA (mm)	Source
Team sport athletes												
Volleyball players	36	15	53.7 ± 3.7				88 ± 14	9.4 ± 1.0				Pelliccia, et al. 1991
Water polo players	21		54.7 ± 3.4				110 ± 15	10.7 ± 0.6				Pelliccia, et al. 1991
Strength and power athletes												
Alpine skiers	24	8	52.1 ± 3.6				87 ± 15	9.0 ± 0.7				Pelliccia, et al.1991
Bobsledders	21		55 ± 2.4			197 ± 21	94 ± 9.7	9.4 ± 0.5	9.8 ± 0.7		37 ± 2.9	Pelliccia et al. 1993
Bobsledders	16		55.1 ± 2.1				96 ± 7	9.7 ± 0.5				Pelliccia, et al. 1991
Bodybuilders	17	1	57 ± 3.8			204 ± 30	102 ± 12.1	9.2 ± 0.8	9.6 ± 0.6		38 ± 3.5	Pelliccia et al. 1993
Bodybuilders	15		53.3 ± 3.4	138 ± 20	41 ± 13.4	270 ± 52	134 ± 19.6	10.2 ± 1.2	10.8 ± 1.2	97 ± 18	36.8 ± 3.8	Deligiannis et al. 1988
Boxers	14		52.5 ± 4.0				101 ± 16	9.8 ± 1.1				Spirito et al. 1994
Cyclists (sprinting)	13	2	54.3 ± 4.5					10.1 ± 0.9				Spirito et al. 1994
Powerlifters	9	1	55 ± 4.7			170 ± 26.3	90 ± 11.7	9.0 ± 0.6	9.8 ± 0.8		36 ± 4.1	Pelliccia et al. 1993
Powerlifters	11		54 ± 7				165 ± 42					Colan et al. 1985
Sprinters	6		49.9 ± 2.6					11.2 ± 1.5	8.5 ± 0.8	88 ± 10		Lusiani et al. 1986
Sprinters	25	15	49.3 ± 4.1					9.1 ± 1.0				Spirito et al. 1994
Taekwondo practitioners	14	3	50.6 ± 4.0				85 ± 17	8.7 ± 1.3				Pelliccia, Maron, et al. 1991
Track throwers	15		57 ± 3.2			211 ± 33	93 ± 8.2	9.6 ± 0.4	10 ± 0.5		37 ± 3.1	Pelliccia et al. 1993
Weightlifters	13		51.5 ± 1.2					9.7 ± 0.4	13.9 ± 0.6			Menapace et al. 1982
Weightlifters	15		52 ± 4.2			177 ± 38	92 ± 12.5	9.2 ± 0.7	9.6 ± 0.9		33 ± 4.3	Pelliccia et al. 1993
Weightlifters	6		44.5 ± 1.9					10.9 ± 1.2	8.7 ± 0.7	74 ± 8.2		Lusiani et al. 1986
Weightlifters	16		56 ± 6.0	181 ± 50		241 ± 70	114 ± 29	9.0 ± 2.0	10.0 ± 2.0	122 ± 30		Pearson et al. 1986
Weightlifters	15		50.3 ± 5.2	122 ± 29	38 ± 13.4	265 ± 57	136 ± 21.1	10.9 ± 1.5	11.2 ± 1.4	84 ± 23	33.9 ± 3.2	Deligiannis et al. 1988
Weightlifters	16			96 ± 7	33 ± 6	220 ± 26		11.0 ± 0.5	10.5 ± 0.4	63 ± 5		Fisman, et al. 1997
Weightlifters	7		53.3 ± 4.0				100 ± 9	10.5 ± 0.7				Pelliccia, et al. 1991
Wrestlers	21		55 ± 4.7			192 ± 48	101 ± 14				36 ± 3.3	Pelliccia, et al. 1993
Wrestlers (collegiate)	10		48.8 ± 2.9			326 ± 46		12.9 ± 1.0	13.5 ± 1.2			Cohen and Segal, 1985

ID = internal diameter; EDV = end-diastolic volume; ESV = end-systolic volume; LV = left ventricle; IVS = intraventricular septum; SV = stroke volume; LA = left atrium dimension.

differences in left ventricular dimension and function seen within an athletic group may relate to methodological differences in the studies, especially in the earlier studies reported. For instance, some investigators measured wall thickness from the outer borders of the septal image while others used the Penn convention. However, most of the studies in table 10.5 used the common two-dimensional and M-mode echocardiogram according to recommendations from the American Society of Echocardiography. Table 10.6 provides cardiac dimensions in male and female athletes from 25 different sports, with soccer, rowing, cycling, and track being the most common. Large gender differences are seen in all variables.

Table 10.7 depicts the influence of the sport impact factor (the difference between the average left ventricular cavity dimension of a sport and the average left ventricular cavity dimension in the reference sport of table tennis), body surface area, and gender on left ventricular dimensions. In their study, Pelliccia and colleagues (1999) reported that 45% of the 1,300 athletes examined had left ventricular cavity dimensions that exceeded the normal limits (≤54 mm) (Henry, Gardin, and Ware 1980; Devereux et al. 1984) and that 14% were categorized as having left ventricles that were substantially enlarged (≥60 mm).

In athletes, left ventricular hypertrophy (LVH) is generally regarded as a physiological adaptation to training (Douglas et al. 1997). Yet, in the normal population LVH is considered a pathological adaptation associated with an increased risk for sudden cardiac death. Table 10.8 compares left ventricular function in untrained controls, athletes, and hypertensive patients with LVH. The data, adapted from Schannwell and colleagues (2002), show that despite possessing similar LVH levels, the athletic and hypertensive populations show differences in left ventricular function that clearly

TABLE 10.6 Cardiac Dimensions in Male and Female Elite Athletes

Cardiac measurement	Males (n = 738)	Range	Females (n = 209)	Range
LVEDD (mm)	54.2 ± 4	44-66	48.4 ± 3.7	40-61
Ventricle septal thickness (mm)	10.1 ± 1.2	7-16	8.4 ± 0.9	6-11
Posterior wall thickness (mm)	9.4 ± 0.9	7-13	7.9 ± 0.8	6-10
LV mass (g)	206 ± 46	108-359	133 ± 29	84-239
LV mass index (g/m^2)	105 ± 20	62-176	80 ± 16	52-138
Left atrial dimension (mm)	36.9 ± 3	27-45	33.5 ± 3	24-38

LVEDD = left ventricular end-diastolic dimension; LV = left ventricle.

TABLE 10.7 Left Ventricular Dimension in Male and Female Athletes Stratified by Sport and Body Surface Area

Effect of sport on LV cavity size	Gender	n	BSA (m^2)	LVD (mm)
High effect	M	52	≤1.80	54.6 ± 3.5
		179	1.81-2.00	56.3 ± 3.6
		86	>2.00	59.0 ± 3.2
	F	7	≤1.50	48.0 ± 3.6
		43	1.51-1.70	49.9 ± 3.4
		16	>1.70	54.8 ± 3.0
Medium effect	M	71	≤1.80	50.9 ± 2.7
		135	1.81-2.00	54.5 ± 3.3
		177	>2.00	58.5 ± 4.2
	F	63	≤1.50	44.0 ± 2.5
		76	1.51-1.70	48.6 ± 2.6
		62	>1.70	52.1 ± 4.1

(continued)

TABLE 10.7   Left Ventricular Dimension in Male and Female Athletes Stratified by Sport and Body Surface Area *(continued)*

Effect of sport on LV cavity size	Gender	n	BSA (m²)	LVD (mm)
Low effect	M	24	≤1.80	51.2 ± 3.0
		74	1.81-2.00	52.6 ± 2.8
		60	>2.00	55.9 ± 3.5
	F	4	≤1.50	45.3 ± 2.8
		27	1.51-1.70	48.1 ± 2.2
		33	>1.70	49.8 ± 3.2

Adapted, by permission, from A. Pellicia et al., 1999, "Physiologic left ventricular cavity dilatation in elite athletes," *Ann Intern Med.* 130: 23-31.

TABLE 10.8   Left Ventricular Function in Physiological and Pathological Hypertrophy

Cardiac measurement	Untrained controls (n = 26)	Endurance athletes (n = 49)	Hypertensive patients (n = 49)
Age (y)	27 ± 4	26 ± 6	28 ± 9
BSA (kg/cm²)	2.29 ± 0.3	2.28 ± 0.4	2.28 ± 0.5
RHR (beats/min)	63 ± 6	56 ± 6	66 ± 4
SBP (mmHg)	135 ± 6	127 ± 8	135 ± 7
DBP (mmHg)	79 ± 8	78 ± 6	82 ± 7
LA (mm)	35 ± 3	33 ± 5	35 ± 6
LVEDD (mm)	48 ± 3	50 ± 4	47 ± 5
FS (%)	43 ± 6	44 ± 5	42 ± 5
IVS (mm)	9 ± 2*	15 ± 3	15 ± 2
LVW (mm)	8 ± 1*	14 ± 2	14 ± 3
LVM (g)	119 ± 12*	225 ± 18	216 ± 16
LVM index (g/m²)	52 ± 7*	99 ± 10	95 ± 11
VE (m/s)	0.67 ± 0.1	0.65 ± 0.08	0.44 ± 0.09#
VA (m/s)	0.52 ± 0.2	0.51 ± 0.09	0.54 ± 0.1
VE/VA	1.28 ± 0.09	1.27 ± 0.11	0.83 ± 0.08#
AT (m · s)	67 ± 6	69 ± 4	66 ± 7
DT (m · s)	177 ± 14	182 ± 14	237 ± 15#
IVRT (m · s)	83 ± 7	76 ± 7	129 ± 9#

* = significantly ($p < .05$) different than athletes and hypertensive patients; # = significantly ($p < .05$) different than controls and athletes; BSA = body surface area; RHR = resting heart rate; SBP = systolic blood pressure; DBP = diastolic blood pressure; LA = left atrium diameter; LVEDD = left ventricular end-diastolic dimension; FS = fractional shortening; IVS = intraventricular septum; LVW = left ventricular posterior wall; LVM = left ventricular mass; VE = peak mitral flow velocity in early diastole; VA = peak mitral flow velocity in late diastole; VE/VA = ratio of peak mitral flow velocity to early and late diastole; AT = acceleration time; DT = deceleration time; IVRT = isovolumetric relaxation time.

Adapted from *American Journal of Hypertension*, Vol. 15, C.M. Schannwell, M. Schneppenheim, G. Plehn, R. Marx and B.E. Strauer, "Left ventricular diastolic function in physiologic and pathologic hypertrophy," pages 513-517, Copyright 2002, with permission from American Journal of Hypertension, Ltd.

demonstrate that in athletes LVH is a normal physiological adaptation to training and not a pathological condition.

Summary

⊃ Accurately measuring blood pressure is critical for assessing the risk for cardiovascular disease.

⊃ The cardiovascular system specifically adapts to the stresses placed on it.

⊃ In an athletic population left ventricular hypertrophy is considered a normal physiological adaptation to training, while in the sedentary population it likely represents a pathological condition.

CHAPTER 11

Lipid Profiles

For the past 40 years epidemiological researchers have attempted to identify risk factors that can be used to predict coronary heart disease (CHD). Numerous risk factors have been associated with an elevated risk for disease. The presence of multiple risk factors magnifies this risk. Hyperlipidemia, cigarette smoking, hypertension, obesity, diabetes, a sedentary lifestyle, and a family history of heart disease are all well-accepted factors associated with a high risk for heart disease. This chapter focuses on blood lipid profiles in healthy and clinical populations and examines the influence of age and fitness on those profiles.

Blood Lipids

Lipids are fats, a class of organic compounds with limited water solubility. In the body they exist in several forms such as triglycerides, fatty acids, phospholipids, and sterols. Most of the stored fat in the body is stored as triglycerides. Triglycerides are the highest concentrated source of energy that we have, and it is comprised of three fatty acids and a glycerol molecule. Triglycerides are a simple, or neutral, fat. These neutral fats can combine with another substance to create compound fats such as phospholipids and lipoproteins. Cholesterol is a derived fat that is produced endogenously in the body but may also be consumed in large quantities. Cholesterol is essential for normal biological function through its presence in cell membranes and its role in the synthesis of bile acids and steroid hormones.

When lipids are combined with another substance, the created compound may be water soluble. For instance, lipids combined with proteins become a lipoprotein that allows fat to be transported in the blood. There are five types of lipoproteins that circulate in the blood: chylomicrons, very low-density lipoproteins (VLDL), intermediate-density lipoproteins, low-density lipoproteins (LDL), and high-density lipoproteins (HDL). Only LDL and HDL are of major concern for CHD.

LDL consists of an apoprotein called apoB, a small quantity of triglycerides, and a large amount of cholesterol. LDL transports 60% to 70% of the total cholesterol in the body to all cells except those in the liver. LDL is the major atherogenic lipoprotein, and high levels of both cholesterol and LDL place an individual at high risk for CHD. As a result, LDL is the primary target of cholesterol-lowering therapies.

The major proteins of HDL are apoA-I and apoA-II. HDL also consists of small amounts of triglycerides and cholesterol. HDL transports 20% to 30% of the total cholesterol in the body to the liver. Since HDL transports cholesterol to the liver for removal, it has an inverse relationship with CHD. HDL protects against the atherogenic effects of cholesterol by reducing its concentration in the blood. Low levels of HDL are also a risk factor for CHD.

VLDL is a triglyceride-rich lipoprotein that contains about 10% to 15% of the total cholesterol in the body. The major lipoproteins of VLDL are apoB-100, apoCs, and apoE. VLDL is a precursor of LDL and has similar atherogenic properties. Intermediate lipoproteins have some remnant lipoproteins but are often included in the LDL fraction during clinical study. Chylomicrons are similar to VLDL except that they include apoB-48 instead of apoB-100. Chylomicrons generally appear in the blood following a meal high in fat, and they have some atherogenic potential.

For years multivariate analyses failed to identify the direct association of elevated triglycerides with heart disease. An indirect association is obvious considering the composition of lipoproteins. However, triglycerides were recently accepted as an independent risk factor for CHD (NCEP 2002) due to research identifying triglyceride-rich lipoprotein remnants as highly atherogenic. These lipoprotein remnants include VLDL and intermediate-density lipoproteins. They share many of the properties of LDL but are independent predictors of CHD (Austin, Hokanson, and Edwards 1998; Krauss 1998; Steiner et al. 1987). As a result, elevated serum triglyceride concentrations indicate a higher risk for atherosclerosis.

Lipid Norms

Table 11.1 classifies total cholesterol, LDL cholesterol, HDL cholesterol, and triglyceride concentrations in the blood of adult populations. It summarizes the *Third Report* of the National Cholesterol Education Program (2002). Individuals should strive for low concentrations of total cholesterol, LDL cholesterol, and triglycerides and for a high concentration of HDL cholesterol.

Using clinical measurements of lipid concentrations to predict CHD has been well accepted by the medical community. However, several studies

TABLE 11.1 Blood Lipid Concentrations in the Blood

Lipid and category	Adult concentrations (mg/dl)
Total cholesterol	
Desirable	<200
Borderline	200-239
High	>240
LDL cholesterol	
Optimal	<100
Near optimal	100-129
Borderline high	130-159
High	160-189
Very high	≥190
HDL cholesterol	
Low	<40
High	≥60
Triglycerides	
Normal	<150
Borderline high	150-199
High	200-499
Very high	≥500

To convert mg/dl to SI units (mmol · L⁻¹), multiply by 0.02586.

From the National Institutes of Health (NIH), and the National Heart, Lung, and Blood Institute (NHLBI), 2002, *Third Report of the Expert Panel on Detection, Evaluation, and Treatment of High Blood Cholesterol in Adults (Adult Treatment Panel III)* (Washington, DC: U.S. Government Printing Office).

have indicated that the ratio of total cholesterol to HDL (TC/HDL) may be superior to total or LDL cholesterol in predicting CHD (Kinosian, Glick, and Garland 1994; Linn et al. 1991). Table 11.2 shows the TC/HDL and the associated likelihood for CHD in men and women. Table 11.3 shows HDL and CHD relative risk and table 11.4 shows HDL ratios and CHD relative risk in men and women. Data are from individuals enrolled in the Framingham heart study. The likelihood ratio (reported by Kinosian, Glick, and Garland 1994) in table 11.2 was calculated as

number of individuals with CHD in each ratio level /
total number with CHD,

number without CHD in each ratio level /
total number without CHD.

From table 11.3 it is apparent that HDL concentrations ≤40 mg/dl are a major risk factor for CHD. Average levels of HDL are 40 to 50 mg/dl in men and 50 to 60 mg/dl in women. As a general rule,

TABLE 11.2 TC/HDL and Likelihood for CHD in Men and Women

TC/HDL	% population	Risk for CHD (%)	Likelihood ratio
Men			
<3	5.6	5.3	0.32
≥3-5	46.7	12.9	0.86
≥5-7	33.9	17.6	1.24
≥7-9	11.8	14.9	1.01
≥9	2.0	35.0	3.12
Women			
<3	12.4	5.6	0.59
≥3-5	58.9	7.8	0.84
≥5-7	22.8	11.9	1.33
≥7-9	4.1	18.9	2.32
≥9	1.8	23.1	2.98

CHD = coronary heart disease.

Adapted, by permission, from B. Kinosian, et al., 1994, "Cholesterol and coronary heart disease: Predicting risks by levels and ratios," *Ann Intern Med.* 121:641-647.

TABLE 11.3 HDL and CHD Risk: Framingham Heart Study

HDL (mg/dl)	RELATIVE RISK Men	Women
25	2.00	—
30	1.80	—
35	1.50	—
40	1.22	1.94
45	1.00	1.55
50	0.82	1.25
55	0.67	1.00
60	0.55	0.80
65	0.45	0.64
70	—	0.52
75	Protection threshold against CHD	

Reprinted, by permission, from R.K. Dishman, R.A. Washburn and G.W. Heath, 2004, *Physical activity epidemiology* (Champaign, IL: Human Kinetics), 146.

TABLE 11.4 HDL Ratios and CHD Risk: Framingham Heart Study

Relative Risk	TC/HDL	LDL/HDL
Men		
0.50	3.43	1.00
1.00	4.97	3.55
2.00	9.55	6.35
3.00	24.00	8.00
Women		
0.50	3.27	1.47
1.00	4.44	3.22
2.00	7.05	5.00
3.00	11.04	6.14

Adapted, by permission, from R.K. Dishman, R.A. Washburn and G.W. Heath, 2004, *Physical activity epidemiology* (Champaign, IL: Human Kinetics), 146.

every 1% change in HDL concentration is associated with a 3% change in CHD risk (Dishman, Washburn, and Heath 2004).

The distribution of serum total cholesterol, LDL cholesterol, HDL cholesterol, and triglycerides in the United States adult population can be seen in tables 11.5 to 11.8. The values included in these tables are from the NHANES III data collected between 1988 and 1994 and reported in the *Third Report* of the National Cholesterol Education

Program on *Detection, Evaluation and Treatment of High Blood Cholesterol* (2002). Tables 11.5 to 11.8 provide selected percentiles examining age, gender, and ethnicity.

Numerous interventions can be used to lower undesirable lipid levels. Often changes in dietary habits, exercise patterns, and pharmaceutical prescriptions are recommended. Most of these interventions, if adhered to, positively change the lipid profile. Figure 11.1 on page 132 compares total cholesterol levels across body fatness and fitness categories. Subjects were 21,925 men ages 30

TABLE 11.5 Serum Total Cholesterol (mg/dl) of Individuals 20 y and Older

Gender/ age/ethnicity	$\bar{X}$	SELECTED PERCENTILE								
		5th	10th	15th	25th	50th	75th	85th	90th	95th
Men										
All	202	139	151	160	173	200	228	244	255	273
20-34	186	131	142	148	161	183	209	223	233	253
35-44	206	143	154	163	180	205	232	247	257	267
45-54	216	154	167	178	191	214	242	255	266	283
55-64	216	154	167	174	189	214	243	258	270	282
65-74	212	149	163	175	186	209	237	248	263	284
>75	205	145	155	164	176	203	230	246	255	273
Women										
All	206	143	153	161	175	201	233	251	265	284
20-34	184	132	141	148	158	181	205	219	231	248
35-44	195	144	153	160	171	192	215	234	243	257
45-54	217	157	166	174	187	212	243	259	274	298
55-64	235	167	184	191	204	229	261	276	286	307
65-74	233	170	181	189	204	232	258	276	289	308
>75	229	161	174	185	198	228	258	274	286	305
Mexican American										
Men	199	137	150	157	171	197	224	241	253	272
Women	198	139	148	156	167	193	223	238	249	274
Non-Hispanic Black										
Men	198	136	147	155	169	195	222	239	251	275
Women	201	136	148	157	170	196	226	246	261	284
Non-Hispanic White										
Men	203	141	153	162	174	201	229	244	256	272
Women	208	144	155	163	177	203	235	252	267	284

From the National Institutes of Health (NIH), and the National Heart, Lung, and Blood Institute (NHLBI), 2002, *Third Report of the Expert Panel on Detection, Evaluation, and Treatment of High Blood Cholesterol in Adults (Adult Treatment Panel III)* (Washington, DC: U.S. Government Printing Office).

TABLE 11.6 Serum LDL Cholesterol (mg/dl) of Individuals 20 y and Older

Gender/ age/ethnicity	$\bar{X}$	SELECTED PERCENTILE								
		5th	10th	15th	25th	50th	75th	85th	90th	95th
Men										
All	130	76	87	93	105	128	153	166	177	194
20-34	119	72	81	87	97	119	139	151	156	170
35-44	135	82	91	96	111	132	156	171	186	205
45-54	140	76	95	106	117	140	164	178	188	195
55-64	138	82	90	99	115	135	162	174	182	200
65-74	136	83	92	103	113	133	158	171	182	196
>75	132	86	92	97	109	128	151	167	177	194
Women										
All	125	69	81	89	98	121	147	162	172	190
20-34	111	63	71	79	90	109	130	142	152	170
35-44	118	70	83	90	96	115	137	147	159	171

Gender/age/ethnicity	$\bar{X}$	5th	10th	15th	25th	50th	75th	85th	90th	95th
SELECTED PERCENTILE										
Women										
45-54	131	70	85	93	106	129	153	166	177	190
55-64	144	80	93	107	121	143	167	184	192	209
65-74	143	76	95	106	119	144	166	182	188	203
>75	145	83	102	106	119	144	167	186	196	209
Mexican American										
Men	124	71	78	85	98	121	144	160	171	188
Women	117	67	75	83	93	115	137	152	161	178
Non-Hispanic Black										
Men	127	71	79	86	100	124	149	165	179	200
Women	122	63	77	84	97	119	145	161	172	193
Non-Hispanic White										
Men	131	79	88	95	106	129	154	167	177	194
Women	126	70	81	89	98	122	149	164	173	189

From the National Institutes of Health (NIH), and the National Heart, Lung, and Blood Institute (NHLBI), 2002, *Third Report of the Expert Panel on Detection, Evaluation, and Treatment of High Blood Cholesterol in Adults (Adult Treatment Panel III)* (Washington, DC: U.S. Government Printing Office).

TABLE 11.7 Serum HDL Cholesterol (mg/dl) of Individuals 20 y and Older

Gender/age/ethnicity	$\bar{X}$	5th	10th	15th	25th	50th	75th	85th	90th	95th
SELECTED PERCENTILE										
Men										
All	46	28	30	34	37	44	53	58	62	72
20-34	46	28	32	34	38	45	53	59	62	69
35-44	45	28	30	32	36	43	52	57	61	73
45-54	45	26	30	32	35	42	52	58	66	75
55-64	45	28	31	34	36	42	51	57	61	71
65-74	46	28	30	32	36	43	54	58	64	73
>75	47	28	31	34	37	44	54	61	66	75
Women										
All	55	34	38	41	44	53	64	70	75	83
20-34	55	34	38	41	45	53	64	69	74	83
35-44	54	34	38	41	44	53	64	68	72	79
45-54	56	36	38	41	45	55	65	72	77	84
55-64	56	33	37	40	44	53	65	73	78	89
65-74	56	33	37	40	45	54	65	71	76	84
>75	56	32	37	40	44	55	65	71	76	86
Mexican American										
Men	46	28	32	34	37	44	52	58	61	67
Women	52	33	36	38	42	51	60	66	71	77
Non-Hispanic Black										
Men	52	32	34	37	41	50	60	68	74	85
Women	57	35	39	42	46	55	66	73	79	86
Non-Hispanic White										
Men	45	27	30	33	36	43	52	57	61	71
Women	56	34	38	41	45	54	64	70	76	84

From the National Institutes of Health (NIH), and the National Heart, Lung, and Blood Institute (NHLBI), 2002, *Third Report of the Expert Panel on Detection, Evaluation, and Treatment of High Blood Cholesterol in Adults (Adult Treatment Panel III)* (Washington, DC: U.S. Government Printing Office).

TABLE 11.8 Serum Triglycerides (mg/dl) of Individuals 20 y and Older

Gender/ age/ethnicity	$\bar{X}$	SELECTED PERCENTILE								
		5th	10th	15th	25th	50th	75th	85th	90th	95th
Men										
All	148	53	62	69	83	118	173	218	253	318
20-34	118	46	55	60	70	94	139	171	204	256
35-44	150	53	62	70	82	126	180	213	242	307
45-54	182	62	72	82	100	135	201	269	296	366
55-64	176	64	80	87	101	144	228	276	311	396
65-74	160	64	76	83	99	137	190	226	256	319
>75	144	64	71	82	96	125	175	200	220	304
Women										
All	128	48	56	61	72	102	152	193	226	273
20-34	101	43	49	55	61	84	117	147	177	226
35-44	123	43	53	57	67	93	132	170	215	288
45-54	136	49	59	66	76	114	163	201	239	277
55-64	166	62	72	82	96	135	203	251	313	396
65-74	157	70	76	85	99	134	182	228	253	283
>75	150	64	74	79	94	130	178	211	235	274
Mexican American										
Men	152	53	60	69	83	120	184	225	259	361
Women	140	55	63	72	85	118	170	210	237	293
Non-Hispanic Black										
Men	114	45	51	56	64	89	135	164	192	245
Women	96	41	46	51	58	79	113	142	162	207
Non-Hispanic White										
Men	152	55	64	71	85	123	181	223	258	319
Women	130	49	56	63	75	104	156	196	229	274

From the National Institutes of Health (NIH), and the National Heart, Lung, and Blood Institute (NHLBI), 2002, *Third Report of the Expert Panel on Detection, Evaluation, and Treatment of High Blood Cholesterol in Adults (Adult Treatment Panel III)* (Washington, DC: U.S. Government Printing Office).

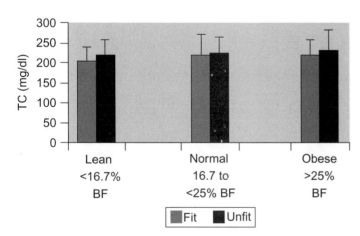

FIGURE 11.1 Total cholesterol levels across body fatness and fitness categories. Data are presented as mean ± standard deviation. BF = Body fat %; TC = total cholesterol.

From C.D. Lee, S.N. Blair and A.S. Jackson, 1999, "Cardiorespiratory fitness, body composition, and all-cause and cardiovascular disease mortality in men," *American Journal of Clinical Nutrition* 69:373-380. Adapted with permission by the *American Journal of Clinical Nutrition*. © Am J Clin Nutr. American Society for Clinical Nutrition.

to 83 ($\bar{X} \pm SD$, 43.8 ± 8.9 y) tested at the Cooper Clinic in Dallas, Texas. Lean, normal, and obese categories of body fatness corresponded to < 25th, 25th to 75th, and ≥75th percentile scores. Cardiorespiratory fitness was categorized as unfit (lower 20% of each age group) or fit (upper 20% of each age group) according to treadmill run times.

The effects of 20 wk of endurance training on lipids and lipoproteins in 502 men and women ($\bar{X} \pm SD$, 34.1 ± 13.3 y) can be seen in figure 11.2. Pre-to-post values are reported for total cholesterol, HDL cholesterol, HDL_2 cholesterol (a subfraction of HDL that is thought to interfere with the disposition of cholesterol to the arterial wall), LDL cholesterol, VLDL cholesterol, triglycerides, and apoB. Twenty weeks of endurance training (3 d/wk ranging from 30-50 min each session) significantly increased total cholesterol, HDL cholesterol, and

HDL$_2$ cholesterol. The increase in HDL cholesterol is an obvious positive adaptation. Interestingly, when data were grouped into quartiles according to fitness improvement, the high responders (those with the greatest improvement in $\dot{V}O_2$max) did not show greater change in these blood lipid variables than the low responders. This finding is consistent with suggestions from the Centers for Disease Control and the American College of Sports Medicine that in achieving health benefits from exercise, the volume (i.e., amount) is more important than the intensity of the activity used to improve aerobic capacity (Pate et al. 1995).

Summary

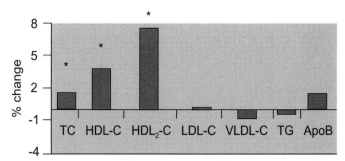

FIGURE 11.2 Relative (%) changes in lipid and lipoprotein values following 20 wk of endurance training. * = significant change from pretraining values. ApoB = apoprotein B; HDL$_2$ = high density lipoprotein 2 ; HDL-C = high density lipoprotein; LDL-C = low density lipoprotein; TC = total cholesterol; TG = triglycerides; VLDL-C = very low density lipoprotein.

Reprinted from *Metabolism*, 11, Wilmore et al, "Relationship of changes in maximal and submaximal aerobic fitness to changes in cardiovascular disease and non-insulin-dependent diabetes mellitus risk factors with endurance training: The Heritage Family study," 1255-1263, Copyright 2001, with permission from Elsevier.

⊃ Measuring blood lipids is important as hyperlipidemia is a known risk factor of cardiovascular disease.

⊃ Most stored fat in the body is stored as triglycerides, simple fats that can combine with other substances to create compound fats such as phospholipids and lipoproteins.

⊃ Cholesterol is a derived fat that is produced endogenously in the body but may also be consumed in large quantities.

⊃ Exercise is a potent stimulus for lowering blood lipid concentrations.

CHAPTER 12

Bone Density

The material composition and structural properties of bone respond to both increases and decreases in mechanical stress and strain. The ability of bone to adapt to physical demands has been accepted for over 100 years. The work of Julius Wolf demonstrated the ability of bone to adapt to specific stresses and thus provide for greater functional loading and efficiency of locomotion (Heinonen 2001). Bone responds positively to the stress and strain of mechanical loading by increasing its density and strength, but it also becomes porous and weaker during disuse. This maladaptation increases the risk for osteoporosis, a debilitating disease that afflicts both elderly men and women but is more prevalent among women.

Bone measurements are both clinically and scientifically important. Clinically they provide information for predicting fracture risk, while scientifically they provide objective evidence of the adaptability of bone to various physical, nutritional, or other lifestyle interventions. The most widely used method for bone mineral assessment is dual energy X ray absorptiometry (DEXA). DEXA uses photon emission by X ray tubes and bases its measurements on the decreases in the energy of the photon beam as it scans bone and nonbone tissue. DEXA results provide information on bone mineral content (BMC) and bone mineral density (BMD). BMC refers to the total grams (g) of bone mineral within a bone region. BMD refers to the grams of bone mineral per unit of bone area (g/cm²). A large individual has a greater BMC due to a greater absolute size, yet he may have a lower BMD than a smaller individual.

When DEXA measurements are used to screen or diagnose for osteoporosis, the clinician interprets the results using a standardized score. A *T* score is generally reported, but results may also be expressed as a *Z* score. These standard scores, developed by the World Health Organization (WHO) (1994), are based on raw BMD values of 25- to 35-year-old healthy, sex-matched individuals. Results are not compared to age-matched controls, as doing so would limit the ability to assess fracture risk due to the reduction of BMD that occurs with age. Table 12.1 provides the WHO diagnostic categories of BMD for assessing fracture risk.

TABLE 12.1 Bone Health Diagnostic Categories Based on Bone Density Values Relative to the Young Adult Mean

Normal	<1 standard deviation (SD) below the mean
Osteopenia	1-2.5 SD below the mean
Osteoporosis	>2.5 SD below the mean
Severe osteoporosis	>2.5 SD below the mean, plus one or more fragility fractures

Data from the World Health Organization (WHO), 1994, "Assessment of fracture risk and its application to screening for postmenopausal osteoporosis," *WHO Technical Report Series* 843: 1-129.

This chapter displays the BMD and BMC of various populations and explores the influence of gender, age, race, athletic background, and nationality on these variables. When possible, the results of multiple studies examining similar populations are listed side by side for comparison purposes. Due to the overwhelming popularity of DEXA in both clinical and scientific studies, the BMD and BMC data in this chapter are only from studies that utilized the DEXA scan.

Bone Mineral Density and Bone Mineral Content of Children and Adolescents

The BMD of children and adolescents can be seen in table 12.2. The results reported from Maynard and colleagues (1998) and van der Sluis and colleagues (2002) are on Caucasian children and adolescents. Boot and colleagues (1997) included various ethnicities in their data, and they reported that ethnicity has no significant association with BMD in boys but does in girls. Girls of Asian descent had significantly lower BMD than Caucasian girls, but no differences in BMD were seen between Blacks and Caucasian girls. Specific ethnic comparisons are discussed later in this chapter. Table 12.3 shows the BMC of male and female children and adolescents.

TABLE 12.2 BMD of Children and Adolescents

Age (y)	TOTAL BODY (G/CM^2)			LUMBAR SPINE (G/CM^2)		
	Maynard et al. 1998	Van der Sluis et al. 2002	Boot et al. 1997	Maynard et al. 1998	Van der Sluis et al. 2002	Boot et al. 1997
Males						
4	—	0.799 ± 0.03	0.781 ± 0.05	—	0.592 ± 0.06	0.591 ± 0.09
5	—	0.819 ± 0.03	0.826 ± 0.02	—	0.631 ± 0.07	0.625 ± 0.06
6	—	0.839 ± 0.04	0.843 ± 0.03	—	0.665 ± 0.07	0.656 ± 0.07
7	—	0.859 ± 0.04	0.866 ± 0.03	—	0.694 ± 0.08	0.720 ± 0.06
8	0.856 ± 0.02	0.880 ± 0.05	0.870 ± 0.04	0.685 ± 0.02	0.719 ± 0.08	0.685 ± 0.05
9	0.900 ± 0.05	0.900 ± 0.05	0.892 ± 0.05	0.723 ± 0.05	0.742 ± 0.09	0.755 ± 0.08
10	0.916 ± 0.04	0.920 ± 0.06	0.894 ± 0.05	0.734 ± 0.06	0.764 ± 0.10	0.726 ± 0.08
11	0.944 ± 0.06	0.942 ± 0.06	0.929 ± 0.04	0.752 ± 0.06	0.791 ± 0.10	0.791 ± 0.07
12	0.943 ± 0.05	0.967 ± 0.07	0.961 ± 0.07	0.742 ± 0.05	0.828 ± 0.11	0.846 ± 0.08
13	0.990 ± 0.08	1.000 ± 0.07	0.998 ± 0.10	0.807 ± 0.09	0.886 ± 0.11	0.868 ± 0.13
14	1.039 ± 0.09	1.045 ± 0.08	1.030 ± 0.09	0.881 ± 0.11	0.968 ± 0.12	0.977 ± 0.17
15	1.098 ± 0.11	1.103 ± 0.08	1.111 ± 0.04	0.956 ± 0.13	1.064 ± 0.12	1.058 ± 0.10
16	1.168 ± 0.09	1.158 ± 0.09	1.133 ± 0.11	1.041 ± 0.14	1.152 ± 0.13	1.119 ± 0.12
17	1.198 ± 0.09	1.200 ± 0.09	1.187 ± 0.08	1.082 ± 0.15	1.214 ± 0.13	1.204 ± 0.11
18	1.236 ± 0.09	1.229 ± 0.10	1.202 ± 0.11	1.111 ± 0.13	1.251 ± 0.14	1.238 ± 0.16
19	—	1.251 ± 0.10	—	—	1.271 ± 0.15	—
Females						
4	—	0.790 ± 0.04	0.781 ± 0.05	—	0.631 ± 0.05	0.591 ± 0.09
5	—	0.809 ± 0.05	0.826 ± 0.02	—	0.660 ± 0.06	0.625 ± 0.06
6	—	0.827 ± 0.05	0.843 ± 0.03	—	0.689 ± 0.07	0.656 ± 0.07
7	—	0.845 ± 0.06	0.866 ± 0.03	—	0.718 ± 0.08	0.720 ± 0.06
8	0.856 ± 0.02	0.864 ± 0.06	0.870 ± 0.04	0.730 ± 0.05	0.747 ± 0.09	0.685 ± 0.05
9	0.900 ± 0.05	0.886 ± 0.06	0.892 ± 0.05	0.739 ± 0.05	0.779 ± 0.09	0.755 ± 0.08
10	0.916 ± 0.04	0.913 ± 0.06	0.894 ± 0.05	0.734 ± 0.06	0.819 ± 0.10	0.726 ± 0.08

Age (y)	TOTAL BODY (G/CM^2)			LUMBAR SPINE (G/CM^2)		
	Maynard et al. 1998	Van der Sluis et al. 2002	Boot et al. 1997	Maynard et al. 1998	Van der Sluis et al. 2002	Boot et al. 1997
	Females					
11	0.944 ± 0.06	0.947 ± 0.07	0.929 ± 0.04	0.786 ± 0.10	0.876 ± 0.11	0.791 ± 0.07
12	0.943 ± 0.05	0.990 ± 0.07	0.961 ± 0.07	0.844 ± 0.11	0.957 ± 0.12	0.846 ± 0.08
13	0.990 ± 0.08	1.036 ± 0.07	0.998 ± 0.10	0.907 ± 0.12	1.049 ± 0.13	0.868 ± 0.13
14	1.039 ± 0.09	1.079 ± 0.07	1.030 ± 0.09	0.973 ± 0.12	1.128 ± 0.13	0.977 ± 0.17
15	1.098 ± 0.11	1.114 ± 0.08	1.111 ± 0.04	1.012 ± 0.13	1.181 ± 0.14	1.058 ± 0.10
16	1.168 ± 0.09	1.139 ± 0.08	1.133 ± 0.11	1.027 ± 0.11	1.214 ± 0.15	1.119 ± 0.12
17	1.198 ± 0.09	1.156 ± 0.08	1.187 ± 0.08	1.047 ± 0.08	1.236 ± 0.16	1.204 ± 0.11
18	1.236 ± 0.09	1.168 ± 0.08	1.202 ± 0.11	1.037 ± 0.09	1.252 ± 0.16	1.238 ± 0.16
19	—	1.177 ± 0.09	—	—	1.265 ± 0.17	—

TABLE 12.3 BMC (g) in Children and Adolescents

Age (y)	FEMALES		MALES	
	Maynard et al. 1998	Van der Sluis et al. 2002	Maynard et al. 1998	Van der Sluis et al. 2002
4	—	714 ± 112	—	708 ± 69
5	—	832 ± 134	—	839 ± 99
6	—	939 ± 156	—	965 ± 129
7	—	1,039 ± 179	—	1,084 ± 159
8	1,059 ± 145	1,147 ± 201	1,059 ± 101	1,197 ± 190
9	1,167 ± 122	1,275 ± 223	1,215 ± 108	1,310 ± 220
10	1,244 ± 147	1,438 ± 246	1,297 ± 126	1,438 ± 250
11	1,438 ± 235	1,640 ± 268	1,447 ± 222	1,599 ± 280
12	1,673 ± 325	1,871 ± 290	1,514 ± 251	1,813 ± 310
13	1,835 ± 331	2,104 ± 313	1,805 ± 413	2,087 ± 340
14	2,004 ± 335	2,313 ± 335	2,151 ± 480	2,406 ± 370
15	2,123 ± 351	2,477 ± 357	2,455 ± 521	2,725 ± 400
16	2,142 ± 31	2,595 ± 379	2,747 ± 379	2,997 ± 430
17	2,249 ± 278	2,673 ± 402	2,904 ± 464	3,200 ± 460
18	2,258 ± 243	2,723 ± 424	3,057 ± 396	3,336 ± 490
19	—	2,753 ± 446	—	3,419 ± 521

Although slight differences in BMD and BMC may be apparent among the studies, similar patterns of bone acquisition are seen throughout childhood. Steady increases in BMC were seen in both girls and boys until age 12. In boys, BMC and BMD increase rapidly after the age of 12, whereas in girls BMC and BMD plateau at age 14 or 15. Girls have higher BMC and BMD values between the ages of 11 and 14 but are surpassed by boys as they reach 16 to 18.

Total-body BMC and BMD and the BMD of the lumbar spine per Tanner stage are reported in table 12.4. Tanner stages represent phases of maturity in children. As a child reaches each stage of maturity, the BMC and BMD are significantly elevated above the previous Tanner stage.

TABLE 12.4 BMC and BMD per Tanner Stage

	BMC (G)	TOTAL BODY (G/CM²)		LUMBAR SPINE (G/CM²)	
Tanner stage	Van der Sluis et al. 2002	Van der Sluis et al. 2002	Boot et al. 1997	Van der Sluis et al. 2002	Boot et al. 1997
Males					
I	1,178 ± 341	0.88 ± 0.07	0.86 ± 0.06	0.71 ± 0.10	0.69 ± 0.09
II	1,785 ± 307	0.96 ± 0.07	0.94 ± 0.07	0.83 ± 0.09	0.82 ± 0.10
III	2,099 ± 508	1.00 ± 0.09	1.02 ± 0.10	0.88 ± 0.14	0.91 ± 0.15
IV	2,823 ± 655	1.12 ± 0.12	1.11 ± 0.12	1.09 ± 0.17	1.08 ± 0.17
V	3,224 ± 509	1.21 ± 0.11	1.15 ± 0.09	1.21 ± 0.16	1.17 ± 0.14
Females					
I	1,067 ± 242	0.85 ± 0.06	0.84 ± 0.05	0.72 ± 0.09	0.71 ± 0.08
II	1,539 ± 296	0.94 ± 0.06	0.93 ± 0.05	0.84 ± 0.09	0.83 ± 0.07
III	1,836 ± 295	0.97 ± 0.07	0.97 ± 0.08	0.96 ± 0.14	0.96 ± 0.15
IV	2,369 ± 477	1.09 ± 0.09	1.08 ± 0.09	1.14 ± 0.15	1.14 ± 0.15
V	2,724 ± 469	1.17 ± 0.08	1.15 ± 0.08	1.25 ± 0.16	1.22 ± 0.14

Bone Mineral Density and Bone Mineral Content of Adults

The BMDs of male and female adults are seen in tables 12.5 and 12.6, respectively. Data ranging from the second or third to the eighth decade of life are reported. When possible, data from large clinical or epidemiological studies are utilized. However, when data from a particular decade were limited, the data incorporated into the tables are from sedentary control subjects in various intervention studies. The tables were formatted using the sites of highest prevalence in BMD measurements: the total body, the lumbar spine (L2-L4), and the femoral neck, greater trochanter, and Wards triangle from the hip. Not all the studies provided measurements for each of these sites. BMC appears to peak in the third decade of life for both men and women. It then declines at about 1% per year in women until age 75, at which point bone loss slows to about 3% per decade (Khan et al. 2001). The rate of bone loss in men is similar to that in women; however, the initial bone strength of men is greater.

TABLE 12.5 BMD (g/cm²) of Men

Age (y)	n	Total body	Lumbar spine	Femoral neck	Greater trochanter	Wards triangle	Source
17	11		1.06 ± 0.21	1.05 ± 0.12	0.89 ± 0.12	0.99 ± 0.16	Conroy et al. 1993
22	13	1.2 ± 0.09	1.19 ± 0.14				Smith and Rutherford 1993
28	37	1.26 ± 0.09	1.29 ± 0.14	1.09 ± 0.19	1.00 ± 0.14	1.09 ± 0.19	Karlsson et al. 1993
33	52	1.24 ± 0.09	1.26 ± 0.15	1.08 ± 0.16	0.97 ± 0.14	1.02 ± 0.21	Karlsson et al. 1993
41	26	1.22 ± 0.1	1.23 ± 0.24	1.02 ± 0.13	0.92 ± 0.12	0.93 ± 0.12	Karlsson et al. 1993
51	247		1.05 ± 0.17	0.86 ± 0.15	0.79 ± 0.14	0.67 ± 0.19	Greendale et al. 2003
75	345			0.88 ± 0.15	0.85 ± 0.15	0.69 ± 0.17	Tucker et al. 2002

TABLE 12.6 BMD (g/cm²) of Women

Age (y)	n	Total body	Lumbar spine	Femoral neck	Greater trochanter	Wards triangle	Source
22	247	1.13 ± 0.09					Teegarden et al. 1995
23	25		1.07 ± 0.10	0.98 ± 0.11			Heinonen et al. 1993
24	26	1.16 ± 0.07					Adams et al. 1992
34	34	1.15 ± 0.07		0.96 ± 0.13	0.76 ± 0.10	0.89 ± 0.16	Lohman et al. 1995
40	195		1.07 ± 0.13	0.83 ± 0.12	0.73 ± 0.10	0.72 ± 0.15	Jorgensen et al. 2001
46	1,044		1.06 ± 0.13	0.83 ± 0.12			Greendale et al. 2003
62	209		0.91 ± 0.15	0.70 ± 0.13	0.63 ± 0.11	0.53 ± 0.15	Jorgensen et al. 2001
69	40	1.02 ± 0.08	0.95 ± 0.15	0.66 ± 0.10	0.60 ± 0.10	0.48 ± 0.11	Taaffe et al. 1995
75	53			0.72 ± 0.12	0.63 ± 0.13	0.56 ± 0.13	Tucker et al. 2002

Race and Ethnic Comparisons

Race and ethnicity cannot be overlooked when examining BMD. Table 12.7 shows data from studies on American Caucasians, African Americans, Asians, and American Asians. Results consistently show that Blacks have a greater BMD than Whites and that Whites have a greater BMD than Asians. Interestingly, Kin and colleagues (1993) showed that Japanese born in America have greater BMD than Japanese born in Japan. These differences between native Japanese and Japanese born in America likely reflect cultural differences in weight-bearing activities in various countries.

TABLE 12.7 Effect of Ethnicity on BMD (g/cm²)

Ethnic group	Gender	Age (y)	n	Total body	Lumbar spine	Femoral neck	Source
African American	F	23.6	26	1.25 ± 0.05			Greendale et al. 2003
African American	F	46.1	544		1.14 ± 0.15	0.94 ± 0.14	Greendale et al. 2003
Caucasian	F	22.5	26	1.16 ± 0.07			Cote and Adams 1993
Caucasian	F	46.3	1044		1.06 ± 0.13	0.83 ± 0.12	Greendale et al. 2003
Chinese	F	46.5	230		1.04 ± 0.13	0.77 ± 0.10	Greendale et al. 2003
Japanese	F	46.6	238		1.02 ± 0.12	0.76 ± 0.09	Greendale et al. 2003
Japanese, Japan born	F	30-39 40-49 50-59 60-69	10 31 48 42	1.09 ± 0.06 1.10 ± 0.06 1.03 ± 0.09 0.95 ± 0.07			Kin et al. 1993
Japanese, U.S. born	F	20-29 30-39 40-49 50-59 60-69 70-79	19 30 26 11 39 20	1.12 ± 0.10 1.12 ± 0.07 1.10 ± 0.07 1.06 ± 0.10 1.00 ± 0.09 0.93 ± 0.05			Kin et al. 1993

Effect of Athletic Participation on Bone Mineral Density

Sport participation appears to increase BMD. Strength and power athletes have the highest BMD, while athletes of endurance sports have the lowest. The investigation by Conroy and colleagues (1993) of the American Junior Olympic weightlifting team demonstrated the ability of even young athletes to increase BMD during their training programs. The data from studies examining the BMD of male and female athletes can be seen in tables 12.8 and 12.9. The importance of maintaining physical activity during aging can be seen in table 12.10. The studies in 12.10 examined master athletes and consistently showed the benefits of exercise on maintaining high BMD. Interestingly, endurance training in the master athlete appears to maintain BMD or help it exceed that of age-matched controls. However, reports in the literature suggest that highly trained, master endurance athletes have a low BMD compared to that of their age-matched peers (Nichols, Palmer, and Levy 2003). Despite their physical activity, these endurance athletes may be at a high risk for fractures with advancing age. Although table 12.10 reports on master athletes, the benefits of exercise for maintaining bone health in older populations have been well documented in a number of intervention studies (Greendale et al. 2003; Heinonen et al. 1996; Lohman et al. 1995).

TABLE 12.8 Effect of Athletic Participation on BMD (g/cm²) in Men Ages 17 to 29

Sport	n	Total body	Lumbar spine	Femoral neck	Greater trochanter	Wards triangle	Arm	Leg	Pelvis	Ribs	Source
American football	26						1.20 ± 0.10	1.64 ± 0.08	1.49 ± 0.10	0.88 ± 0.04	Hoffman, unpublished research
Cycling	14	1.21 ± 0.07	0.96 ± 0.11				0.84 ± 0.04	1.42 ± 0.12			Stewart and Hannon 2000
Judo	12	1.40 ± 0.06					1.18 ± 0.06	1.55 ± 0.07			Andreoli et al. 2001
Karate	14	1.36 ± 0.08					1.07 ± 0.07	1.58 ± 0.12			Andreoli et al. 2001
Rowing	12	1.27 ± 0.07	1.32 ± 0.10				1.12 ± 0.07	1.39 ± 0.10	1.30 ± 0.12	0.81 ± 0.05	Smith and Rutherford 1993
Running	31	1.10 ± 0.11					0.88 ± 0.05	1.33 ± 0.11			Bennell et al. 1997
Running	12	1.32 ± 0.07	1.09 ± 0.10				0.86 ± 0.04	1.60 ± 0.13			Stewart and Hannon 2000
Track throwing	27		1.24 ± 0.14				0.94 ± 0.07	1.39 ± 0.12			Bennell et al. 1997
Triathlon	8	1.21 ± 0.04	1.17 ± 0.09				1.07 ± 0.07	1.34 ± 0.08	1.13 ± 0.08	0.71 ± 0.03	Smith and Rutherford 1993
Water polo	24	1.31 ± 0.09					1.09 ± 0.07	1.46 ± 0.12			Andreoli et al. 2001
Weight-lifting	21	1.38 ± 0.25	1.46 ± 0.18	1.30 ± 0.29	1.14 ± 0.18	1.29 ± 0.29					Karlsson, Johnell, and Obrant 1993
Weight-lifting, junior	25	—	1.41 ± 0.20	1.30 ± 0.15	1.05 ± 0.13	1.26 ± 0.20					Conroy et al. 1993

TABLE 12.9 Effect of Athletic Participation on BMD (g/cm²) in Women

Sport	Age	n	Total body	Lumbar spine	Femoral neck	Arms	Legs	Source
Cycling	24	29		1.07 ± 0.12	0.96 ± 0.11			Heinonen et al. 1993
Gymnastics	10	16	0.78 ± 0.05	0.65 ± 0.06	0.70 ± 0.06			Dyson et al. 1997
Running	21	30		1.04 ± 0.13		0.78 ± 0.04	1.19 ± 0.10	Bennell et al. 1997
Running	21	28		1.07 ± 0.10	1.04 ± 0.12			Heinonen et al. 1993
Track throwing	20	23		1.17 ± 0.12		0.81 ± 0.04	1.22 ± 0.10	Bennell et al. 1997
Weightlifting	25	18		1.23 ± 0.13	1.08 ± 0.16			Heinonen et al. 1993

TABLE 12.10 Effect of Athletic Participation on BMD (g/cm²) in Master Athletes

Sport	Age	n	Total body	Lumbar spine	Femoral neck	Greater trochanter	Wards triangle	Arms	Legs	Source
Basketball and netball	45	20	1.15 ± 0.08					0.73 ± 0.05	1.20 ± 0.09	Dook et al. 1997
Field hockey and running	46	20	1.12 ± 0.08					0.71 ± 0.05	0.71 ± 0.05	Dook et al. 1997
Swimming	46	20	1.06 ± 0.07					1.18 ± 0.09	1.11 ± 0.09	Dook et al. 1997
Weightlifting	41	19	1.33 ± 0.11	1.38 ± 0.19	1.16 ± 0.18	1.04 ± 0.18	1.05 ± 0.18			Karlsson, Johnell, and Obrant 1993

Bilateral Comparison

Bone adaptation to exercise and sport may be specific to the dominant limb of action. Figures 12.1 through 12.4 compare the right and left arms and legs of male and female athletes. Surprisingly, in sports that are not single-arm dominant (e.g., baseball), differences ranging from 4% to 10% occur between the upper limbs in both males and females (McClanahan et al. 2002). Such differences likely relate to adaptations resulting from activities associated with daily living.

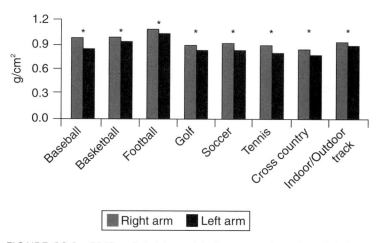

FIGURE 12.1   BMD of right and left arms of male athletes. * = significant difference (p < .05).

Adapted from B.S. McClanahan, et al., 2002, "Side to side comparisons of bone mineral density in upper and lower limbs of collegiate athletes," *Journal of Strength and Conditioning Research* 16:586-590.

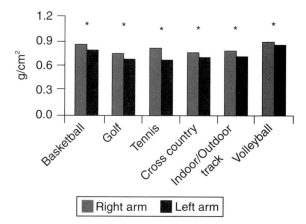

FIGURE 12.2   BMD of right and left arms of female athletes. * = significant difference (p < .05).

Adapted from B.S. McClanahan, et al., 2002, "Side to side comparisons of bone mineral density in upper and lower limbs of collegiate athletes," *Journal of Strength and Conditioning Research* 16:586-590.

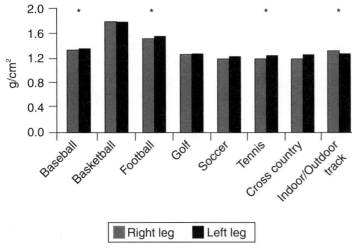

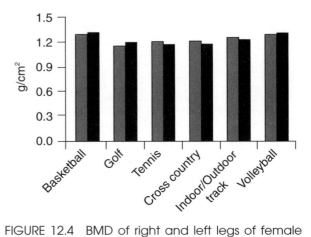

FIGURE 12.4   BMD of right and left legs of female athletes.

Adapted from B.S. McClanahan, et al., 2002, "Side to side comparisons of bone mineral density in upper and lower limbs of collegiate athletes," *Journal of Strength and Conditioning Research* 16:586-590.

FIGURE 12.3   BMD of right and left legs of male athletes. * = significant difference *(p < .05)*.

Adapted from B.S. McClanahan, et al., 2002, "Side to side comparisons of bone mineral density in upper and lower limbs of collegiate athletes," *Journal of Strength and Conditioning Research* 16:586-590.

BMD differences between lower limbs are generally not seen in women athletes (McClanahan et al. 2002). Lee and colleagues (1995), though, did see significant differences between the legs of female volleyball players. Interestingly, the nondominant leg had significantly greater BMD. This finding is similar to reports on BMD differences in the lower limbs of males playing football and tennis (McClanahan et al. 2002). Although the mechanisms that result in a greater BMD in nondominant lower limbs are unclear, they likely relate to forces that are exerted on the nondominant support leg when the dominant leg leads. In American football the stances of linemen are generally staggered, meaning the dominant foot aligns with the middle of the nondominant foot and the body weight is disproportionately placed on the nondominant limb. As the player comes out of his stance, the initial forces are exerted with that nondominant limb, which may disproportionately increase the ground reaction forces experienced by the nondominant leg. Ground reaction forces play an important role in bone remodeling (Bassey and Ramsdale 1994).

Summary

- Bone loss occurs with age, yet exercise programs may reduce the risk of fractures in the elderly.
- Gender, race, and ethnic differences in bone strength need to be acknowledged when comparing various populations.
- A bilateral difference in BMD is often seen in athletes who use a dominant limb.

CHAPTER 13

Hematological Profiles

Blood variables indicate the health status of individuals and the function of various physiological systems within the body. In an athletic population such measures may also inform us of physiological adaptation or of maladaptation during high-intensity training that suggests stress, fatigue, and possible overtraining. This chapter provides normative data and commonly used hematological profiles for both sedentary and athletic populations.

Blood Chemistry and Hematology

Commonly used blood chemistry and hematology measurements are reviewed in table 13.1. Nearly all of these tests are used for screening or diagnostic purposes. Screening is used to detect a disease when symptoms are not present, while diagnostic testing confirms a suspected disease. Blood lipid profiles (see chapter 11) may be used to screen for potential heart disease, whereas creatine kinase measurements may be used to diagnose a heart attack. Reference ranges for the tests in table 13.1 can be seen in table 13.2. Reference ranges are also referred to as *normal ranges* and typically represent the 95% confidence limits of values observed in a healthy population. Although these values depend on the methods and conditions used for the analysis, most laboratories use standardized methods. Regardless, differences between laboratories may exist. Results from blood tests may also be affected by the time of day or the time of month (specifically for women) of the test, by what food or drink was consumed before the test, and by whether the individual was rested after exercise or other strenuous activity.

In athletes the primary purpose of biochemical monitoring is to describe the intensity of exercise and the stress of training. Exercise scientists compare training measurements to baseline values (obtained at the beginning of training program). Changes may suggest training stress or a positive physiological adaptation, but they are not expected to indicate disease or severity of disease. Changes in hematological values do not need to be outside the normal range to indicate training adaptation or stress.

TABLE 13.1 Specific Blood Tests

Test	Purpose
Albumin	Screen for liver or kidney disease or to evaluate nutritional status.
Alkaline phosphatase (ALP)	Monitor treatment for a liver or bone disorder. Elevations may be normal in children, reflecting bone growth.
Ammonia	Index ATP resynthesis and indirectly index fast-twitch fiber activity.
Amylase	Diagnose pancreatic diseases.
Anion gap	Examine electrolyte profile. It is a calculated value that has more than one formula: (a) $(Na^+) - ((Cl^-) + (HCO_3^-))$ and (b) $(Na^+ + K^+) - (Cl^- + HCO_3^-)$, where Na^+ = sodium, Cl^- = chloride, HCO_3^- = bicarbonate, and K^+ = potassium. An abnormal anion gap is nonspecific but may suggest metabolic abnormalities such as starvation or diabetes or the presence of a toxic substance such as oxalate, glycolate, or aspirin.
Bicarbonate (CO_2 content)	Calculated from pH and PCO_2, it measures the metabolic component of acid–base balance. HCO_3^- is excreted and reabsorbed by the kidneys in response to pH imbalances and directly relates to pH level.
Billirubin	Screen and monitor liver disorders such as jaundice or liver diseases such as cirrhosis.
Calcium	Determine if calcium concentrations in blood are normal. It is also part of a routine metabolic panel in persons with kidney, bone, or nerve disease.
Chloride	Examine acid–base balance and monitor treatment. Part of standard electrolyte or metabolic panel.
Creatine kinase	Clinically used to determine a heart attack; also a common marker used in exercise science to assess muscle damage.
Creatinine	Screen kidney function and monitor treatment for kidney disease. Part of standard electrolyte or metabolic panel. Also provides information concerning changes in skeletal muscle.
Ferritin	Examine ability of body to store iron. It is the main protein that stores iron for areas that need it, especially the liver and bone marrow. May become elevated during acute infection and inflammation.
Gamma-glutamyl transpeptidase (GGT)	Screen for liver disease and alcohol abuse and to differentiate between liver and bone disease as a cause for elevated alkaline phosphatase (ALP).
Glucose	Screen or monitor diabetes mellitus. Often used in exercise science to index carbohydrate use; is a factor of metabolite control.
Hematocrit	Measure proportion of red blood cells to the total volume of blood.
Hemoglobin	Measure amount of oxygen carrying protein in red blood cells.
Iron (Fe)	Measure iron concentrations in blood and potential iron deficiency. Its role in binding oxygen to hemoglobin makes it an important marker of anemia. May also indicate chronic bleeding.
Iron binding capacity	Measure transferrin, a blood protein that transports iron from the gut to the cells that use it.
Lactate	Used primarily in exercise science as an indicator of intensity of anaerobic or anaerobic-aerobic exercise. Is used to assess anaerobic threshold and anaerobic working capacity.
Lactate dehydrogenase (LDH)	Indicate muscle damage. At one time it was an important indicator of heart attack, but it has been replaced by more effective markers.
Lipase	Diagnose pancreatitis or other pancreatic disease.
Magnesium	Evaluate the level of magnesium in blood and help determine the cause of abnormal calcium or potassium levels. Elevations or decreases in magnesium may result in weakness, irritability, cardiac arrhythmia, nausea, or diarrhea.
Mean corpuscular hemoglobin (MCH)	Measure volume of hemoglobin in the average cell. Calculated by dividing the total hemoglobin by total red blood cells.
Mean corpuscular hemoglobin concentration (MCHC)	Measure percentage of hemoglobin in the average red blood cell. Decreased values point to hypochromasia, or decreased oxygen-carrying capacity, because of decreased hemoglobin inside the cell.
Mean corpuscular volume (MCV)	Estimate the volume of red blood cells. Calculated by dividing the hematocrit by the total red blood cells.
Phosphorus	Evaluate phosphorus concentrations in blood for information about digestion, storage, and utilization of carbohydrates.

Test	Purpose
Platelet count	Number of platelets in a volume of blood. Provides information concerning blood clotting function.
Potassium	Evaluate potassium concentrations in blood for information concerning kidney function and other organ function.
Red blood cell	Number of red blood cells. An indicator of anemia when reduced; elevated numbers may compromise circulation due to decrease in blood flow.
Sodium	Evaluate sodium concentrations in blood to investigate salt/water balance, fluid control, and kidney and adrenal function.
Thyroid stimulating hormone (TSH)	Screen and diagnose thyroid disorders; monitor treatment of hyperthyroidism.
Thyroxin	Diagnose hypothyroidism or hyperthyroidism in adults.
Total protein	Determine nutritional status or screen for certain liver and kidney disorders as well as other diseases.
Transaminases (AST, ALT)	Screen and diagnose liver damage.
Transferrin	Evaluate ability of body to transport iron.
Triiodothyronine	Diagnose hyperthyroidism.
Urea nitrogen (BUN)	Evaluate kidney function. Rises during dehydration and kidney or heart failure. Elevated levels may also indicate liver or thyroid inactivity, while decreased levels may indicate pancreatic or adrenal inactivity. May also be elevated by a high-protein diet or recent exercise. In exercise science may be used to assess overtraining.
Uric acid	Screen for gout, an end product of protein digestion. Its concentration depends on liver production and kidney elimination. Increases during prolonged aerobic exercise.
Vitamin B$_{12}$	Diagnose the cause of anemia and neuropathy and evaluate nutritional status.
White blood cell count (WBC)	Measure number of white blood cells in a volume of blood.

TABLE 13.2 Blood Test Reference Ranges

Test	Population	Conventional range
Albumin		3.5-5.0 g/dl
Alkaline phosphatase (ALP)	Adult (nonpregnant)	25-100 units/L
	Growing children	70-300 units/L
Ammonia		15-50 μg of nitrogen/dl
Amylase		53-123 units/L
Anion gap		8-16 meq/L
Ascorbic acid		0.4-1.5 mg/dl
Bicarbonate (CO$_2$ content)		18-23 meq/L
Billirubin	Direct	0-0.4 mg/dl
	Total	0.1-1.0 mg/dl
Calcium		8.5-10.5 mg/dl
Chloride		98-106 meq/L
Creatine kinase	Males	38-174 units/L
	Females	96-140 units/L
Creatinine		0.6-1.2 mg/dl
Ferritin	Males	30-300 μg/L
	Females	15-200 μg/L
Gamma-glutamyl transpeptidase (GGT)		9-85 units/L
Glucose	Fasting	70-110 mg/dl

(continued)

TABLE 13.2 Blood Test Reference Ranges *(continued)*

Test	Population	Conventional range
Hematocrit	Males	
	12-18 y	37%-49%
	18+ y	38%-50%
	Females	
	12–18 y	36%-45%
	18+ y	36%-45%
Hemoglobin	Males	
	12-18 y	13-15.5 g/dl
	18+ y	13-18 g/dl
	Females	
	12-18 y	12-15.5 g/dl
	18+ y	11.5-15.5 g/dl
Iron (Fe)		60-160 µg/dl
Iron binding capacity		250-460 µg/dl
Lactate dehydrogenase (LDH)		50-150 units/L
Lipase		10-150 units/L
Magnesium		1.5-2.0 mg/dl
Mean corpuscular hemoglobin (MCH)	12-18 y	25-35 pg
	18+ y	27.3-33.6 pg
Mean corpuscular hemoglobin concentration (MCHC)		32.3-35.7 g/dl
Mean corpuscular volume (MCV)		80-100 fl
Phosphorus		3.0-4.5 g/dl (inorganic)
Platelet count		$150\text{-}400 \times 10^3\ \mu\text{L}$
Potassium		3.5-5.0 meq/L
Red blood cell	Males	
	12-18 y	$4.5\text{-}5.3 \times 10^6\ \mu\text{L}$
	18+ y	$4.4\text{-}5.6 \times 10^6\ \mu\text{L}$
	Females	
	12-18 y	$4.1\text{-}5.1 \times 10^6\ \mu\text{L}$
	18+ y	$3.8\text{-}5.0 \times 10^6\ \mu\text{L}$
Sodium		135-145 meq/L
Thyroxin	Total (T4)	85-160 nmol/L
	Free (FT4)	10-25 pmol/L
Thyroid stimulating hormone (TSH)		0.5-6.0 units/mL
Total protein		6.0-8.4 g/dl
Transaminases	Alanine (ALT)	1-21 units/L
	Aspartate (AST)	7-27 units/L
Transferrin		2.1-3.6 g/L
Triiodothyronine	Total (T3)	1.5-2.6 nmol/L
	Free (FT3)	4-8 pmol/L
Urea nitrogen (BUN)		8-20 mg/dl
Uric acid	Males	2.1-8.5 mg/dl
	Females	2.0-7.0 mg/dl
Vitamin B_{12}		120-680 pmol/L
White blood cell count (WBC)		$4.3\text{-}10 \times 10^3\ \mu\text{L}$

IMMUNE CELLS

Table 13.3 presents information on the major types of leukocytes (white blood cells) in the circulation. These cells are involved in immune response and inform on an individual's ability to combat disease, infection, and inflammation. Many of these cells display surface proteins, or *clusters of differentiation (CD)*, which signify the cells' roles. The cluster of differentiation is a number assigned to each cell that is arbitrary and indicates their order of discovery, but they have no scientific meaning. In exercise science the measurement of these cells may indicate overreaching during stressful training in athletes (Fry et al. 1991).

BLOOD LACTATE

The most frequent blood measurement made in exercise science is for lactate. Blood lactate is used to assess anaerobic capacity, anaerobic threshold, and intensity of training (Viru and Viru 2001). Lactate responses positively relate to exercise intensity. Elevations in lactic acid indicate the onset of anaerobic exercise, and further increases in lactic acid reflect a greater intensity of training. Since lactate levels represent anaerobic metabolism, they inversely relate to concentrations of free fatty acids. Free fatty acids indicate the use of lipid as an energy substrate during exercise. Increases in free fatty acids suggest that a greater

TABLE 13.3 Circulating Leukocytes and Lymphocytes

Cell	% of circulating leukocytes	Normal cell number per liter of blood	Primary functions
Leukocytes			
Granulocytes	60-70		
Neutrophils	90% of granulocytes	3.00-5.55	Phagocytosis, primary defense against bacterial infection
Eosinophils	2.5% of granulocytes	0.05-0.25	Phagocytosis of parasites, production of the antiinflammatory protein histamine
Basophils	0.2% of granulocytes	0.02	Chemotactic factor production, respond to allergic reactions, control inflammation and damage of body tissues
Monocytes	10-15	0.15-0.60	Phagocytosis, act as germ-eating cells, decrease risk of infection
Lymphocytes	20-25	1.0-2.5	Protect against pathogens (bacteria, viruses, and fungi)

Subset	% lymphocytes	Normal number per liter blood	Major CD antigens	Primary functions
Lymphocytes				
T cell	60-75	1.0-2.5	CD2, CD4, CD8	Lymphocyte regulation
Helper T and inflammatory T	60-70 of T cells	0.5-1.6	CD4	Cytokine secretion, antigen recognition, B cell activation
Cytotoxic T	30-40 of T cells	0.3-0.9	CD8	Cytotoxicity, lymphocyte regulation
B cell	5-15	0.3	CD19-CD23	Antibody production, memory
Large granular lymphocytes/ natural killer cells	10-20	0.1-0.5	CD16, CD56	Cytotoxicity, cytokine production

aerobic metabolism is fueling exercise. Table 13.4 compares the concentrations of blood lactate and free fatty acids during various types of exercise. The use of blood lactate to assess various endurance workouts can be seen in table 13.5. Table 13.5 should only be used as a guide, but it demonstrates how lactate can provide information to coaches of endurance athletes.

ELECTROLYTES

Electrolyte measurements are commonly used in clinical settings to screen for electrolyte and pH imbalances or to monitor the treatment of a known imbalance. They may also be used to diagnose for edema or for cardiac arrhythmias. However,

electrolyte measurements are also important in human performance studies examining hydration and sweating during exercise in both mild and temperate environments. Often, electrolyte measurements made during exercise are made from sweat. The concentrations of these minerals in sweat are much lower than those in plasma or other body fluids (see table 13.6). Electrolyte changes vary among individuals and depend on sweat rate, physical condition, and state of heat acclimatization (Maughan 1991). Changes in electrolyte balance may significantly affect exercise performance by altering the membrane potential of the motor unit (the nerve and the muscle fibers it innervates) (Sjogaard 1986).

TABLE 13.4 Effect of Exercise Type on Blood Lactate and Free Fatty Acid Response

Exercise type	Anaerobic	Aerobic-anaerobic		Aerobic		
Duration (min)	1-2	3-10	11-35	36-90	90-360	>360
% $\dot{V}O_2$ max	95-100	95-100	90-95	80-95	60-85	50-60
Aerobic/anaerobic ratio	50:50	80:20	85:15	95:5	98:2	99:1
Blood lactate (mmol · L⁻¹)	18	20	14	8	4	2
Free fatty acids in plasma (mmol · L⁻¹)	0.5	0.5	0.8	1.0	2.0	2.5

Adapted, by permission, from G. Neumann, 1992, Cycling. In *Endurance in sport*, edited by R.J. Shephard and P.O. Åstrand (London: Blackwell Scientific), 582-596.

TABLE 13.5 Lactate Values of Running Exercises in Top Marathon Runners

Exercise	Blood lactate (mmol/L)	Exercise intensity (% of marathon velocity)
Recovery workout	1.0	<80
Extensive endurance	1.0-1.1	80-90
Intensive endurance	1.3	90-97
Tempo endurance	2.0	100
Extensive intervals (fartlek)	3.0	105
Intensive intervals	>8.0	

Adapted, by permission, from H. Liesen, 1985, "Trainingsteierung im Hochleistungssport einge Aspekte und Beispiele," *Deutsche Zeitschrift fur Sportmedizin* 1:8-18.

TABLE 13.6 Major Electrolytes in Sweat, Plasma, and Muscle

Electrolyte	ELECTROLYTE CONCENTRATIONS (MEQ/L)		
	Plasma	Sweat	Muscle
Sodium (Na⁺)	137-144	40-80	10
Chloride (Cl⁻)	100-108	30-70	2
Calcium (Ca²⁺)	4.4-5.2	3-4	0-2
Potassium (K⁺)	3.5-4.9	4-8	148
Magnesium (Mg²⁺)	1.5-2.1	1-4	30-40

Adapted from R.J. Maughan, 1991, "Fluid and electrolyte loss and replacement," *Journal of Sport Sciences* 9: 117-142, with permission of Taylor & Francis Ltd. www.tandf.co.uk/journals.

Summary

➲ Blood chemistry and hematological measurements assess health status in a normal, healthy population.

➲ These measurements can also be used to monitor training programs for changes suggestive of normal physiological adaptation or of maladaptation indicating overtraining syndrome.

CHAPTER 14

Energy Expenditure

In this chapter the energy expenditures for various activities are listed. These activities include recreational and competitive sporting and exercise events, household chores, and occupations. These values are based on data compiled by Ainsworth and colleagues (2000), who reported the metabolic equivalents (METs) for these specific activities in their compendium of physical activities. A MET is the amount of energy the body utilizes during activity that is in proportion to the amount of energy it uses at rest. At rest the body uses approximately 3.5 milliliters of oxygen per kilogram of body mass per minute ($3.5 \ ml \cdot kg^{-1} \cdot min^{-1}$). This resting metabolic rate is known as 1.0 MET. If an activity increases energy expenditure by threefold, it is said to be at a 3 MET intensity level. If the MET level of any activity is known, it can be converted into units of oxygen consumption by multiplying by 3.5. As seen earlier, this calculation provides $\dot{V}O_2$ in relative units ($ml \cdot kg^{-1} \cdot min^{-1}$). Thus, if an activity is a 4 MET activity, the energy it requires is four times greater than that expended at rest, or $14 \ ml \cdot kg^{-1} \cdot min^{-1}$.

Metabolic Equations

Metabolic equations can be used to calculate the caloric consumption (expressed in kcal/min) of an activity. The initial step is to convert the $\dot{V}O_2$ of the activity into absolute terms ($L \cdot min^{-1}$). This is accomplished by multiplying the $\dot{V}O_2$ by body mass (kg) and dividing by 1000 (because there are 1000 ml in 1 L). The next step is to multiply by 5 kcal/min to obtain the caloric expenditure. Energy expenditure can be calculated from the MET value as follows:

Energy expenditure (kcal/min) = (METs × 3.5 × body mass) / 200,

where body mass is in kg.

MET Values for Energy Costs

Table 14.1 provides the MET intensity and associated energy expenditures for a host of physical activities. The table is divided into several sections and is categorized by activity level. These categories include dancing, exercise, home activities, home repair, lawn and gardening, music playing, occupation, running, sports, walking, water activities, and winter activities. The second column lists the MET intensity level of the activity, and the subsequent columns provide the energy expenditures (kcal/min) for a range of body weights for the specific activity. To determine the total energy expenditure for a particular activity, select the activity level, find its energy expenditure in kcal/min, and multiply the energy expenditure by the total number of minutes the activity was performed. For instance, if a 209 lb (94.8 kg) man ran for 30 min at 5 mph (8.0 km/h or 12 min/mi), the total energy expended was 420 kcal·min^{-1} (14 kcal·min^{-1} × 30 min).

There are some inherent limitations to using MET values to determine the energy cost of an activity. For example, the terrain or surface on which the activity is performed can affect energy expenditure. Running or walking on sand may increase energy expenditure almost twofold, while performing these same activities in soft snow elevates the energy cost even more (Smolander et al. 1989). Walking on a treadmill may increase energy cost as compared to walking at the same speed on a floor (Pearce et al. 1983). In addition, table 14.1 does not account for differences in energy expenditure relating to body composition, age, sex, movement efficiency, and environmental conditions. All of these factors may result in an over- or underestimation of energy expenditure. Although differences in the energy cost for a particular activity may be large, the information in this table does provide the most effective indirect method of estimating the energy cost of an activity.

Table 14.1 Energy Expenditures for Various Sports and Activities

Dancing	lb	99	110	121	132	143	154	165	176	187	198	209	220	231	242	253	264
	kg	45	50	55	60	65	70	75	80	85	90	95	100	105	110	115	120
	METs																
Aerobic, general	6.5	5.1	5.7	6.3	6.8	7.4	8.0	8.5	9.1	9.7	10.2	10.8	11.4	11.9	12.5	13.1	13.7
Aerobic, high impact	7.0	5.5	6.1	6.7	7.4	8.0	8.6	9.2	9.8	10.4	11.0	11.6	12.3	12.9	13.5	14.1	14.7
Aerobic, low impact	5.0	3.9	4.4	4.8	5.3	5.7	6.1	6.6	7.0	7.4	7.9	8.3	8.8	9.2	9.6	10.1	10.5
Aerobic, step with 10-12 in. (25.4-30.5 cm) step	10.0	7.9	8.8	9.6	10.5	11.4	12.3	13.1	14.0	14.9	15.8	16.6	17.5	18.4	19.3	20.1	21.0
Aerobic, step with 6-8 in. (15.2-20.3 cm) step	8.5	6.7	7.4	8.2	8.9	9.7	10.4	11.2	11.9	12.6	13.4	14.1	14.9	15.6	16.4	17.1	17.9
Ballet or modern	4.8	3.8	4.2	4.6	5.0	5.5	5.9	6.3	6.7	7.1	7.6	8.0	8.4	8.8	9.2	9.7	10.1
Ballroom, fast (disco, folk, square)	4.5	3.5	3.9	4.3	4.7	5.1	5.5	5.9	6.3	6.7	7.1	7.5	7.9	8.3	8.7	9.1	9.5
Ballroom, slow	3.0	2.4	2.6	2.9	3.2	3.4	3.7	3.9	4.2	4.5	4.7	5.0	5.3	5.5	5.8	6.0	6.3
General	4.5	3.5	3.9	4.3	4.7	5.1	5.5	5.9	6.3	6.7	7.1	7.5	7.9	8.3	8.7	9.1	9.5

Exercise	lb	99	110	121	132	143	154	165	176	187	198	209	220	231	242	253	264
	kg	45	50	55	60	65	70	75	80	85	90	95	100	105	110	115	120
	METs																
BMX or mountain biking	8.5	6.7	7.4	8.2	8.9	9.7	10.4	11.2	11.9	12.6	13.4	14.1	14.9	15.6	16.4	17.1	17.9
General biking	8.0	6.3	7.0	7.7	8.4	9.1	9.8	10.5	11.2	11.9	12.6	13.3	14.0	14.7	15.4	16.1	16.8
<10 mph (16.09 km/h), leisure cycling	4.0	3.2	3.5	3.9	4.2	4.6	4.9	5.3	5.6	6.0	6.3	6.7	7.0	7.4	7.7	8.1	8.4

Exercise	lb	99	110	121	132	143	154	165	176	187	198	209	220	231	242	253	264
	kg	45	50	55	60	65	70	75	80	85	90	95	100	105	110	115	120
	METs																
10-11.9 mph (16.09-19.15 km/h), leisure cycling, slow, light effort	6.0	4.7	5.3	5.8	6.3	6.8	7.4	7.9	8.4	8.9	9.5	10.0	10.5	11.0	11.6	12.1	12.6
12-13.9 mph (19.31-22.37 km/h), leisure cycling, moderate effort	8.0	6.3	7.0	7.7	8.4	9.1	9.8	10.5	11.2	11.9	12.6	13.3	14.0	14.7	15.4	16.1	16.8
14-15.9 mph (22.5-25.58 km/h), racing or leisure cycling, fast	10.0	7.9	8.8	9.6	10.5	11.4	12.3	13.1	14.0	14.9	15.8	16.6	17.5	18.4	19.3	20.1	21.0
16-19 mph (25.7-30.6 km/h), racing, not drafting	12.0	9.5	10.5	11.6	12.6	13.7	14.7	15.8	16.8	17.9	18.9	20.0	21.0	22.1	23.1	24.2	25.2
>20 mph (32.2 km/h), racing, not drafting	16.0	12.6	14.0	15.4	16.8	18.2	19.6	21.0	22.4	23.8	25.2	26.6	28.0	29.4	30.8	32.2	33.6
Bicycling, stationary, general	7.0	5.5	6.1	6.7	7.4	8.0	8.6	9.2	9.8	10.4	11.0	11.6	12.3	12.9	13.5	14.1	14.7
Bicycling, stationary, 50 W, very light effort	3.0	2.4	2.6	2.9	3.2	3.4	3.7	3.9	4.2	4.5	4.7	5.0	5.3	5.5	5.8	6.0	6.3
Bicycling, stationary, 100 W, light effort	5.5	4.3	4.8	5.3	5.8	6.3	6.7	7.2	7.7	8.2	8.7	9.1	9.6	10.1	10.6	11.1	11.6
Bicycling, stationary, 150 W, moderate effort	7.0	5.5	6.1	6.7	7.4	8.0	8.6	9.2	9.8	10.4	11.0	11.6	12.3	12.9	13.5	14.1	14.7
Bicycling, stationary, 200 W, vigorous effort	10.5	8.3	9.2	10.1	11.0	11.9	12.9	13.8	14.7	15.6	16.5	17.5	18.4	19.3	20.2	21.1	22.1
Bicycling, stationary, 250 W, very vigorous effort	12.5	9.8	10.9	12.0	13.1	14.2	15.3	16.4	17.5	18.6	19.7	20.8	21.9	23.0	24.1	25.2	26.3
Calisthenics (push-ups, sit-ups), heavy vigorous effort	8.0	6.3	7.0	7.7	8.4	9.1	9.8	10.5	11.2	11.9	12.6	13.3	14.0	14.7	15.4	16.1	16.8
Calisthenics, light or moderate effort	3.5	2.8	3.1	3.4	3.7	4.0	4.3	4.6	4.9	5.2	5.5	5.8	6.1	6.4	6.7	7.0	7.4
Circuit training	8.0	6.3	7.0	7.7	8.4	9.1	9.8	10.5	11.2	11.9	12.6	13.3	14.0	14.7	15.4	16.1	16.8
Powerlifting or bodybuilding	6.0	4.7	5.3	5.8	6.3	6.8	7.4	7.9	8.4	8.9	9.5	10.0	10.5	11.0	11.6	12.1	12.6
Rowing, stationary ergometer, general	7.0	5.5	6.1	6.7	7.4	8.0	8.6	9.2	9.8	10.4	11.0	11.6	12.3	12.9	13.5	14.1	14.7
Rowing, stationary, 50 W, light effort	3.5	2.8	3.1	3.4	3.7	4.0	4.3	4.6	4.9	5.2	5.5	5.8	6.1	6.4	6.7	7.0	7.4
Rowing, stationary, 100 W, moderate effort	7.0	5.5	6.1	6.7	7.4	8.0	8.6	9.2	9.8	10.4	11.0	11.6	12.3	12.9	13.5	14.1	14.7
Rowing, stationary, 150 W, vigorous effort	8.5	6.7	7.4	8.2	8.9	9.7	10.4	11.2	11.9	12.6	13.4	14.1	14.9	15.6	16.4	17.1	17.9
Rowing, stationary, 200 W, very vigorous effort	12.0	9.5	10.5	11.6	12.6	13.7	14.7	15.8	16.8	17.9	18.9	20.0	21.0	22.1	23.1	24.2	25.2
Ski machine, general	7.0	5.5	6.1	6.7	7.4	8.0	8.6	9.2	9.8	10.4	11.0	11.6	12.3	12.9	13.5	14.1	14.7

(continued)

TABLE 14.1   Energy Expenditures for Various Sports and Activities *(continued)*

Exercise	lb	99	110	121	132	143	154	165	176	187	198	209	220	231	242	253	264
	kg	45	50	55	60	65	70	75	80	85	90	95	100	105	110	115	120
	METs																
Slimnastics, jazzercise	6.0	4.7	5.3	5.8	6.3	6.8	7.4	7.9	8.4	8.9	9.5	10.0	10.5	11.0	11.6	12.1	12.6
Stretching	2.5	2.0	2.2	2.4	2.6	2.8	3.1	3.3	3.5	3.7	3.9	4.2	4.4	4.6	4.8	5.0	5.3
Teaching aerobic exercise class	6.0	4.7	5.3	5.8	6.3	6.8	7.4	7.9	8.4	8.9	9.5	10.0	10.5	11.0	11.6	12.1	12.6
Water aerobics, water calisthenics	4.0	3.2	3.5	3.9	4.2	4.6	4.9	5.3	5.6	6.0	6.3	6.7	7.0	7.4	7.7	8.1	8.4
Weightlifting	3.0	2.4	2.6	2.9	3.2	3.4	3.7	3.9	4.2	4.5	4.7	5.0	5.3	5.5	5.8	6.0	6.3

Home activities	lb	99	110	121	132	143	154	165	176	187	198	209	220	231	242	253	264
	kg	45	50	55	60	65	70	75	80	85	90	95	100	105	110	115	120
	METs																
Carrying groceries upstairs	7.5	5.9	6.6	7.2	7.9	8.5	9.2	9.8	10.5	11.2	11.8	12.5	13.1	13.8	14.4	15.1	15.8
Cleaning, vigorous effort	3.0	2.4	2.6	2.9	3.2	3.4	3.7	3.9	4.2	4.5	4.7	5.0	5.3	5.5	5.8	6.0	6.3
Cooking	2.0	1.6	1.8	1.9	2.1	2.3	2.5	2.6	2.8	3.0	3.2	3.3	3.5	3.7	3.9	4.0	4.2
Household tasks, light effort	2.5	2.0	2.2	2.4	2.6	2.8	3.1	3.3	3.5	3.7	3.9	4.2	4.4	4.6	4.8	5.0	5.3
Household tasks, moderate effort	3.5	2.8	3.1	3.4	3.7	4.0	4.3	4.6	4.9	5.2	5.5	5.8	6.1	6.4	6.7	7.0	7.4
Household tasks, vigorous effort	4.0	3.2	3.5	3.9	4.2	4.6	4.9	5.3	5.6	6.0	6.3	6.7	7.0	7.4	7.7	8.1	8.4
Ironing	2.3	1.8	2.0	2.2	2.4	2.6	2.8	3.0	3.2	3.4	3.6	3.8	4.0	4.2	4.4	4.6	4.8
Mopping	3.5	2.8	3.1	3.4	3.7	4.0	4.3	4.6	4.9	5.2	5.5	5.8	6.1	6.4	6.7	7.0	7.4
Moving furniture	6.0	4.7	5.3	5.8	6.3	6.8	7.4	7.9	8.4	8.9	9.5	10.0	10.5	11	11.6	12.1	12.6
Scrubbing floors	3.8	3.0	3.3	3.7	4.0	4.3	4.7	5.0	5.3	5.7	6.0	6.3	6.7	7.0	7.3	7.6	8.0
Sweeping	3.3	2.6	2.9	3.2	3.5	3.8	4	4.3	4.6	4.9	5.2	5.5	5.8	6.1	6.4	6.6	6.9
Vacuuming	3.5	2.8	3.1	3.4	3.7	4.0	4.3	4.6	4.9	5.2	5.5	5.8	6.1	6.4	6.7	7.0	7.4
Washing dishes	2.3	1.8	2.0	2.2	2.4	2.6	2.8	3.0	3.2	3.4	3.6	3.8	4.0	4.2	4.4	4.6	4.8

Home repair	lb	99	110	121	132	143	154	165	176	187	198	209	220	231	242	253	264
	kg	45	50	55	60	65	70	75	80	85	90	95	100	105	110	115	120
	METs																
Automobile body work	4.0	3.2	3.5	3.9	4.2	4.6	4.9	5.3	5.6	6.0	6.3	6.7	7.0	7.4	7.7	8.1	8.4
Automobile repair	3.0	2.4	2.6	2.9	3.2	3.4	3.7	3.9	4.2	4.5	4.7	5.0	5.3	5.5	5.8	6.0	6.3
Carpentry, general, workshop	3.0	2.4	2.6	2.9	3.2	3.4	3.7	3.9	4.2	4.5	4.7	5.0	5.3	5.5	5.8	6.0	6.3
Carpentry, outside house	6.0	4.7	5.3	5.8	6.3	6.8	7.4	7.9	8.4	8.9	9.5	10.0	10.5	11.0	11.6	12.1	12.6
Carpentry, refinishing furniture	4.5	3.5	3.9	4.3	4.7	5.1	5.5	5.9	6.3	6.7	7.1	7.5	7.9	8.3	8.7	9.1	9.5
Carpentry, sawing hardwood	7.5	5.9	6.6	7.2	7.9	8.5	9.2	9.8	10.5	11.2	11.8	12.5	13.1	13.8	14.4	15.1	15.8
Caulking	5.0	3.9	4.4	4.8	5.3	5.7	6.1	6.6	7.0	7.4	7.9	8.3	8.8	9.2	9.6	10.1	10.5
Cleaning gutters	5.0	3.9	4.4	4.8	5.3	5.7	6.1	6.6	7.0	7.4	7.9	8.3	8.8	9.2	9.6	10.1	10.5

Home repair	lb	99	110	121	132	143	154	165	176	187	198	209	220	231	242	253	264
	kg	45	50	55	60	65	70	75	80	85	90	95	100	105	110	115	120
	METs																
Hanging storm windows	5.0	3.9	4.4	4.8	5.3	5.7	6.1	6.6	7.0	7.4	7.9	8.3	8.8	9.2	9.6	10.1	10.5
Laying or removing carpet	4.5	3.5	3.9	4.3	4.7	5.1	5.5	5.9	6.3	6.7	7.1	7.5	7.9	8.3	8.7	9.1	9.5
Laying tile	4.5	3.5	3.9	4.3	4.7	5.1	5.5	5.9	6.3	6.7	7.1	7.5	7.9	8.3	8.7	9.1	9.5
Plastering, scraping, hanging sheetrock	3.0	2.4	2.6	2.9	3.2	3.4	3.7	3.9	4.2	4.5	4.7	5.0	5.3	5.5	5.8	6.0	6.3
Painting	4.5	3.5	3.9	4.3	4.7	5.1	5.5	5.9	6.3	6.7	7.1	7.5	7.9	8.3	8.7	9.1	9.5
Roofing	6.0	4.7	5.3	5.8	6.3	6.8	7.4	7.9	8.4	8.9	9.5	10.0	10.5	11.0	11.6	12.1	12.6
Sanding floors	4.5	3.5	3.9	4.3	4.7	5.1	5.5	5.9	6.3	6.7	7.1	7.5	7.9	8.3	8.7	9.1	9.5
Wiring, plumbing	3.0	2.4	2.6	2.9	3.2	3.4	3.7	3.9	4.2	4.5	4.7	5.0	5.3	5.5	5.8	6.0	6.3

Lawn and gardening	lb	99	110	121	132	143	154	165	176	187	198	209	220	231	242	253	264
	kg	45	50	55	60	65	70	75	80	85	90	95	100	105	110	115	120
	METs																
Carrying or stacking lumber	5.0	3.9	4.4	4.8	5.3	5.7	6.1	6.6	7.0	7.4	7.9	8.3	8.8	9.2	9.6	10.1	10.5
Chopping wood	6.0	4.7	5.3	5.8	6.3	6.8	7.4	7.9	8.4	8.9	9.5	10	10.5	11.0	11.6	12.1	12.6
Clearing land	5.0	3.9	4.4	4.8	5.3	5.7	6.1	6.6	7.0	7.4	7.9	8.3	8.8	9.2	9.6	10.1	10.5
Digging sandbox	5.0	3.9	4.4	4.8	5.3	5.7	6.1	6.6	7.0	7.4	7.9	8.3	8.8	9.2	9.6	10.1	10.5
Fertilizing or seeding a lawn	2.5	2.0	2.2	2.4	2.6	2.8	3.1	3.3	3.5	3.7	3.9	4.2	4.4	4.6	4.8	5.0	5.3
Gardening with power tools	6.0	4.7	5.3	5.8	6.3	6.8	7.4	7.9	8.4	8.9	9.5	10.0	10.5	11.0	11.6	12.1	12.6
Gardening, general	4.0	3.2	3.5	3.9	4.2	4.6	4.9	5.3	5.6	6.0	6.3	6.7	7.0	7.4	7.7	8.1	8.4
Laying sod	5.0	3.9	4.4	4.8	5.3	5.7	6.1	6.6	7.0	7.4	7.9	8.3	8.8	9.2	9.6	10.1	10.5
Mowing lawn, general	5.5	4.3	4.8	5.3	5.8	6.3	6.7	7.2	7.7	8.2	8.7	9.1	9.6	10.1	10.6	11.1	11.6
Operating snow blower	4.5	3.5	3.9	4.3	4.7	5.1	5.5	5.9	6.3	6.7	7.1	7.5	7.9	8.3	8.7	9.1	9.5
Picking fruit	3.0	2.4	2.6	2.9	3.2	3.4	3.7	3.9	4.2	4.5	4.7	5.0	5.3	5.5	5.8	6.0	6.3
Planting	4.5	3.5	3.9	4.3	4.7	5.1	5.5	5.9	6.3	6.7	7.1	7.5	7.9	8.3	8.7	9.1	9.5
Raking lawn	4.3	3.4	3.8	4.1	4.5	4.9	5.3	5.6	6.0	6.4	6.8	7.1	7.5	7.9	8.3	8.7	9.0
Sacking grass, leaves	4.0	3.2	3.5	3.9	4.2	4.6	4.9	5.3	5.6	6.0	6.3	6.7	7.0	7.4	7.7	8.1	8.4
Trimming with power cutter	3.5	2.8	3.1	3.4	3.7	4.0	4.3	4.6	4.9	5.2	5.5	5.8	6.1	6.4	6.7	7.0	7.4
Trimming manually	4.5	3.5	3.9	4.3	4.7	5.1	5.5	5.9	6.3	6.7	7.1	7.5	7.9	8.3	8.7	9.1	9.5
Watering lawn	1.5	1.2	1.3	1.4	1.6	1.7	1.8	2.0	2.1	2.2	2.4	2.5	2.6	2.8	2.9	3.0	3.2

Music playing	lb	99	110	121	132	143	154	165	176	187	198	209	220	231	242	253	264
	kg	45	50	55	60	65	70	75	80	85	90	95	100	105	110	115	120
	METs																
Accordion	1.8	1.4	1.6	1.7	1.9	2.0	2.2	2.4	2.5	2.7	2.8	3.0	3.2	3.3	3.5	3.6	3.8
Cello	2.0	1.6	1.8	1.9	2.1	2.3	2.5	2.6	2.8	3.0	3.2	3.3	3.5	3.7	3.9	4.0	4.2
Conducting	2.5	2.0	2.2	2.4	2.6	2.8	3.1	3.3	3.5	3.7	3.9	4.2	4.4	4.6	4.8	5.0	5.3
Drums	4.0	3.2	3.5	3.9	4.2	4.6	4.9	5.3	5.6	6.0	6.3	6.7	7.0	7.4	7.7	8.1	8.4

(continued)

TABLE 14.1 Energy Expenditures for Various Sports and Activities *(continued)*

Music playing	lb	99	110	121	132	143	154	165	176	187	198	209	220	231	242	253	264
	kg	45	50	55	60	65	70	75	80	85	90	95	100	105	110	115	120
	METs																
Flute (sitting)	2.0	1.6	1.8	1.9	2.1	2.3	2.5	2.6	2.8	3.0	3.2	3.3	3.5	3.7	3.9	4.0	4.2
Horn	2.0	1.6	1.8	1.9	2.1	2.3	2.5	2.6	2.8	3.0	3.2	3.3	3.5	3.7	3.9	4.0	4.2
Piano or organ	2.5	2.0	2.2	2.4	2.6	2.8	3.1	3.3	3.5	3.7	3.9	4.2	4.4	4.6	4.8	5.0	5.3
Trombone	3.5	2.8	3.1	3.4	3.7	4.0	4.3	4.6	4.9	5.2	5.5	5.8	6.1	6.4	6.7	7.0	7.4
Trumpet	2.5	2.0	2.2	2.4	2.6	2.8	3.1	3.3	3.5	3.7	3.9	4.2	4.4	4.6	4.8	5.0	5.3
Violin	2.5	2.0	2.2	2.4	2.6	2.8	3.1	3.3	3.5	3.7	3.9	4.2	4.4	4.6	4.8	5.0	5.3
Woodwind	2.0	1.6	1.8	1.9	2.1	2.3	2.5	2.6	2.8	3.0	3.2	3.3	3.5	3.7	3.9	4.0	4.2
Guitar, classical, folk (sitting)	2.0	1.6	1.8	1.9	2.1	2.3	2.5	2.6	2.8	3.0	3.2	3.3	3.5	3.7	3.9	4.0	4.2
Guitar, rock 'n' roll (standing)	3.0	2.4	2.6	2.9	3.2	3.4	3.7	3.9	4.2	4.5	4.7	5.0	5.3	5.5	5.8	6.0	6.3
Marching band	4.0	3.2	3.5	3.9	4.2	4.6	4.9	5.3	5.6	6.0	6.3	6.7	7.0	7.4	7.7	8.1	8.4

Occupation	lb	99	110	121	132	143	154	165	176	187	198	209	220	231	242	253	264
	kg	45	50	55	60	65	70	75	80	85	90	95	100	105	110	115	120
	METs																
Baking, moderate effort	4.0	3.2	3.5	3.9	4.2	4.6	4.9	5.3	5.6	6.0	6.3	6.7	7.0	7.4	7.7	8.1	8.4
Baking, light effort	2.5	2.0	2.2	2.4	2.6	2.8	3.1	3.3	3.5	3.7	3.9	4.2	4.4	4.6	4.8	5.0	5.3
Book binding	2.3	1.8	2.0	2.2	2.4	2.6	2.8	3.0	3.2	3.4	3.6	3.8	4.0	4.2	4.4	4.6	4.8
Building roads	6.0	4.7	5.3	5.8	6.3	6.8	7.4	7.9	8.4	8.9	9.5	10.0	10.5	11.0	11.6	12.1	12.6
Carpentry, general	3.5	2.8	3.1	3.4	3.7	4.0	4.3	4.6	4.9	5.2	5.5	5.8	6.1	6.4	6.7	7.0	7.4
Carrying heavy loads	8.0	6.3	7.0	7.7	8.4	9.1	9.8	10.5	11.2	11.9	12.6	13.3	14.0	14.7	15.4	16.1	16.8
Carrying moderate loads (16-40 lb or 7.3-18.1 kg)	8.0	6.3	7.0	7.7	8.4	9.1	9.8	10.5	11.2	11.9	12.6	13.3	14.0	14.7	15.4	16.1	16.8
Chambermaid, making bed (nursing)	2.5	2.0	2.2	2.4	2.6	2.8	3.1	3.3	3.5	3.7	3.9	4.2	4.4	4.6	4.8	5.0	5.3
Coal mining, general	6.0	4.7	5.3	5.8	6.3	6.8	7.4	7.9	8.4	8.9	9.5	10.0	10.5	11.0	11.6	12.1	12.6
Construction, outside, remodeling	5.5	4.3	4.8	5.3	5.8	6.3	6.7	7.2	7.7	8.2	8.7	9.1	9.6	10.1	10.6	11.1	11.6
Custodial work	3.5	2.8	3.1	3.4	3.7	4.0	4.3	4.6	4.9	5.2	5.5	5.8	6.1	6.4	6.7	7.0	7.4
Electrical work, plumbing	3.5	2.8	3.1	3.4	3.7	4.0	4.3	4.6	4.9	5.2	5.5	5.8	6.1	6.4	6.7	7.0	7.4
Farming, vigorous effort	8.0	6.3	7.0	7.7	8.4	9.1	9.8	10.5	11.2	11.9	12.6	13.3	14.0	14.7	15.4	16.1	16.8
Farming, driving tractor	2.5	2.0	2.2	2.4	2.6	2.8	3.1	3.3	3.5	3.7	3.9	4.2	4.4	4.6	4.8	5.0	5.3
Farming, feeding	4.0	3.2	3.5	3.9	4.2	4.6	4.9	5.3	5.6	6.0	6.3	6.7	7.0	7.4	7.7	8.1	8.4
Farming, forking straw bales	8.0	6.3	7.0	7.7	8.4	9.1	9.8	10.5	11.2	11.9	12.6	13.3	14.0	14.7	15.4	16.1	16.8
Farming, milking by hand	3.0	2.4	2.6	2.9	3.2	3.4	3.7	3.9	4.2	4.5	4.7	5.0	5.3	5.5	5.8	6.0	6.3
Farming, shoveling grain	5.5	4.3	4.8	5.3	5.8	6.3	6.7	7.2	7.7	8.2	8.7	9.1	9.6	10.1	10.6	11.1	11.6
Firefighter, general	12.0	9.5	10.5	11.6	12.6	13.7	14.7	15.8	16.8	17.9	18.9	20.0	21.0	22.1	23.1	24.2	25.2
Forestry, chopping, fast	17.0	13.4	14.9	16.4	17.9	19.3	20.8	22.3	23.8	25.3	26.8	28.3	29.8	31.2	32.7	34.2	35.7

Occupation	lb	99	110	121	132	143	154	165	176	187	198	209	220	231	242	253	264
	kg	45	50	55	60	65	70	75	80	85	90	95	100	105	110	115	120
	METs																
Forestry, chopping, slow	5.0	3.9	4.4	4.8	5.3	5.7	6.1	6.6	7.0	7.4	7.9	8.3	8.8	9.2	9.6	10.1	10.5
Forestry, barking trees	7.0	5.5	6.1	6.7	7.4	8.0	8.6	9.2	9.8	10.4	11.0	11.6	12.3	12.9	13.5	14.1	14.7
Forestry, carrying logs	11.0	8.7	9.6	10.6	11.6	12.5	13.5	14.4	15.4	16.4	17.3	18.3	19.3	20.2	21.2	22.1	23.1
Forestry, felling trees	8.0	6.3	7.0	7.7	8.4	9.1	9.8	10.5	11.2	11.9	12.6	13.3	14.0	14.7	15.4	16.1	16.8
Forestry, general	8.0	6.3	7.0	7.7	8.4	9.1	9.8	10.5	11.2	11.9	12.6	13.3	14.0	14.7	15.4	16.1	16.8
Forestry, hoeing	5.0	3.9	4.4	4.8	5.3	5.7	6.1	6.6	7.0	7.4	7.9	8.3	8.8	9.2	9.6	10.1	10.5
Forestry, planting	6.0	4.7	5.3	5.8	6.3	6.8	7.4	7.9	8.4	8.9	9.5	10.0	10.5	11.0	11.6	12.1	12.6
Forestry, hand sawing	7.0	5.5	6.1	6.7	7.4	8.0	8.6	9.2	9.8	10.4	11.0	11.6	12.3	12.9	13.5	14.1	14.7
Forestry, power sawing	4.5	3.5	3.9	4.3	4.7	5.1	5.5	5.9	6.3	6.7	7.1	7.5	7.9	8.3	8.7	9.1	9.5
Forestry, trimming trees	9.0	7.1	7.9	8.7	9.5	10.2	11.0	11.8	12.6	13.4	14.2	15.0	15.8	16.5	17.3	18.1	18.9
Forestry, weeding	4.0	3.2	3.5	3.9	4.2	4.6	4.9	5.3	5.6	6.0	6.3	6.7	7.0	7.4	7.7	8.1	8.4
Locksmith	3.5	2.8	3.1	3.4	3.7	4.0	4.3	4.6	4.9	5.2	5.5	5.8	6.1	6.4	6.7	7.0	7.4
Machine tooling, machining	2.5	2.0	2.2	2.4	2.6	2.8	3.1	3.3	3.5	3.7	3.9	4.2	4.4	4.6	4.8	5.0	5.3
Machine tooling, tapping and drilling	4.0	3.2	3.5	3.9	4.2	4.6	4.9	5.3	5.6	6.0	6.3	6.7	7.0	7.4	7.7	8.1	8.4
Machine tooling, welding	3.0	2.4	2.6	2.9	3.2	3.4	3.7	3.9	4.2	4.5	4.7	5.0	5.3	5.5	5.8	6.0	6.3
Masonry	7.0	5.5	6.1	6.7	7.4	8.0	8.6	9.2	9.8	10.4	11.0	11.6	12.3	12.9	13.5	14.1	14.7
Masseur, masseuse	4.0	3.2	3.5	3.9	4.2	4.6	4.9	5.3	5.6	6.0	6.3	6.7	7.0	7.4	7.7	8.1	8.4
Operating heavy duty equipment	2.5	2.0	2.2	2.4	2.6	2.8	3.1	3.3	3.5	3.7	3.9	4.2	4.4	4.6	4.8	5.0	5.3
Orange grove work	4.5	3.5	3.9	4.3	4.7	5.1	5.5	5.9	6.3	6.7	7.1	7.5	7.9	8.3	8.7	9.1	9.5
Printing (standing)	2.3	1.8	2.0	2.2	2.4	2.6	2.8	3.0	3.2	3.4	3.6	3.8	4.0	4.2	4.4	4.6	4.8
Shoveling, digging ditches	8.5	6.7	7.4	8.2	8.9	9.7	10.4	11.2	11.9	12.6	13.4	14.1	14.9	15.6	16.4	17.1	17.9
Shoveling, >16 lb/min (7.3 kg/min)	9.0	7.1	7.9	8.7	9.5	10.2	11.0	11.8	12.6	13.4	14.2	15.0	15.8	16.5	17.3	18.1	18.9
Shoveling <10 lb/min (4.5 kg/min)	6.0	4.7	5.3	5.8	6.3	6.8	7.4	7.9	8.4	8.9	9.5	10.0	10.5	11.0	11.6	12.1	12.6
Shoveling, 10-15 lb/min (4.5-6.8 kg/min)	7.0	5.5	6.1	6.7	7.4	8.0	8.6	9.2	9.8	10.4	11.0	11.6	12.3	12.9	13.5	14.1	14.7
Standing, light (bartender, store clerk)	2.3	1.8	2.0	2.2	2.4	2.6	2.8	3.0	3.2	3.4	3.6	3.8	4.0	4.2	4.4	4.6	4.8
Steel mill, general	8.0	6.3	7.0	7.7	8.4	9.1	9.8	10.5	11.2	11.9	12.6	13.3	14.0	14.7	15.4	16.1	16.8
Tailoring, general	2.5	2.0	2.2	2.4	2.6	2.8	3.1	3.3	3.5	3.7	3.9	4.2	4.4	4.6	4.8	5.0	5.3
Using heavy power tools (jackhammers)	6.0	4.7	5.3	5.8	6.3	6.8	7.4	7.9	8.4	8.9	9.5	10.0	10.5	11.0	11.6	12.1	12.6
Using heavy tools (not power)	8.0	6.3	7.0	7.7	8.4	9.1	9.8	10.5	11.2	11.9	12.6	13.3	14.0	14.7	15.4	16.1	16.8
Teaching physical education	4.0	3.2	3.5	3.9	4.2	4.6	4.9	5.3	5.6	6.0	6.3	6.7	7.0	7.4	7.7	8.1	8.4

(continued)

TABLE 14.1 Energy Expenditures for Various Sports and Activities *(continued)*

Running	lb	99	110	121	132	143	154	165	176	187	198	209	220	231	242	253	264
	kg	45	50	55	60	65	70	75	80	85	90	95	100	105	110	115	120
	METs																
Jogging, general	7.0	5.5	6.1	6.7	7.4	8.0	8.6	9.2	9.8	10.4	11.0	11.6	12.3	12.9	13.5	14.1	14.7
Jogging, on a minitrampoline	4.5	3.5	3.9	4.3	4.7	5.1	5.5	5.9	6.3	6.7	7.1	7.5	7.9	8.3	8.7	9.1	9.5
Running, 5 mph (8.0 km/h or 12 min/mi)	8.0	6.3	7.0	7.7	8.4	9.1	9.8	10.5	11.2	11.9	12.6	13.3	14.0	14.7	15.4	16.1	16.8
Running, 5.2 mph (8.37 km/h or 11.5 min/mi)	9.0	7.1	7.9	8.7	9.5	10.2	11.0	11.8	12.6	13.4	14.2	15.0	15.8	16.5	17.3	18.1	18.9
Running, 6 mph (9.6 km/h or 10 min/mi)	10.0	7.9	8.8	9.6	10.5	11.4	12.3	13.1	14.0	14.9	15.8	16.6	17.5	18.4	19.3	20.1	21.0
Running, 6.7 mph (10.78 km/h or 9 min/mi)	11.0	8.7	9.6	10.6	11.6	12.5	13.5	14.4	15.4	16.4	17.3	18.3	19.3	20.2	21.2	22.1	23.1
Running, 7 mph (11.3 km/h or 8.5 min/mi)	11.5	9.1	10.1	11.1	12.1	13.1	14.1	15.1	16.1	17.1	18.1	19.1	20.1	21.1	22.1	23.1	24.2
Running, 7.5 mph (12.07 km/h or 8 min/mi)	12.5	9.8	10.9	12.0	13.1	14.2	15.3	16.4	17.5	18.6	19.7	20.8	21.9	23.0	24.1	25.2	26.3
Running, 8 mph (12.8 km/h or 7.5 min/mi)	13.5	10.6	11.8	13.0	14.2	15.4	16.5	17.7	18.9	20.1	21.3	22.4	23.6	24.8	26.0	27.2	28.4
Running, 8.6 mph (13.84 km/h or 7 min/mi)	14.0	11.0	12.3	13.5	14.7	15.9	17.2	18.4	19.6	20.8	22.1	23.3	24.5	25.7	27.0	28.2	29.4
Running, 9 mph (14.5 km/h or 6.5 min/mi)	15.0	11.8	13.1	14.4	15.8	17.1	18.4	19.7	21.0	22.3	23.6	24.9	26.3	27.6	28.9	30.2	31.5
Running, 10 mph (16.1 km/h or 6 min/mi)	16.0	12.6	14.0	15.4	16.8	18.2	19.6	21.0	22.4	23.8	25.2	26.6	28.0	29.4	30.8	32.2	33.6
Running, 10.9 mph (17.54 km/h or 5.5 min/mi)	18.0	14.2	15.8	17.3	18.9	20.5	22.1	23.6	25.2	26.8	28.4	29.9	31.5	33.1	34.7	36.2	37.8
Running, cross country	9.0	7.1	7.9	8.7	9.5	10.2	11.0	11.8	12.6	13.4	14.2	15.0	15.8	16.5	17.3	18.1	18.9
Running, stairs	15.0	11.8	13.1	14.4	15.8	17.1	18.4	19.7	21.0	22.3	23.6	24.9	26.3	27.6	28.9	30.2	31.5
Running, track practice	10.0	7.9	8.8	9.6	10.5	11.4	12.3	13.1	14.0	14.9	15.8	16.6	17.5	18.4	19.3	20.1	21.0

Sports	lb	99	110	121	132	143	154	165	176	187	198	209	220	231	242	253	264
	kg	45	50	55	60	65	70	75	80	85	90	95	100	105	110	115	120
	METs																
Archery (nonhunting)	3.5	2.8	3.1	3.4	3.7	4.0	4.3	4.6	4.9	5.2	5.5	5.8	6.1	6.4	6.7	7.0	7.4
Badminton, competitive	7.0	5.5	6.1	6.7	7.4	8.0	8.6	9.2	9.8	10.4	11.0	11.6	12.3	12.9	13.5	14.1	14.7
Badminton, recreational	4.5	3.5	3.9	4.3	4.7	5.1	5.5	5.9	6.3	6.7	7.1	7.5	7.9	8.3	8.7	9.1	9.5
Basketball, game	8.0	6.3	7.0	7.7	8.4	9.1	9.8	10.5	11.2	11.9	12.6	13.3	14.0	14.7	15.4	16.1	16.8
Basketball, officiating	7.0	5.5	6.1	6.7	7.4	8.0	8.6	9.2	9.8	10.4	11.0	11.6	12.3	12.9	13.5	14.1	14.7
Basketball, shooting baskets	4.5	3.5	3.9	4.3	4.7	5.1	5.5	5.9	6.3	6.7	7.1	7.5	7.9	8.3	8.7	9.1	9.5

Sports	lb	99	110	121	132	143	154	165	176	187	198	209	220	231	242	253	264
	kg	45	50	55	60	65	70	75	80	85	90	95	100	105	110	115	120
	METs																
Basketball, wheelchair	6.5	5.1	5.7	6.3	6.8	7.4	8.0	8.5	9.1	9.7	10.2	10.8	11.4	11.9	12.5	13.1	13.7
Billiards	2.5	2.0	2.2	2.4	2.6	2.8	3.1	3.3	3.5	3.7	3.9	4.2	4.4	4.6	4.8	5.0	5.3
Bowling	3.0	2.4	2.6	2.9	3.2	3.4	3.7	3.9	4.2	4.5	4.7	5.0	5.3	5.5	5.8	6.0	6.3
Boxing, punching bag	6.0	4.7	5.3	5.8	6.3	6.8	7.4	7.9	8.4	8.9	9.5	10.0	10.5	11.0	11.6	12.1	12.6
Boxing, sparring	9.0	7.1	7.9	8.7	9.5	10.2	11.0	11.8	12.6	13.4	14.2	15.0	15.8	16.5	17.3	18.1	18.9
Coaching	4.0	3.2	3.5	3.9	4.2	4.6	4.9	5.3	5.6	6.0	6.3	6.7	7.0	7.4	7.7	8.1	8.4
Cricket	5.0	3.9	4.4	4.8	5.3	5.7	6.1	6.6	7.0	7.4	7.9	8.3	8.8	9.2	9.6	10.1	10.5
Croquet	2.5	2.0	2.2	2.4	2.6	2.8	3.1	3.3	3.5	3.7	3.9	4.2	4.4	4.6	4.8	5.0	5.3
Curling	4.0	3.2	3.5	3.9	4.2	4.6	4.9	5.3	5.6	6.0	6.3	6.7	7.0	7.4	7.7	8.1	8.4
Darts	2.5	2.0	2.2	2.4	2.6	2.8	3.1	3.3	3.5	3.7	3.9	4.2	4.4	4.6	4.8	5.0	5.3
Fencing	6.0	4.7	5.3	5.8	6.3	6.8	7.4	7.9	8.4	8.9	9.5	10.0	10.5	11.0	11.6	12.1	12.6
Football, competitive	9.0	7.1	7.9	8.7	9.5	10.2	11.0	11.8	12.6	13.4	14.2	15.0	15.8	16.5	17.3	18.1	18.9
Football, touch, flag	8.0	6.3	7.0	7.7	8.4	9.1	9.8	10.5	11.2	11.9	12.6	13.3	14.0	14.7	15.4	16.1	16.8
Football or baseball, playing catch	2.5	2.0	2.2	2.4	2.6	2.8	3.1	3.3	3.5	3.7	3.9	4.2	4.4	4.6	4.8	5.0	5.3
Frisbee, catch	3.0	2.4	2.6	2.9	3.2	3.4	3.7	3.9	4.2	4.5	4.7	5.0	5.3	5.5	5.8	6.0	6.3
Frisbee, ultimate	8.0	6.3	7.0	7.7	8.4	9.1	9.8	10.5	11.2	11.9	12.6	13.3	14.0	14.7	15.4	16.1	16.8
Golf	4.5	3.5	3.9	4.3	4.7	5.1	5.5	5.9	6.3	6.7	7.1	7.5	7.9	8.3	8.7	9.1	9.5
Golf, miniature, driving range	3.0	2.4	2.6	2.9	3.2	3.4	3.7	3.9	4.2	4.5	4.7	5.0	5.3	5.5	5.8	6.0	6.3
Gymnastics	4.0	3.2	3.5	3.9	4.2	4.6	4.9	5.3	5.6	6.0	6.3	6.7	7.0	7.4	7.7	8.1	8.4
Handball	12.0	9.5	10.5	11.6	12.6	13.7	14.7	15.8	16.8	17.9	18.9	20.0	21.0	22.1	23.1	24.2	25.2
Handball, team	8.0	6.3	7.0	7.7	8.4	9.1	9.8	10.5	11.2	11.9	12.6	13.3	14.0	14.7	15.4	16.1	16.8
Hang gliding	3.5	2.8	3.1	3.4	3.7	4.0	4.3	4.6	4.9	5.2	5.5	5.8	6.1	6.4	6.7	7.0	7.4
Hockey, field	8	6.3	7.0	7.7	8.4	9.1	9.8	10.5	11.2	11.9	12.6	13.3	14.0	14.7	15.4	16.1	16.8
Hockey, ice	8.0	6.3	7.0	7.7	8.4	9.1	9.8	10.5	11.2	11.9	12.6	13.3	14.0	14.7	15.4	16.1	16.8
Horseback riding	4.0	3.2	3.5	3.9	4.2	4.6	4.9	5.3	5.6	6.0	6.3	6.7	7.0	7.4	7.7	8.1	8.4
In-line skating	12.5	9.8	10.9	12.0	13.1	14.2	15.3	16.4	17.5	18.6	19.7	20.8	21.9	23.0	24.1	25.2	26.3
Kickball	7.0	5.5	6.1	6.7	7.4	8.0	8.6	9.2	9.8	10.4	11.0	11.6	12.3	12.9	13.5	14.1	14.7
Lacrosse	8.0	6.3	7.0	7.7	8.4	9.1	9.8	10.5	11.2	11.9	12.6	13.3	14.0	14.7	15.4	16.1	16.8
Martial arts	10.0	7.9	8.8	9.6	10.5	11.4	12.3	13.1	14.0	14.9	15.8	16.6	17.5	18.4	19.3	20.1	21.0
Motor cross	4.0	3.2	3.5	3.9	4.2	4.6	4.9	5.3	5.6	6.0	6.3	6.7	7.0	7.4	7.7	8.1	8.4
Orienteering	9.0	7.1	7.9	8.7	9.5	10.2	11.0	11.8	12.6	13.4	14.2	15.0	15.8	16.5	17.3	18.1	18.9
Paddleball, recreational	6.0	4.7	5.3	5.8	6.3	6.8	7.4	7.9	8.4	8.9	9.5	10.0	10.5	11.0	11.6	12.1	12.6
Paddleball, competitive	10.0	7.9	8.8	9.6	10.5	11.4	12.3	13.1	14.0	14.9	15.8	16.6	17.5	18.4	19.3	20.1	21.0
Polo	8.0	6.3	7.0	7.7	8.4	9.1	9.8	10.5	11.2	11.9	12.6	13.3	14.0	14.7	15.4	16.1	16.8
Racquetball, recreational	7.0	5.5	6.1	6.7	7.4	8.0	8.6	9.2	9.8	10.4	11.0	11.6	12.3	12.9	13.5	14.1	14.7
Racquetball, competitive	10.0	7.9	8.8	9.6	10.5	11.4	12.3	13.1	14.0	14.9	15.8	16.6	17.5	18.4	19.3	20.1	21.0
Rappeling	8.0	6.3	7.0	7.7	8.4	9.1	9.8	10.5	11.2	11.9	12.6	13.3	14.0	14.7	15.4	16.1	16.8

(continued)

TABLE 14.1 Energy Expenditures for Various Sports and Activities (*continued*)

Sports	lb	99	110	121	132	143	154	165	176	187	198	209	220	231	242	253	264
	kg	45	50	55	60	65	70	75	80	85	90	95	100	105	110	115	120
	METs																
Rock climbing	11.0	8.7	9.6	10.6	11.6	12.5	13.5	14.4	15.4	16.4	17.3	18.3	19.3	20.2	21.2	22.1	23.1
Rope jumping, fast	12.0	9.5	10.5	11.6	12.6	13.7	14.7	15.8	16.8	17.9	18.9	20.0	21.0	22.1	23.1	24.2	25.2
Rope jumping, moderate	10.0	7.9	8.8	9.6	10.5	11.4	12.3	13.1	14.0	14.9	15.8	16.6	17.5	18.4	19.3	20.1	21.0
Rope jumping, slow	8.0	6.3	7.0	7.7	8.4	9.1	9.8	10.5	11.2	11.9	12.6	13.3	14.0	14.7	15.4	16.1	16.8
Rugby	10.0	7.9	8.8	9.6	10.5	11.4	12.3	13.1	14.0	14.9	15.8	16.6	17.5	18.4	19.3	20.1	21.0
Shuffleboard	3.0	2.4	2.6	2.9	3.2	3.4	3.7	3.9	4.2	4.5	4.7	5.0	5.3	5.5	5.8	6.0	6.3
Skateboarding	5.0	3.9	4.4	4.8	5.3	5.7	6.1	6.6	7.0	7.4	7.9	8.3	8.8	9.2	9.6	10.1	10.5
Skating, roller	7.0	5.5	6.1	6.7	7.4	8.0	8.6	9.2	9.8	10.4	11.0	11.6	12.3	12.9	13.5	14.1	14.7
Skydiving	3.5	2.8	3.1	3.4	3.7	4.0	4.3	4.6	4.9	5.2	5.5	5.8	6.1	6.4	6.7	7.0	7.4
Soccer, competitive	10.0	7.9	8.8	9.6	10.5	11.4	12.3	13.1	14.0	14.9	15.8	16.6	17.5	18.4	19.3	20.1	21.0
Soccer, recreational	7.0	5.5	6.1	6.7	7.4	8.0	8.6	9.2	9.8	10.4	11.0	11.6	12.3	12.9	13.5	14.1	14.7
Softball or baseball	5.0	3.9	4.4	4.8	5.3	5.7	6.1	6.6	7.0	7.4	7.9	8.3	8.8	9.2	9.6	10.1	10.5
Softball, pitching	6.0	4.7	5.3	5.8	6.3	6.8	7.4	7.9	8.4	8.9	9.5	10.0	10.5	11.0	11.6	12.1	12.6
Squash	12.0	9.5	10.5	11.6	12.6	13.7	14.7	15.8	16.8	17.9	18.9	20.0	21.0	22.1	23.1	24.2	25.2
Table tennis, ping pong	4.0	3.2	3.5	3.9	4.2	4.6	4.9	5.3	5.6	6.0	6.3	6.7	7.0	7.4	7.7	8.1	8.4
Tai chi	4.0	3.2	3.5	3.9	4.2	4.6	4.9	5.3	5.6	6.0	6.3	6.7	7.0	7.4	7.7	8.1	8.4
Tennis, general	7.0	5.5	6.1	6.7	7.4	8.0	8.6	9.2	9.8	10.4	11.0	11.6	12.3	12.9	13.5	14.1	14.7
Tennis, doubles	6.0	4.7	5.3	5.8	6.3	6.8	7.4	7.9	8.4	8.9	9.5	10.0	10.5	11.0	11.6	12.1	12.6
Tennis, singles	8.0	6.3	7.0	7.7	8.4	9.1	9.8	10.5	11.2	11.9	12.6	13.3	14.0	14.7	15.4	16.1	16.8
Track and field, jumpers	6.0	4.7	5.3	5.8	6.3	6.8	7.4	7.9	8.4	8.9	9.5	10.0	10.5	11.0	11.6	12.1	12.6
Track and field, steeplechase, hurdles	10.0	7.9	8.8	9.6	10.5	11.4	12.3	13.1	14.0	14.9	15.8	16.6	17.5	18.4	19.3	20.1	21.0
Track and field, throwing	4.0	3.2	3.5	3.9	4.2	4.6	4.9	5.3	5.6	6.0	6.3	6.7	7.0	7.4	7.7	8.1	8.4
Trampoline	3.5	2.8	3.1	3.4	3.7	4.0	4.3	4.6	4.9	5.2	5.5	5.8	6.1	6.4	6.7	7.0	7.4
Volleyball	4.0	3.2	3.5	3.9	4.2	4.6	4.9	5.3	5.6	6.0	6.3	6.7	7.0	7.4	7.7	8.1	8.4
Volleyball, beach	8.0	6.3	7.0	7.7	8.4	9.1	9.8	10.5	11.2	11.9	12.6	13.3	14.0	14.7	15.4	16.1	16.8
Volleyball, competitive	8.0	6.3	7.0	7.7	8.4	9.1	9.8	10.5	11.2	11.9	12.6	13.3	14.0	14.7	15.4	16.1	16.8
Volleyball, recreational	3.0	2.4	2.6	2.9	3.2	3.4	3.7	3.9	4.2	4.5	4.7	5.0	5.3	5.5	5.8	6.0	6.3
Wallyball	7.0	5.5	6.1	6.7	7.4	8.0	8.6	9.2	9.8	10.4	11.0	11.6	12.3	12.9	13.5	14.1	14.7
Wrestling	6.0	4.7	5.3	5.8	6.3	6.8	7.4	7.9	8.4	8.9	9.5	10.0	10.5	11.0	11.6	12.1	12.6

Walking	lb	99	110	121	132	143	154	165	176	187	198	209	220	231	242	253	264
	kg	45	50	55	60	65	70	75	80	85	90	95	100	105	110	115	120
	METs																
Backpacking	7.0	5.5	6.1	6.7	7.4	8.0	8.6	9.2	9.8	10.4	11.0	11.6	12.3	12.9	13.5	14.1	14.7
Carrying 1-15 lb (0.5-6.8 kg) load	5.0	3.9	4.4	4.8	5.3	5.7	6.1	6.6	7.0	7.4	7.9	8.3	8.8	9.2	9.6	10.1	10.5

Walking	lb	99	110	121	132	143	154	165	176	187	198	209	220	231	242	253	264
	kg	45	50	55	60	65	70	75	80	85	90	95	100	105	110	115	120
	METs																
Carrying 16-24 lb (7.3-10.9 kg) load	6.0	4.7	5.3	5.8	6.3	6.8	7.4	7.9	8.4	8.9	9.5	10.0	10.5	11.0	11.6	12.1	12.6
Carrying 25-49 lb (11.3-22.2 kg) load	8.0	6.3	7.0	7.7	8.4	9.1	9.8	10.5	11.2	11.9	12.6	13.3	14.0	14.7	15.4	16.1	16.8
Carrying 50-74 lb (22.7-33.6 kg) load	10.0	7.9	8.8	9.6	10.5	11.4	12.3	13.1	14.0	14.9	15.8	16.6	17.5	18.4	19.3	20.1	21.0
Carrying 74+ lb (33.6+ kg) load	12.0	9.5	10.5	11.6	12.6	13.7	14.7	15.8	16.8	17.9	18.9	20.0	21.0	22.1	23.1	24.2	25.2
Climbing hills with 0-9 lb (0-4.1 kg) load	7.0	5.5	6.1	6.7	7.4	8.0	8.6	9.2	9.8	10.4	11.0	11.6	12.3	12.9	13.5	14.1	14.7
Climbing hills with 10-20 lb (4.5-9.1 kg) load	7.5	5.9	6.6	7.2	7.9	8.5	9.2	9.8	10.5	11.2	11.8	12.5	13.1	13.8	14.4	15.1	15.8
Climbing hills with 21-42 lb (9.5-19.1 kg) load	8.0	6.3	7.0	7.7	8.4	9.1	9.8	10.5	11.2	11.9	12.6	13.3	14.0	14.7	15.4	16.1	16.8
Climbing hills with 42+ lb (19.1+ kg) load	9.0	7.1	7.9	8.7	9.5	10.2	11.0	11.8	12.6	13.4	14.2	15.0	15.8	16.5	17.3	18.1	18.9
Hiking, cross country	6.0	4.7	5.3	5.8	6.3	6.8	7.4	7.9	8.4	8.9	9.5	10.0	10.5	11.0	11.6	12.1	12.6
Marching rapidly	6.5	5.1	5.7	6.3	6.8	7.4	8.0	8.5	9.1	9.7	10.2	10.8	11.4	11.9	12.5	13.1	13.7
Racewalking	6.5	5.1	5.7	6.3	6.8	7.4	8.0	8.5	9.1	9.7	10.2	10.8	11.4	11.9	12.5	13.1	13.7
Rock or mountain climbing	8.0	6.3	7.0	7.7	8.4	9.1	9.8	10.5	11.2	11.9	12.6	13.3	14.0	14.7	15.4	16.1	16.8
Walking, <2.0 mph (3.22 km/h)	2.0	1.6	1.8	1.9	2.1	2.3	2.5	2.6	2.8	3.0	3.2	3.3	3.5	3.7	3.9	4.0	4.2
Walking, 2.0 mph (3.22 km/h), level	2.5	2.0	2.2	2.4	2.6	2.8	3.1	3.3	3.5	3.7	3.9	4.2	4.4	4.6	4.8	5.0	5.3
Walking, 2.5 mph (4.02 km/h)	2.8	2.2	2.5	2.7	2.9	3.2	3.4	3.7	3.9	4.2	4.4	4.7	4.9	5.1	5.4	5.6	5.9
Walking, 3.0 mph (4.83 km/h)	3.3	2.6	2.9	3.2	3.5	3.8	4.0	4.3	4.6	4.9	5.2	5.5	5.8	6.1	6.4	6.6	6.9
Walking, 3.5 mph (5.63 km/h)	3.8	3.0	3.3	3.7	4.0	4.3	4.7	5.0	5.3	5.7	6.0	6.3	6.7	7.0	7.3	7.6	8.0
Walking, 3.5 mph (5.63 km/h), uphill	6.0	4.7	5.3	5.8	6.3	6.8	7.4	7.9	8.4	8.9	9.5	10.0	10.5	11.0	11.6	12.1	12.6
Walking, 4.0 mph (6.44 km/h)	5.0	3.9	4.4	4.8	5.3	5.7	6.1	6.6	7.0	7.4	7.9	8.3	8.8	9.2	9.6	10.1	10.5
Walking, 4.5 mph (7.24 km/h)	6.3	5.0	5.5	6.1	6.6	7.2	7.7	8.3	8.8	9.4	9.9	10.5	11.0	11.6	12.1	12.7	13.2
Walking, 5.0 mph (8.05 km/h)	8.0	6.3	7.0	7.7	8.4	9.1	9.8	10.5	11.2	11.9	12.6	13.3	14.0	14.7	15.4	16.1	16.8
Walking, for pleasure	3.5	2.8	3.1	3.4	3.7	4.0	4.3	4.6	4.9	5.2	5.5	5.8	6.1	6.4	6.7	7.0	7.4
Walking, household	2.0	1.6	1.8	1.9	2.1	2.3	2.5	2.6	2.8	3.0	3.2	3.3	3.5	3.7	3.9	4.0	4.2
Walking, grass track	5.0	3.9	4.4	4.8	5.3	5.7	6.1	6.6	7.0	7.4	7.9	8.3	8.8	9.2	9.6	10.1	10.5
Walking the dog	3.0	2.4	2.6	2.9	3.2	3.4	3.7	3.9	4.2	4.5	4.7	5.0	5.3	5.5	5.8	6.0	6.3
Walking to work or class	4.0	3.2	3.5	3.9	4.2	4.6	4.9	5.3	5.6	6.0	6.3	6.7	7.0	7.4	7.7	8.1	8.4

(continued)

TABLE 14.1 Energy Expenditures for Various Sports and Activities (continued)

Water activities	lb	99	110	121	132	143	154	165	176	187	198	209	220	231	242	253	264
	kg	45	50	55	60	65	70	75	80	85	90	95	100	105	110	115	120
	METs																
Canoeing, on camping trip	4.0	3.2	3.5	3.9	4.2	4.6	4.9	5.3	5.6	6.0	6.3	6.7	7.0	7.4	7.7	8.1	8.4
Canoeing, rowing 2.0-3.9 mph (3.22-6.28 km/h), light effort	3.0	2.4	2.6	2.9	3.2	3.4	3.7	3.9	4.2	4.5	4.7	5.0	5.3	5.5	5.8	6.0	6.3
Canoeing, rowing 4.0-5.9 mph (6.44-9.49 km/h), moderate effort	7.0	5.5	6.1	6.7	7.4	8.0	8.6	9.2	9.8	10.4	11.0	11.6	12.3	12.9	13.5	14.1	14.7
Canoeing, rowing >6 mph (9.65 km/h)	12.0	9.5	10.5	11.6	12.6	13.7	14.7	15.8	16.8	17.9	18.9	20.0	21.0	22.1	23.1	24.2	25.2
Canoeing, rowing for pleasure	3.5	2.8	3.1	3.4	3.7	4.0	4.3	4.6	4.9	5.2	5.5	5.8	6.1	6.4	6.7	7.0	7.4
Canoeing, rowing for competition or crew	12.0	9.5	10.5	11.6	12.6	13.7	14.7	15.8	16.8	17.9	18.9	20.0	21.0	22.1	23.1	24.2	25.2
Diving, springboard	3.0	2.4	2.6	2.9	3.2	3.4	3.7	3.9	4.2	4.5	4.7	5.0	5.3	5.5	5.8	6.0	6.3
Kayaking	5.0	3.9	4.4	4.8	5.3	5.7	6.1	6.6	7.0	7.4	7.9	8.3	8.8	9.2	9.6	10.1	10.5
Paddleboating	4.0	3.2	3.5	3.9	4.2	4.6	4.9	5.3	5.6	6.0	6.3	6.7	7.0	7.4	7.7	8.1	8.4
Sailing, windsurfing	3.0	2.4	2.6	2.9	3.2	3.4	3.7	3.9	4.2	4.5	4.7	5.0	5.3	5.5	5.8	6.0	6.3
Sailing, in competition	5.0	3.9	4.4	4.8	5.3	5.7	6.1	6.6	7.0	7.4	7.9	8.3	8.8	9.2	9.6	10.1	10.5
Sailing	3.0	2.4	2.6	2.9	3.2	3.4	3.7	3.9	4.2	4.5	4.7	5.0	5.3	5.5	5.8	6.0	6.3
Skiing, water	6.0	4.7	5.3	5.8	6.3	6.8	7.4	7.9	8.4	8.9	9.5	10.0	10.5	11.0	11.6	12.1	12.6
Skimobiling	7.0	5.5	6.1	6.7	7.4	8.0	8.6	9.2	9.8	10.4	11.0	11.6	12.3	12.9	13.5	14.1	14.7
Skin diving, scuba diving	7.0	5.5	6.1	6.7	7.4	8.0	8.6	9.2	9.8	10.4	11.0	11.6	12.3	12.9	13.5	14.1	14.7
Snorkeling	5.0	3.9	4.4	4.8	5.3	5.7	6.1	6.6	7.0	7.4	7.9	8.3	8.8	9.2	9.6	10.1	10.5
Surfing, body or board	3.0	2.4	2.6	2.9	3.2	3.4	3.7	3.9	4.2	4.5	4.7	5.0	5.3	5.5	5.8	6.0	6.3
Swimming laps, freestyle	10.0	7.9	8.8	9.6	10.5	11.4	12.3	13.1	14.0	14.9	15.8	16.6	17.5	18.4	19.3	20.1	21.0
Swimming, backstroke	7.0	5.5	6.1	6.7	7.4	8.0	8.6	9.2	9.8	10.4	11.0	11.6	12.3	12.9	13.5	14.1	14.7
Swimming, breaststroke	10.0	7.9	8.8	9.6	10.5	11.4	12.3	13.1	14.0	14.9	15.8	16.6	17.5	18.4	19.3	20.1	21.0
Swimming, butterfly	11.0	8.7	9.6	10.6	11.6	12.5	13.5	14.4	15.4	16.4	17.3	18.3	19.3	20.2	21.2	22.1	23.1
Swimming, crawl, fast (75 yd/min or 68.6 m/min)	11.0	8.7	9.6	10.6	11.6	12.5	13.5	14.4	15.4	16.4	17.3	18.3	19.3	20.2	21.2	22.1	23.1
Swimming, crawl, slow (50 yd/min or 45.7 m/min)	8.0	6.3	7.0	7.7	8.4	9.1	9.8	10.5	11.2	11.9	12.6	13.3	14.0	14.7	15.4	16.1	16.8
Swimming, leisurely, not lap	6.0	4.7	5.3	5.8	6.3	6.8	7.4	7.9	8.4	8.9	9.5	10.0	10.5	11.0	11.6	12.1	12.6
Swimming, sidestroke	8.0	6.3	7.0	7.7	8.4	9.1	9.8	10.5	11.2	11.9	12.6	13.3	14.0	14.7	15.4	16.1	16.8
Swimming, synchronized	8.0	6.3	7.0	7.7	8.4	9.1	9.8	10.5	11.2	11.9	12.6	13.3	14.0	14.7	15.4	16.1	16.8
Swimming, treading water	10.0	7.9	8.8	9.6	10.5	11.4	12.3	13.1	14.0	14.9	15.8	16.6	17.5	18.4	19.3	20.1	21.0
Water aerobics, water calisthenics	4.0	3.2	3.5	3.9	4.2	4.6	4.9	5.3	5.6	6.0	6.3	6.7	7.0	7.4	7.7	8.1	8.4

Water activities	lb	99	110	121	132	143	154	165	176	187	198	209	220	231	242	253	264
	kg	45	50	55	60	65	70	75	80	85	90	95	100	105	110	115	120
	METs																
Water jogging	8.0	6.3	7.0	7.7	8.4	9.1	9.8	10.5	11.2	11.9	12.6	13.3	14.0	14.7	15.4	16.1	16.8
Water polo	10.0	7.9	8.8	9.6	10.5	11.4	12.3	13.1	14.0	14.9	15.8	16.6	17.5	18.4	19.3	20.1	21.0
Water volleyball	3.0	2.4	2.6	2.9	3.2	3.4	3.7	3.9	4.2	4.5	4.7	5.0	5.3	5.5	5.8	6.0	6.3
White-water rafting, kayaking	5.0	3.9	4.4	4.8	5.3	5.7	6.1	6.6	7.0	7.4	7.9	8.3	8.8	9.2	9.6	10.1	10.5

Winter activities	lb	99	110	121	132	143	154	165	176	187	198	209	220	231	242	253	264
	kg	45	50	55	60	65	70	75	80	85	90	95	100	105	110	115	120
	METs																
Skating, ice, 9 mph (14.5 km/h) or less	5.0	3.9	4.4	4.8	5.3	5.7	6.1	6.6	7.0	7.4	7.9	8.3	8.8	9.2	9.6	10.1	10.5
Skating, ice	7.0	5.5	6.1	6.7	7.4	8.0	8.6	9.2	9.8	10.4	11.0	11.6	12.3	12.9	13.5	14.1	14.7
Skating, ice, >9 mph (14.5 km/h)	9.0	7.1	7.9	8.7	9.5	10.2	11.0	11.8	12.6	13.4	14.2	15.0	15.8	16.5	17.3	18.1	18.9
Skating, speed, competitive	15.0	11.8	13.1	14.4	15.8	17.1	18.4	19.7	21.0	22.3	23.6	24.9	26.3	27.6	28.9	30.2	31.5
Ski jumping	7.0	5.5	6.1	6.7	7.4	8.0	8.6	9.2	9.8	10.4	11.0	11.6	12.3	12.9	13.5	14.1	14.7
Skiing, cross country, 2.5 mph (4.02 km/h)	7.0	5.5	6.1	6.7	7.4	8.0	8.6	9.2	9.8	10.4	11.0	11.6	12.3	12.9	13.5	14.1	14.7
Skiing, cross country, 4.0 mph (6.44km/h)	8.0	6.3	7.0	7.7	8.4	9.1	9.8	10.5	11.2	11.9	12.6	13.3	14.0	14.7	15.4	16.1	16.8
Skiing, cross country, 5.0-7.9 mph (8.05-12.71 km/h)	9.0	7.1	7.9	8.7	9.5	10.2	11.0	11.8	12.6	13.4	14.2	15.0	15.8	16.5	17.3	18.1	18.9
Skiing, cross country, >8.0 mph (12.8 km/h)	14.0	11.0	12.3	13.5	14.7	15.9	17.2	18.4	19.6	20.8	22.1	23.3	24.5	25.7	27.0	28.2	29.4
Skiing, cross country, uphill	16.5	13.0	14.4	15.9	17.3	18.8	20.2	21.7	23.1	24.5	26.0	27.4	28.9	30.3	31.8	33.2	34.7
Skiing, downhill, light effort	5.0	3.9	4.4	4.8	5.3	5.7	6.1	6.6	7.0	7.4	7.9	8.3	8.8	9.2	9.6	10.1	10.5
Skiing, downhill, moderate effort	6.0	4.7	5.3	5.8	6.3	6.8	7.4	7.9	8.4	8.9	9.5	10.0	10.5	11.0	11.6	12.1	12.6

Adapted, by permission, from Ainsworth et al., 2000, "Compendium of physical activities: An update of activity codes and MET intensities," *Med. Sci. Sports Exerc.* 32: S498-504.

Summary

⊃ At rest the body consumes 3.5 milliliters of oxygen per kilogram of body mass per minute. This resting metabolic rate is known as 1.0 MET.

⊃ The energy cost of an activity can be expressed in METs or as relative oxygen consumed.

⊃ By knowing the energy expenditure of an exercise, one can easily calculate the calories consumed during the activity.

CHAPTER 15

Caloric Values

In this chapter the nutritive values for various food groups are listed. These values were accumulated primarily from data compiled by the United States Department of Agriculture (USDA 2002). Values for specific sport drinks and other food items were attained from the Web sites of various companies.

Caloric Consumption

The simplest method for determining the caloric consumption of a diet is to use a dietary recall log to record food consumption. An example of a dietary recall log can be seen on page 166. All the food consumed in a single day is recorded. Boxes separate breakfast, lunch, and dinner. In addition, a box is available for recording between-meal snacks or other food items consumed during the day. Individuals can use the dietary recall on a daily basis or perhaps provide a three day recall (e.g., food consumption is recorded for three consecutive days) to estimate average daily energy intake. The individual (whether yourself, your athlete, or your client) should be as specific as possible concerning the amount of food consumed. Table 15.1 provides helpful hints on estimating the amount of food consumed. Once the recall is completed, table 15.2 or a computerized dietary analysis can be used to calculate the nutritive value of the diet. The example on page 166 shows the caloric value of the food consumed per meal, including the quantities of protein, fat, and carbohydrate. At the bottom of the dietary recall log, the caloric and macronutrient intakes are summed and the macronutrient composition is computed.

Dietary Recall Log

Name: *Frank Sweet*

Food/beverage description	Cal	Protein (g)	Fat (g)	CHO (g)
Breakfast				
1 bowl of Wheaties	110	3	1	24
6 oz (177 ml) of 2% milk	84	6	3	9
1 banana	109	1	1	28
1 cup of coffee	1	0	0	0
6 oz (177 ml) orange juice	84	1.5	0	18
Lunch				
2 pieces of roasted chicken breast	284	54	6	0
10 leaves of iceberg lettuce	10	0	0	0
1 tomato	26	1	0	6
1 cucumber	34	2	0	7
1 oz (28 g) ketchup	30	0.5	0	7
2 oz (57 g) Italian dressing, low calorie	32	0	2	2
12 oz (355 ml) water	0	0	0	0
Dinner				
12 oz (340 g) sirloin	684	96	30	0
6 oz (170 g) mashed potatoes	223	4	9	35
4 oz (113 g) freshly cooked green beans	40	2	0	8
1 slice of apple pie	277	2	13	40
12 oz (355 ml) ginger ale	120	0	0	30
Other meals or snacks				
12 oz (355 ml) ruby red grapefruit juice	204	0	0	51
1 cup of coffee	1	0	0	0
1 slice of pizza	140	8	3	21
TOTALS	2493	181	68	286
PERCENT OF TOTAL CALORIES		29%	25%	46%

TABLE 15.1 Hints on Estimating the Amount of Food Consumed

Food	Serving	Estimated size
Breads and grains	1/2 cup cereal, pasta, or rice	Volume of cupcake wrapper or half a baseball
	4 oz (113 g) bagel (large)	Diameter of a compact disc
	Medium piece of cornbread	Medium bar of soap
Fruits and vegetables	Medium piece of fruit	Tennis ball
	1/4 cup of dried fruit	Golf ball or handful for average adult
	1/2 cup of fruit or vegetable	Half of a baseball
	1 cup of broccoli	Light bulb
	1/2 cup	6 asparagus spears, 7 or 8 baby carrots
Meat, fish, and poultry	1 oz (28 g)	3 tbsp. meat or poultry
	2 oz (57 g)	Small chicken drumstick or thigh
	3 oz (85 g)	Adult's hand, small chicken breast, or medium pork chop
Cheese	1 oz (28 g)	Average person's thumb, 2 dominoes, or 4 dice

Adapted from USDA (United States Department of Agriculture) 2002, "Nutritive value of foods," *Home and Garden Bulletin* No. 72. (Washington, DC: US Government Printing Office).

TABLE 15.2 Nutritive Value of Various Foods

Beverages (per amount) Soft Drinks (1 oz or 30 ml)	Cal	Protein (g)	Fat (g)	CHO (g)
Cola, regular	12	0	0	3
Cola, diet	0	0	0	0
Club soda	0	0	0	0
Cream soda	15	0	0	4
Diet soda, assorted flavors	0	0	0	0
Fruit-flavored soda	13	0	0	3
Fruit punch	13	Trace	0	3
Ginger ale	10	Trace	0	3
Grape soda	12	0	0	3
Kool-Aid, artificial sweetener	0	0	0	0
Kool-Aid, sugar added	12	0	0	3
Lemon lime soda	12	0	0	3
Lemonade	11	0	0	3
Orange drink	14	0	0	4
Red Bull	14	Trace	0	3
Root beer	12	Trace	0	3
Pineapple grapefruit drink	13	Trace	0	3
Pineapple orange drink	13	Trace	0	3
Tonic water	10	0	0	3

(continued)

TABLE 15.2 Nutritive Value of Various Foods *(continued)*

Coffees, teas, and cocoa (1 oz or 30 ml)	Cal	Protein (g)	Fat (g)	CHO (g)
Coffee, brewed	1	Trace	0	Trace
Coffee, espresso	3	Trace	0	1
Coffee, instant	1	Trace	0	Trace
Cocoa	17	1	Trace	4
Tea, brewed, black	0	0	0	0
Tea, brewed, herbal	0	0	0	0
Tea, instant	0	0	0	0

Fruit juices and sport drinks (1 oz or 30 ml)	Cal	Protein (g)	Fat (g)	CHO (g)
Accelerade	11	0.50	0	2
Apple juice	14	Trace	0	3
Allsport	9	0	0	3
Carrot juice	12	Trace	Trace	3
Cranberry juice	18	0	0	4
Cytomax cool citrus	4	0	0	1
Gatorade	6	0	0	2
Grapefruit juice, fresh	11	Trace	0	3
Grapefruit juice, sweetened	13	Trace	0	3
Grapefruit juice, unsweetened	11	Trace	0	3
Grape juice, bottled or canned	17	Trace	0	4
Grape juice, prep frozen	15	Trace	0	4
Iced tea, original	11	0	0	3
Lemon juice, fresh	7	Trace	0	2
Lemon juice, bottled	6	Trace	0	2
Lemonade	14	0	0	3
Lime juice, fresh	8	Trace	0	3
Lime juice, bottled	6	Trace	0	2
Mixed berry juice	15	0	0	4
Orange juice	14	Trace	0	3
Orange juice, light	9	Trace	0	2
Paradise Blend Juice	15	Trace	0	4
Pineapple juice	15	Trace	0	4
Powerade	9	0	0	2
Prune juice, bottled	20	Trace	0	5
Ruby red grapefruit juice	17	0	0	4
Strawberry kiwi juice	16	0	0	4
White grape juice	20	0	0	5

Alcohols (1 oz or 30 ml)	Cal	Protein (g)	Fat (g)	CHO (g)
Beer, regular	12	Trace	0	1
Beer, light	8	Trace	0	<0.5
Gin, rum, vodka, whiskey—80 proof	64	0	0	0
Gin, rum, vodka, whiskey—86 proof	73	0	0	0

Alcohols (1 oz or 30 ml)	Cal	Protein (g)	Fat (g)	CHO (g)
Gin, rum, vodka, whiskey—90 proof	74	0	0	0
Wine, dessert dry	36	Trace	0	1
Wine, dessert sweet	44	Trace	0	3
Wine, table red	20	Trace	0	1
Wine, table white	19	Trace	0	Trace

Cheeses (1 oz or 30 ml)	Cal	Protein (g)	Fat (g)	CHO (g)
American, processed	106	6.5	9	Trace
American cheese spread	82	5	6	2
Blue	100	6	8	1
Brick	105	6.5	8	1
Brie	95	6	8	Trace
Camembert	85	5.5	7	Trace
Caraway	107	7	8	1
Cheddar	114	7	9	Trace
Colby	112	7	9	1
Cottage	29	3.5	1	1
Cottage, 2% fat	26	4	<1	1
Cottage, 1% fat	21	3.5	Trace	1
Cottage, dry curd	24	5	Trace	0.5
Cream, regular	99	2	10	1
Cream, low fat	18	1	1.5	0.5
Cream, fat free	8	1	Trace	0.5
Feta	75	4	6	1
Gorgonzola	111	7	9	0
Gouda	101	7	7.5	0.5
Gruyere	117	8.5	9	Trace
Limburger	93	5.5	7.5	Trace
Monterey Jack	106	7	8.5	1
Mozzarella, slim, low moisture	80	7.5	4.5	1
Mozzarella, whole milk, regular	80	5.5	5.5	0.5
Mozzarella, whole milk, moist	90	6	7	0.5
Muenster	104	6.5	8.5	0.5
Neufchatel	74	3	6.5	1
Parmesan, hard	111	10	7.5	1
Parmesan, grated	129	12	9	1
Provolone	100	7	7.5	0.5
Ricotta, part skim	39	3	2	1.5
Ricotta, whole milk	49	3	3.5	1
Romano, hard	110	9	7.5	1
Romano, grated	128	10.5	9	1
Roquefort	105	6	9	0.5
Swiss	107	8	8	1
Swiss, processed	95	7	7	0.5

(continued)

TABLE 15.2 Nutritive Value of Various Foods *(continued)*

Milk products (1 oz or 30 ml)	Cal	Protein (g)	Fat (g)	CHO (g)
Milk, 1% fat	12	1	0.5	1.5
Milk, 2% fat	14	1	0.5	1.5
Milk, nonfat	10	1	Trace	1.5
Milk, whole	17	1	1	1.5
Buttermilk	12	1	0.5	1.5
Milk, instant nonfat dry	102	10	Trace	15
Evaporated nonfat milk, canned	22	2	Trace	3
Evaporated whole milk, canned	38	2	2	3
Chocolate milk, 1%	18	1	0.5	3
Chocolate milk, 2%	20	1	0.5	3
Chocolate milk, whole	24	1	1	3
Hot cocoa, whole milk	25	1	1	3
Instant breakfast, 1% milk	23	1.5	Trace	3.5
Instant breakfast, 2% milk	25	1.5	0.5	3.5
Instant breakfast, nonfat milk	22	1.5	Trace	3.5
Instant breakfast, whole milk	28	1.5	1	3.5
Eggnog	38	1	2	4
Milkshake, chocolate	36	1	1	6
Milkshake, strawberry	32	1	1	5.5
Milkshake, vanilla	32	1	1	5
Milk, goat	20	1	1	1.5
Milk, sheep	31	1.5	2	1.5
Milk, soybean	9	1	0.5	0.5
Yogurt, low fat, plain	18	1.5	0.5	2
Yogurt, low fat, fruit	29	1	0.5	5.5
Yogurt, nonfat milk	16	1.5	Trace	2
Yogurt, whole milk	17	1	1	1.5

Eggs (per amount or per egg)	Cal	Protein (g)	Fat (g)	CHO (g)
Egg, whole, medium	66	5	4	1
Egg, whole, large	75	6	5	1
Egg, whole, extra large	86	7	6	1
Egg white, large	17	4	0	Trace
Egg yolk, large	59	3	5	Trace
Egg, fried	92	6	7	1
Egg, hard boiled	78	6	5	1
Egg, poached	75	6	5	1
Egg, scrambled with milk	101	7	7	1
Egg substitute, liquid (1/4 cup)	53	8	2	Trace

Fats (1 tsp.)	Cal	Protein (g)	Fat (g)	CHO (g)
Butter, salted	36	Trace	4	Trace
Margarine, hard, 80% fat	34	Trace	4	Trace
Margarine, soft, 80% fat	34	Trace	4	Trace
Margarine, hard, 60% fat	26	Trace	3	0
Margarine, soft, 60% fat	26	Trace	3	0
Margarine, spread, 40% fat	17	Trace	2	0

Oils (1 tbsp.)	Cal	Protein (g)	Fat (g)	CHO (g)
Canola	124	0	14	0
Corn	120	0	14	0
Olive	119	0	14	0
Peanut	119	0	14	0
Safflower, high oleic	120	0	14	0
Sesame	120	0	14	0
Soybean	120	0	14	0
Sunflower	120	0	14	0

Salad dressings (per tbsp.)	Cal	Protein (g)	Fat (g)	CHO (g)
Blue cheese, regular	77	1	8	1
Blue cheese, light	15	1	1	Trace
Caesar, regular	78	Trace	8	Trace
Caesar, light	17	Trace	1	3
French, regular	67	Trace	6	3
French, light	22	Trace	1	4
Italian, regular	69	Trace	7	1
Italian, light	16	Trace	1	1
Mayonnaise, regular	99	Trace	11	Trace
Mayonnaise, light	49	Trace	5	1
Mayonnaise, fat free	12	0	Trace	2
Russian, regular	76	Trace	8	2
Russian, light	23	Trace	1	4
Thousand Island, regular	59	Trace	6	2
Thousand Island, light	24	Trace	2	2
Vinegar and oil	70	0	8	Trace

Fish and shellfish (1 oz or 28 g)	Cal	Protein (g)	Fat (g)	CHO (g)
Anchovy, raw	37	5.78	1.37	0
Bass, freshwater raw	32	5.5	1	0
Bluefish, baked, broiled	45	7.5	1.5	0
Bluefish, breaded, fried	58	6.5	3	1.5
Bluefish, raw	35	5.5	1	0
Carp, raw	36	5	1.5	0
Catfish, raw	33	5	1	0
Cod, baked with butter	37	6.5	1	0
Cod, batter fried	56	5.5	3	23
Cod, baked, broiled	30	6.5	Trace	0
Cod, poached, steamed	29	6	Trace	0
Cod, smoked	22	5	Trace	0
Cod, Atlantic, raw	23	5	Trace	0
Crab, cooked	24	5	Trace	1
Haddock, breaded, fried	58	5.5	3	2.5
Haddock, smoked	33	7	0.5	0
Haddock, raw	22	5.5	Trace	0
Herring, pickled	74	4	5	2.5

(continued)

TABLE 15.2 Nutritive Value of Various Foods *(continued)*

Fish and shellfish (1 oz or 28 g)	Cal	Protein (g)	Fat (g)	CHO (g)
Herring, smoked, kippered	62	7	3.5	0
Herring, canned, liquid	59	5.5	4	0
Lobster meat, cooked	28	6	Trace	0.5
Mackerel, fried	49	7	2.5	0
Mackerel, Atlantic, baked, broiled	74	7	5	0
Mackerel, Atlantic, raw	58	5.5	4	0
Mackerel, Pacific, raw	45	6	3	0
Northern pike, raw	25	5.5	Trace	0
Ocean perch, breaded, fried	62	5.5	3.5	2.5
Pollock, baked, broiled	28	6.5	0.5	0
Pollock, poached	36	6.5	0.5	0
Salmon, Atlantic, canned	36	5	1.5	0
Salmon, broiled, baked	61	7.5	3	0
Salmon, coho, steamed, poached	52	7.5	2	0
Salmon, pink, raw	33	5.5	1	0
Salmon, smoked	33	5	1	0
Sardines	59	7	3	0
Scampi, fried in crumbs	69	6	3.5	3.5
Sea trout, raw	30	4.5	1	0
Sea trout, cooked	37	6	1.5	0
Shrimp, boiled	28	6	0.5	0
Shrimp, breaded and fried	65	2.5	3.5	5.5
Smelt, rainbow, raw	28	5	0.5	0
Snapper, raw	28	6	0.5	0
Snapper, baked, broiled	36	7.5	0.5	0
Sole/flounder, baked, broiled	33	7	0.5	0
Sole/flounder, batter fried	83	4.5	5	4
Sole/flounder, breaded, fried	53	5	2.5	2.5
Sole/flounder, steamed	26	5.5	0.5	0
Sole/flounder, raw	26	5.5	0.5	0
Sole, lemon, raw	23	5	Trace	0
Sole, lemon, breaded, fried	56	4.5	3	2.5
Sole, lemon, steamed	26	6	Trace	0
Squid (calamari), fried in flour	50	5	2	2
Swordfish, raw	34	5.5	1	0
Swordfish, baked, broiled	44	7	1.5	0
Trout, baked, broiled	43	7.5	1	0
Tuna, in oil	56	8.5	2.5	0
Tuna, in water	37	8.5	Trace	0
Tuna, raw	31	6.5	0.5	0
Whiting, breaded, fried	54	5	1.5	2

Fruits (1 piece, 1 cup, 1 oz, or 28 g)	Cal	Protein (g)	Fat (g)	CHO (g)
Apple, with peel	81	Trace	Trace	21
Apple slices, with peel, fresh	63	Trace	Trace	16
Applesauce, sweetened (1 cup)	194	Trace	Trace	51

| Applesauce, unsweetened (1 cup) | 105 | Trace | Trace | 28 |
Fruits (1 piece, 1 cup, 1 oz, or 28 g)	Cal	Protein (g)	Fat (g)	CHO (g)
Apricot	17	Trace	Trace	4
Apricot halves, heavy syrup (1 cup)	214	1	Trace	55
Apricot nectar, canned (1 cup)	141	1	Trace	36
Avocado (1 oz or 28 g)	41	Trace	4	2.5
Banana	109	1	1	28
Blackberries, fresh (1 cup)	75	1	1	18
Blueberries, fresh (1 cup)	81	1	1	20
Blueberries, frozen, sweetened (1 cup)	186	1	Trace	50
Cantaloupe, cubes (1 cup)	56	1	Trace	13
Cherries, sour (1 cup)	88	2	Trace	22
Cherries, sweet (1 cup)	49	1	1	11
Dates, whole, each	23	Trace	Trace	6
Figs, whole, each	21	Trace	Trace	5.5
Figs, dried, each	49	0.5	Trace	12.5
Fruit cocktail, heavy syrup (1 cup)	181	1	Trace	47
Fruit cocktail, light syrup	109	1	Trace	28
Grapefruit half, pink or red	37	1	Trace	9
Grapefruit half, white	39	1	Trace	10
Grapefruit sections, canned (1 cup)	152	1	Trace	39
Grapes (1 cup)	114	1	1	28
Honeydew melon, cubes (1 cup)	60	1	Trace	16
Kiwi	46	1	Trace	11
Lemon, fresh	17	1	Trace	5
Mango, fresh, slices (1 cup)	107	1	Trace	28
Mango, fresh, whole	135	1	1	35
Mixed fruit, frozen, thawed (1 cup)	245	4	Trace	61
Nectarine	67	1	1	16
Orange	62	1	Trace	15
Orange sections, fresh (1 cup)	85	2	Trace	21
Papaya, whole, fresh	119	2	Trace	30
Papaya, cubed, fresh (1 cup)	55	1	Trace	14
Peaches, fresh	42	1	Trace	11
Peach slices, frozen or thawed (1 cup)	235	2	Trace	60
Peach halves, heavy syrup	73	Trace	Trace	20
Peach halves, light syrup	43	1	Trace	11
Peach halves, dried	31	Trace	Trace	8
Pears	98	1	1	25
Pear halves, heavy syrup	56	Trace	Trace	15
Pear halves, light syrup	38	Trace	Trace	10
Pineapple, diced (1 cup)	76	1	1	19
Pineapple slices, heavy syrup (1 cup)	198	1	Trace	51
Pineapple slices, light syrup (1 cup)	149	1	Trace	39
Plantains	218	2	1	57
Plums	36	1	Trace	9

(continued)

TABLE 15.2 Nutritive Value of Various Foods *(continued)*

Plums, canned, heavy syrup	41	Trace	Trace	11
Fruits (1 piece, 1 cup ·1oz, or 28 g)	**Cal**	**Protein (g)**	**Fat (g)**	**CHO (g)**
Plums, canned, light syrup	27	Trace	Trace	7
Prunes, dried	20	Trace	Trace	5
Raisins, seedless (1 cup)	435	5	1	115
Raspberries, fresh (1 cup)	60	1	1	14
Raspberries, thawed, sweetened (1 cup)	258	2	Trace	65
Strawberries, fresh	5	Trace	Trace	1
Strawberries, frozen (1 cup)	245	1	Trace	66
Tangerine, fresh	37	1	Trace	9
Tangerines, canned, light syrup (1 cup)	154	1	Trace	41
Watermelon (wedge)	92	2	1	21

Grain products (per amount) Breads (per slice unless otherwise indicated)	Cal	Protein (g)	Fat (g)	CHO (g)
Bagel (4 in. or 10 cm), plain	245	9	1	48
Banana bread	196	3	6	33
Biscuit (2.5 in. or 6.4 cm), regular	93	2	4	13
Biscuit (2.5 in. or 6.4 cm), low fat	63	2	1	12
Bread crumbs, dry, grated (1 oz or 28 g)	111	4	1.5	21
Bread crumbs, soft (1 oz or 28 g)	76	2.5	1	14
Cornbread	188	4	6	29
Cracked wheat	65	2	1	12
Croissant	231	5	12	26
Doughnuts	59	1	3	7
English muffin	133	4	1	26
Egg bread (challah)	230	8	4	38
French	138	4	2	26
Italian	54	2	1	10
Mixed grain	65	3	1	12
Oatmeal	74	2.5	1	14
Pita pocket, white (4 in. or 10 cm)	78	3	0.5	15.5
Pumpernickel	80	3	1	15
Raisin	71	2	1	14
Rolls, dinner	84	2	2	14
Rolls, hamburger or hotdog	123	4	2	22
Rolls, hard, kaiser	167	6	2	30
Rolls, sweet	109	2	4	17
Rye	83	3	1	15
Rye, light	47	2	1	9
White	67	2	1	12
Whole wheat	65	2	1	12

Cereals (1 cup without milk)	Cal	Protein (g)	Fat (g)	CHO (g)
All Bran	158	8	2	46
Apple Cinnamon Cheerios	157	2.5	2.5	33.5

Apple Jacks	110	1.5	Trace	25.5
Cereals (1 cup without milk)	**Cal**	**Protein (g)**	**Fat (g)**	**CHO (g)**
Buc Wheats	110	2	1	24
Captain Crunch	143	1.5	1.5	30.5
Captain Crunchberries	139	1.5	1.5	29.5
Captain Crunch, Peanut Butter	149	2.5	2.5	29.5
Cheerios	110	4	2	19.5
Cheerios, Honey Nut	115	3	1	24
Cocoa Krispies	160	2.5	1.5	36
Cocoa Puffs	119	1	1	27
Corn Chex	111	2	Trace	25
Corn Flakes	102	2	Trace	24
Corn Pops	118	1	Trace	28
Crispix	108	2	Trace	25
Farina, cooked	14	0.5	Trace	3
Fruit Loops	117	1	1	26
Frosted Mini-Wheats	173	5	1	42
Golden Grahams	155	2.5	1.5	34.5
Honey Frosted Wheaties	110	2	Trace	26
Honey Nut Clusters	213	5	3	43
Kix	114	2	1	26
Life	161	4	1.5	33.5
Lucky Charms	116	2	1	25
Nature Valley Granola	330	8	13.5	48
100% Natural Cereal with oats and honey	436	10	14	72
100% Natural Cereal with raisins, low fat	390	8	6	72
Product 19	110	3	Trace	25
Puffed Rice	56	1	Trace	13
Puffed Wheat	44	2	Trace	10
Raisin Bran	178	4	1	43
Rice Chex	112	1.5	1	25
Rice Krispies	110	2	Trace	24
Special K	115	6	Trace	22
Sugar Smacks	137	2.5	1.5	32
Total	105	3	0.5	22.5
Trix	122	1	2	26
Wheat Chex	104	3	1	23
Wheaties	110	3	1	24

Cakes (per slice)	**Cal**	**Protein (g)**	**Fat (g)**	**CHO (g)**
Boston crème	232	2	8	39
Brownies	227	3	9	36
Brownies, fat free	89	1	Trace	22
Angel food	129	3	Trace	29
Carrot	103	1	5.5	13
Cheese	257	4	18	20

(continued)

TABLE 15.2 Nutritive Value of Various Foods *(continued)*

Coffee	263	4	15	29

Cakes (per slice)	Cal	Protein (g)	Fat (g)	CHO (g)
Fruit	139	1	4	26
Gingerbread	263	3	12	36
Pound	109	2	6	14
Pound, fat free	79	2	Trace	17
Short	225	4	9	32
Sponge	187	5	3	36
White, coconut	399	5	12	71
White, white frosting	264	4	9	42
Yellow, chocolate frosting	243	2	11	35

Pies (slice)	Cal	Protein (g)	Fat (g)	CHO (g)
Apple	277	2	13	40
Blueberry	271	2	12	41
Cherry	304	2	13	47
Chocolate cream	344	3	22	38
Coconut custard	270	6	14	31
Lemon meringue	303	2	10	53
Pecan	452	5	21	65
Pumpkin	229	4	10	30

Cookies (1 cookie)	Cal	Protein (g)	Fat (g)	CHO (g)
Butter	23	Trace	1	3
Chocolate chip	48	1	2	7
Fig bar	56	1	1	11
Oatmeal	113	2	5	17
Peanut butter	72	1	4	9
Sandwich type, chocolate	47	Trace	2	7
Sandwich type, vanilla	48	Trace	2	7
Shortbread	40	Trace	2	5
Sugar	72	1	3	10
Vanilla wafers	18	Trace	1	3

Additional breakfast foods and pastries	Cal	Protein (g)	Fat (g)	CHO (g)
Éclair	262	6	16	24
Danish pastry, cheese	266	6	16	26
Danish pastry, fruit	263	4	13	34
French toast	149	5	7	16
Granola bar, hard, plain	134	3	6	18
Granola bar, soft, chocolate chip	119	2	5	20
Granola bar, soft, raisin	113	2	5	19
Granola bar, soft, chocolate covered, peanut butter	144	3	9	15
Matzo	112	3	Trace	24

Muffin, blueberry	158	3	4	27
Additional breakfast foods and pastries	**Cal**	**Protein (g)**	**Fat (g)**	**CHO (g)**
Muffin, bran with raisins	106	2	3	19
Muffin, corn	174	3	5	29
Muffin, oat bran	154	4	4	28
Nutri Grain cereal bar, fruit filled	136	2	3	27
Oat Bran (1 cup)	88	7	2	25
Pancakes	83	3	3	11
Toaster pastries, brown sugar cinnamon	206	3	7	34
Toaster pastries, chocolate with frosting	201	3	5	37
Toaster pastries, fruit filled	204	2	5	37
Toaster pastries, low fat	193	2	3	40
Waffles	218	6	11	25
Waffles, low fat	83	2	1	15

Chips and crackers (1 oz or 28 g)	**Cal**	**Protein (g)**	**Fat (g)**	**CHO (g)**
Corn chips, plain	153	2	9	16
Corn chips, barbecue	148	2	9	16
Crackers, cheese (10 crackers)	50	1	3	6
Crackers, graham (2 squares)	59	1	1	11
Melba toast	20	0.5	Trace	4
Rye wafer	37	1	Trace	9
Saltine (4 crackers)	52	1	1	9
Tortilla chips, nacho flavor	139	2	7	18
Tortilla chips, nacho flavor, reduced fat	126	2	4	20
Tortilla chips, regular	142	2	7	18
Tortilla chips, regular, reduced fat	54	2	1	11
Wheat cracker, thin	124	3	5	18
Whole-wheat crackers	124	3	5.5	18

Pasta and noodles (1 cup)	**Cal**	**Protein (g)**	**Fat (g)**	**CHO (g)**
Egg noodles, cooked	213	8	2	40
Egg noodles, spinach, cooked	211	8	3	39
Macaroni, elbows, enriched	197	7	1	40
Noodles, chow mein	237	4	14	26
Pasta, tomato sauce with cheese	192	6	2	39
Pasta, meatballs in tomato sauce	260	11	10	31
Spaghetti, cooked, enriched	197	7	1	40
Spaghetti, whole wheat, cooked	174	7	1	37

Pizza (per slice)	**Cal**	**Protein (g)**	**Fat (g)**	**CHO (g)**
Pizza, cheese	140	8	3	21
Pizza, meat and vegetables	184	13	5	21

(continued)

TABLE 15.2 Nutritive Value of Various Foods (*continued*)

Pizza, pepperoni	181	10	7	20

Popcorn (1 cup)	**Cal**	**Protein (g)**	**Fat (g)**	**CHO (g)**
Popcorn, plain, air popped	31	1	Trace	6
Popcorn, cooked in oil, salted	55	1	3	6
Popcorn, syrup coated	168	3	3	34

Rice (1 cup)	**Cal**	**Protein (g)**	**Fat (g)**	**CHO (g)**
Brown, cooked	216	5	2	45
White, regular, cooked	205	4	Trace	45
White, instant, prepared	162	3	Trace	35
Wild, cooked	166	7	1	35

Legumes, nuts, and seeds (per amount)	**Cal**	**Protein (g)**	**Fat (g)**	**CHO (g)**
Almonds, whole toasted (1 oz or 28 g)	164	6	14.5	6.5
Baked beans, canned (1 cup)	236	12	1	52
Beans, black (1 cup)	227	15	1	41
Beans, kidney (1 cup)	225	15	1	40
Beans, lima (1 cup)	216	15	1	39
Beans, navy (1 cup)	258	16	1	48
Beans, pinto (1 cup)	234	14	1	44
Black-eyed peas (1 cup)	200	13	1	36
Cashews, dry roasted (1 oz or 28 g)	163	4	13	9
Cashews, oil roasted (1 oz or 28 g)	172	5	14	8
Chestnuts (1 cup)	350	5	3	76
Chickpeas (1 cup)	269	15	4	45
Coconut, shredded (1 cup)	283	3	27	12
Hummus, commercial (1 tbsp.)	23	1	1	2
Lentils (1 cup)	230	18	1	40
Macadamia nuts (1 oz or 28 g)	203	2	22	4
Mixed nuts, dry roasted (1 oz or 28 g)	168	5	15	7
Mixed nuts, oil roasted (1 oz or 28 g)	175	5	16	6
Peanuts, dry roasted (1 oz or 28 g)	166	7	14	6
Peanuts, oil roasted (1 oz or 28 g)	165	7	14	5
Peanut butter (1 tbsp.)	95	4	8	3
Peas (1 cup)	231	16	1	41
Pine nuts (1 oz or 28 g)	160	7	14	4
Pistachio nuts (1 oz or 28 g)	161	6	13	8
Pumpkin and squash kernels (1 oz or 28 g)	148	9	12	4
Refried beans (1 cup)	237	14	3	39
Sesame seeds (1 tbsp.)	47	2	4	1
Soybeans (1 cup)	298	29	15	17
Sunflower seeds (1 oz or 28 g)	165	5	14	7
Tahini (1 tbsp.)	89	3	8	3

Walnuts (1 oz or 28 g)	185	4	18	4

Beef (1 oz or 28 g)	Cal	Protein (g)	Fat (g)	CHO (g)
Beef chuck, pot roasted, lean and fat	98	7.5	7.5	0
Beef chuck, pot roasted, lean	77	9	4.5	0
Beef frankfurter (each frank)	142	5	13	1
Beef liver, fried	61	7.5	2.5	2.5
Beef rib, oven roasted, lean	68	7.5	4	0
Beef round, pot roasted, lean and fat	74	8	4.5	0
Beef round, pot roasted, lean	60	9	2.5	0
Beef round, oven roasted, lean	54	8	2	0
Beef rump roast, lean	51	8.5	2	0
Ground beef, lean	77	7	5.5	0
Ground beef, regular	82	6.5	6	0
Sirloin steak, lean and fat	73	8	4.5	0
Sirloin steak, lean	57	8	2.5	0
T-bone steak, lean and fat	92	7	7	0

Lamb (1 oz or 28 g)	Cal	Protein (g)	Fat (g)	CHO (g)
Chops, arm, braised, lean and fat	98	8.5	6.5	0
Chops, arm, braised, lean	55	10	4	0
Leg, roasted, lean and fat	73	7.5	4.5	0
Leg, roasted, lean	54	8	2.5	0
Loin, broiled, lean and fat	90	7	6.5	0
Loin, broiled, lean	61	8.5	2.5	0
Rib roasted, lean an fat	102	6	8.5	0
Rib roasted, lean	66	7.5	3.5	0

Pork (1 oz or 28 g)	Cal	Protein (g)	Fat (g)	CHO (g)
Bacon, regular	36	2	3	Trace
Bacon, Canadian	43	5.5	2	0.5
Beef and pork frankfurter	144	5	13	1
Ham, roasted, lean and fat	69	6	4.5	0
Ham, roasted, lean	44	7	2.5	0
Pork chop, broiled, lean and fat	68	8	3.5	0
Pork chop, broiled, lean	57	8.5	2.5	0
Pork chop, pan fried, lean and fat	78	8.5	4.5	0
Port chop, pan fried, lean	66	9	3	0
Ribs, roasted backribs	105	7	8.5	0
Ribs, country-style braised	84	6.5	6	0
Ribs, spareribs	112	8.5	8.5	0
Sausages (link)	52	2	4.5	0.5

Sandwich meats (1 oz or 28 g)	Cal	Protein (g)	Fat (g)	CHO (g)
Bologna, beef	89	3.5	8	0.5

(continued)

TABLE 15.2 Nutritive Value of Various Foods *(continued)*

Bratwurst	92	4	8	1
Chicken roll, light	45	5.5	2	0.5

Sandwich meats (1 oz or 28 g)	Cal	Protein (g)	Fat (g)	CHO (g)
Ham, regular	52	5	3	1
Ham, extra lean	38	5.5	1.5	0.5
Liverwurst	93	4	8	0.5
Salami, beef and pork	72	4	5.5	0.5
Turkey roll	41	5.5	2	Trace
Turkey bologna	56	4	4.5	Trace
Turkey ham	36	5.5	1.5	0.5
Turkey salami	55	4.5	4	Trace
Turkey pastrami	37	5	2	0.5

Chicken (1 cup, 1 oz, 1 part, or 28 g)	Cal	Protein (g)	Fat (g)	CHO (g)
Chicken, fried, batter dipped, breast	364	35	18	13
Chicken, fried, batter dipped, drumstick	193	16	11	6
Chicken, fried, batter dipped, thigh	238	19	14	8
Chicken, fried, batter dipped, wing	159	10	11	5
Chicken, fried, flour coated, breast	218	31	9	2
Chicken, fried, flour coated, drumstick	120	13	7	1
Chicken, fried, dark meat (1 oz or 28 g)	68	8	3	2
Chicken, fried, light meat (1 oz or 28 g)	54	9.5	1.5	Trace
Chicken, roasted, breast	142	27	3	0
Chicken, roasted, drumstick	76	12	2	0
Chicken, roasted, thigh	109	13	6	0
Chicken meat, stewed (1 cup)	332	43	17	0
Chicken giblets	228	37	7	1
Chicken liver	35	5	1	Trace
Chicken frankfurter	116	6	9	3

Turkey (1 cup, oz, or part or 28 g)	Cal	Protein (g)	Fat (g)	CHO (g)
Turkey, dark meat	53	8	2	0
Turkey, white meat	44	8.5	1	0
Turkey, ground patty	193	22	11	0
Turkey, giblets (1 cup)	242	39	7	3

Soups (1 cup)	Cal	Protein (g)	Fat (g)	CHO (g)
Bean with ham	231	13	9	27
Bean with pork	172	8	6	23
Beef broth	29	5	0	2
Beef noodle	83	5	3	9
Chicken broth	17	3	0	1
Chicken noodle, canned ready	175	13	6	17

| Chicken noodle, prepared with water | 75 | 4 | 2 | 9 |
| Chicken and rice, canned ready | 116 | 7 | 3 | 14 |

Soups (1 cup)	Cal	Protein (g)	Fat (g)	CHO (g)
Chicken and rice, prepared with water	60	4	2	7
Chicken and vegetable	166	12	5	19
Chicken, rice, and vegetable	88	6	1	12
Clam chowder, New England with milk	164	9	7	17
Clam chowder, New England, canned	117	5	2	20
Clam chowder, Manhattan	78	2	2	12
Cream of chicken, milk	191	7	11	15
Cream of chicken, water	117	3	7	9
Cream of mushroom, milk	203	6	14	15
Cream of mushroom, water	129	2	9	9
Lentil	126	8	2	20
Minestrone, prepared with water	82	4	3	11
Minestrone, canned ready	123	5	3	20
Pea, green	165	9	3	27
Tomato, milk	161	6	6	22
Tomato, water	85	2	2	17
Vegetable, prepared with water	72	2	2	12
Vegetable, canned ready	81	4	1	13

Sauces (1 cup, tbsp., or tsp.)	Cal	Protein (g)	Fat (g)	CHO (g)
Barbecue (1 tbsp.)	12	Trace	Trace	2
Hoisin (1 tbsp.)	35	1	1	7
Nacho cheese (1/4 cup)	119	5	10	3
Pepper or hot (1 tsp.)	1	Trace	Trace	Trace
Salsa (1 tbsp.)	4	Trace	Trace	1
Soy (1 tbsp.)	9	1	Trace	1
Spaghetti/marinara/pasta (1 cup)	143	4	5	21
Teriyaki (1 tbsp.)	15	1	0	3
Worchester (1 tbsp.)	11	0	0	3

Gravies (1/4 cup)	Cal	Protein (g)	Fat (g)	CHO (g)
Beef	31	2	1	3
Chicken	47	1	3	3
Country sausage	96	3	8	4
Mushroom	30	1	2	3
Turkey	31	2	1	3

Condiments (1 tbsp. or oz or 28 g)	Cal	Protein (g)	Fat (g)	CHO (g)
Chocolate syrup, thin type (1 tbsp.)	53	Trace	Trace	12
Chocolate syrup, fudge type (1 tbsp.)	67	1	2	12
Ketchup (1 oz or 28 g)	30	0.5	Trace	7
Maple syrup	52	0	0	13

(continued)

TABLE 15.2 Nutritive Value of Various Foods *(continued)*

Mustard (1 oz or 28 g)	21	1.5	1	2

Puddings (1 cup, 1 oz, or 28 g)	Cal	Protein (g)	Fat (g)	CHO (g)
Chocolate, with 2% milk, instant (1/2 cup)	150	5	3	28
Chocolate, with 2% milk, regular (1/2 cup)	151	5	3	28
Vanilla, with 2% milk, instant (1/2 cup)	148	4	2	28
Vanilla, with 2% milk, regular (1/2 cup)	141	4	2	26
Chocolate, ready to eat (1 oz or 28 g)	150	3	5	26
Rice, ready to eat (1 oz or 28 g)	184	2	8	25
Tapioca, ready to eat (1 oz or 28 g)	134	2	4	22
Vanilla, ready to eat (1 oz or 28 g)	147	3	4	25
Chocolate, fat free (1 oz or 28 g)	107	3	Trace	23
Tapioca, fat free (1 oz or 28 g)	98	2	Trace	23
Vanilla, fat free (1 oz or 28 g)	105	2	Trace	24

Candy (bar, piece)	Cal	Protein (g)	Fat (g)	CHO (g)
Caramel	39	Trace	1	8
Chocolate bar, plain	226	3	14	22
Chocolate bar, with almonds	216	4	14	19
Chocolate bar, with peanuts (Mr. Goodbar)	267	5	17	25
Chocolate bar, with rice cereal (Nestle Crunch)	230	3	12	28
Chocolate-covered peanuts (each)	21	0.5	1.5	10
Chocolate-covered raisins (each)	4	Trace	Trace	1.5
Chocolate fudge (piece)	65	Trace	1	14
Chocolate fudge with nuts (piece)	81	1	3	14
Gummy bears (each)	9	0	0	2
Gummy worms (each)	29	0	0	7
Hard candy (each)	24	0	Trace	6
Jelly beans (each)	10	0	Trace	2.5
Kit Kat	216	3	11	27
M&M's, plain (piece)	3	Trace	Trace	0.5
M&M's, peanut (piece)	10	Trace	0.5	1
Milky Way	258	3	10	44
Reese's Peanut Butter Cup	38	1	2	4
Snickers	273	5	14	34
Vanilla fudge	59	Trace	1	13
Vanilla fudge with nuts	62	Trace	2	11

Additional sweets (bar, piece, or 1 tbsp.)	Cal	Protein (g)	Fat (g)	CHO (g)
Fruit and juice bar	63	1	Trace	16
Ice pop	42	0	0	10.5
Italian ices (1/2 cup)	61	Trace	Trace	15

Gelatin dessert, regular (1/2 cup)	80	2	0	19
Gelatin dessert, with aspartame	8	1	0	1

Additional sweets (bar, piece, or 1 tbsp.)	Cal	Protein (g)	Fat (g)	CHO (g)
Jams (1 tbsp.)	56	Trace	Trace	14
Jellies (1 tbsp.)	54	Trace	Trace	13

Vegetables (1 piece, 1 oz, or 28 g)	Cal	Protein (g)	Fat (g)	CHO (g)
Alfalfa sprouts (1 oz or 28 g)	9	1	Trace	1
Artichoke heart, marinated	60	4	Trace	11
Asparagus, raw spear	4	0.5	Trace	1
Asparagus, canned spear	4	0.5	Trace	1
Bamboo shoot, sliced, raw (1 oz or 28 g)	8	0.5	Trace	1.5
Bamboo shoot, sliced, canned (1 oz or 28 g)	5	0.5	Trace	1
Bean sprout, fresh, raw (1 oz or 28 g)	9	1	Trace	1.5
Bean sprout, boiled (1 oz or 28 g)	6	0.5	Trace	1
Bean spout, stir fried (1 oz or 28 g)	14	1	Trace	3
Green beans, raw (1 oz or 28 g)	9	0.5	Trace	2
Green beans, fresh, cooked (1 oz or 28 g)	10	0.5	Trace	2
Green beans, frozen, cooked (1 oz or 28 g)	8	0.5	Trace	1.5
Green beans, canned, drained (1 oz or 28 g)	6	0.5	Trace	1
Lima beans, fresh, cooked (1 oz or 28 g)	35	2	Trace	6.5
Lima beans, dry, small (1 oz or 28 g)	98	6	0.5	18
Lima beans, canned, drained (1 oz or 28 g)	27	1.5	Trace	5
White beans, dry (1 oz or 28 g)	95	6	0.5	18
White beans, dry, cooked (1 oz or 28 g)	40	2.5	Trace	7.5
Yellow wax beans, raw (1 oz or 28 g)	9	0.5	Trace	2
Yellow wax beans, frozen (1 oz or 28 g)	8	0.5	Trace	1.5
Beets, cooked (1 oz or 28 g)	9	0.5	Trace	2
Beets, pickled slices (1 oz or 28 g)	18	Trace	Trace	4.5
Broccoli, raw spears	9	1	Trace	2
Broccoli, cooked spears	10	1	Trace	2
Brussels sprouts, raw (1 oz or 28 g)	12	0.5	Trace	2.5
Brussels sprouts, cooked (1 oz or 28 g)	11	0.5	Trace	2.5
Cabbage, raw, shredded (1 oz or 28 g)	7	0.5	Trace	1.5
Cabbage, cooked (1 oz or 28 g)	6	0.5	Trace	1.5
Bok choy, raw, shredded (1 oz or 28 g)	4	0.5	Trace	0.5
Bok choy, cooked (1 oz or 28 g)	3	0.5	Trace	0.5
Red cabbage, raw (1 oz or 28 g)	8	0.5	Trace	1.5
Red cabbage, cooked (1 oz or 28 g)	6	0.5	Trace	1

(continued)

TABLE 15.2 Nutritive Value of Various Foods *(continued)*

Vegetables (1 piece, 1 oz, or 28 g)	Cal	Protein (g)	Fat (g)	CHO (g)
Carrot, whole, raw	31	1	Trace	7
Carrot, grated, raw (1 oz or 28 g)	6	Trace	Trace	1.5
Carrots, sliced, cooked (1 oz or 28 g)	9	Trace	Trace	2
Carrots, frozen, cooked (1 oz or 28 g)	7	Trace	Trace	2
Carrots, canned, drained (1 oz or 28 g)	5	Trace	Trace	1
Cauliflower, raw	3	Trace	Trace	1
Cauliflower, cooked	4	Trace	Trace	1
Cauliflower, frozen, cooked	4	Trace	Trace	1
Celery, raw, chopped	6	Trace	Trace	1
Collards, fresh, cooked (1 oz or 28 g)	6	1	Trace	0.5
Collards, frozen, cooked (1 oz or 28 g)	8	1	Trace	1
Corn, kernels, frozen (1 oz or 28 g)	16	0.5	Trace	4
Corn on the cob, cooked	83	3	1	19
Corn, canned, drained (1 oz or 28 g)	21	0.5	Trace	5
Corn, canned, cream style (1 oz or 28 g)	23	0.5	Trace	5
Cucumber, whole, peeled	34	2	Trace	7
Cucumber, whole, with peel	39	2	Trace	8
Eggplant, cooked (1 oz or 28 g)	4	Trace	Trace	1
Endive, chopped (1 oz or 28 g)	1	Trace	Trace	1
Jerusalem artichoke, sliced (1 oz or 28 g)	14	0.5	Trace	3
Kale, fresh, chopped (1 oz or 28 g)	5	Trace	Trace	1
Kohlrabi, raw, slices (1 oz or 28 g)	6	0.5	Trace	1
Leeks, chopped, raw (1 oz or 28 g)	4	Trace	Trace	1
Lettuce, butterhead (leaf)	1	Trace	Trace	Trace
Lettuce, iceberg (leaf)	1	Trace	Trace	Trace
Lettuce, romaine (leaf)	1	Trace	Trace	Trace
Mushrooms, raw, sliced (1 oz or 28 g)	2	Trace	Trace	0.5
Mushrooms, cooked (1 oz or 28 g)	5	0.5	Trace	1
Mushrooms, canned, drained (1 oz or 28 g)	5	0.5	Trace	1
Mushroom, shiitake (1 oz or 28 g)	10	Trace	Trace	2.5
Mustard greens, cooked (1 oz or 28 g)	3	0.5	Trace	0.5
Okra, fresh, cooked (1 oz or 28 g)	6	0.5	Trace	1
Okra, frozen, cooked (1 oz or 28 g)	6	0.5	Trace	1
Onions, chopped, raw (1 oz or 28 g)	7	Trace	Trace	1.5
Onion slice, raw	5	Trace	Trace	1
Onion, dehydrated flakes (1 tbsp.)	17	Trace	Trace	4
Onion rings, frozen, heated (each)	24	0.5	1.5	2.5
Parsnips, sliced, raw (1 oz or 28 g)	16	Trace	Trace	4
Peas, raw, cooked	8	0.5	Trace	1.5
Peas, frozen, cooked	10	0.5	Trace	2
Green chili pepper, raw	18	1	Trace	4
Red chili pepper, raw	18	1	Trace	4
Jalapeno pepper, raw	32	1	Trace	8
Jalapeno pepper, ring	3	Trace	Trace	1
Pumpkin, canned (1 cup)	83	3	1	20

Pumpkin, cooked, mashed (1 cup)	49	2	Trace	12
Red radish	1	Trace	Trace	Trace

Vegetables (1 piece, 1 oz, or 28 g)	Cal	Protein (g)	Fat (g)	CHO (g)
Rutabaga, cooked, cubed (1 cup)	66	2	Trace	15
Sauerkraut, canned in liquid (1 cup)	45	2	Trace	10
Spinach, fresh, cooked (1 cup)	41	5	Trace	6
Spinach, canned (1 cup)	49	6	1	7
Summer squash (1 cup)	36	2	1	8
Butternut squash, baked (1 cup)	94	3	Trace	24
Winter squash, boiled (1 cup)	80	2	1	18
Tomato, fresh, whole	26	1	Trace	6
Tomatoes, whole, canned (1 cup)	46	2	Trace	10
Tomatoes, cherry	4	Trace	Trace	1
Turnip, cubed (1 cup)	33	1	Trace	8
Mixed vegetables, frozen, cooked (1 cup)	107	5	Trace	24
Mixed vegetables, canned (1 cup)	77	4	Trace	15
Water chestnuts (1 cup)	70	1	Trace	17

Potatoes (1 cup or piece)	Cal	Protein (g)	Fat (g)	CHO (g)
Baked, with skin	220	5	Trace	51
Baked, flesh only	145	3	Trace	34
Potato skin, oven baked	115	2	Trace	27
Boiled	117	2.5	Trace	27
French fries, oven heated (10 pieces)	100	2	4	16
Hash browns (1 cup)	326	4	22	33
Mashed potatoes, prepared with milk (1 cup)	237	4	12	32
Mashed potatoes, prepared with milk and margarine (1 cup)	223	4	9	35
Potato pancake	207	5	12	22
Potatoes au gratin, homemade (1 cup)	323	12	19	28
Potatoes au gratin, mix	228	6	10	31
Scalloped potatoes, recipe (1 cup)	211	7	9	26
Sweet potato, with skin	150	3	Trace	35
Sweet potato, without skin	164	3	Trace	38

Mexican foods	Cal	Protein (g)	Fat (g)	CHO (g)
Beef taco (large)	568	32	32	41
Beef taco (small)	369	21	21	27
Burrito, beans and cheese	189	8	6	27
Burrito, beans and meat	255	11	9	33
Chimichanga, beef	425	20	20	43
Cheese enchilada	319	10	19	29
Nachos with cheese (6-8 nachos)	346	9	19	36
Taco salad (1.5 cups)	279	31	15	24
Tostada, beans and beef	333	16	17	30
Tostada, with guacamole	181	6	12	16

Adapted from USDA (United States Department of Agriculture) 2002, "Nutritive value of foods," *Home and Garden Bulletin* No. 72. (Washington, DC: US Government Printing Office).

To determine the percentages of protein, fat, and carbohydrate in a diet, the total calories for each of these macronutrients must be computed and then divided by the total caloric intake. The example dietary recall log on page 166 shows that the diet of the fictitious Frank Sweet consisted of 286 g of carbohydrate. This equals 1,144 calories (286 g × 4 kcal/g carbohydrate), and the percentage of carbohydrate in the diet can be calculated by dividing the number of calories of carbohydrate by the total number of calories consumed in the diet. Using this example, 46% of the calories in Mr. Sweet's diet are from carbohydrate. The amounts of calories per gram of macronutrient are as follows:

- Protein—4 cal/g
- Fat—9 cal/g
- Carbohydrate—4 cal/g

For comparison purposes the food and nutrient intakes for children and adults are displayed in table 15.3. Table 15.3 provides the total energy and macronutrient breakdown in calories and grams, respectively. The table also reports the mean intakes of energy and protein as percentages of the recommended daily allowance (RDA) for Americans. The data from these tables were compiled from data collected by the United States Department of Agriculture (USDA 1999a and b). Tables 15.2 and 15.3 provide only the caloric value and macronutrient contribution of each food item. For a more detailed nutrient breakdown the reader should examine the primary sources.

TABLE 15.3　Food and Nutrient Intakes for Children and Adults

Age (y)	Gender	Energy (cal)	% RDA	Protein (g)	% RDA	Fat (g)	CHO (g)
6-9	Males	2,003	103	70	258	74	273
	Females	1,768	91	61	227	64	243
10-11	Males	2,050	101	71	244	75	280
	Females	1,825	91	63	214	67	250
12-19	Males	2,765	99	97	184	103	366
	Females	1,911	87	65	145	69	262
20-39	Males	2,759	95	103	168	104	334
	Females	1,772	79	65	131	65	229
40-59	Males	2,377	89	93	147	91	286
	Females	1,647	79	64	127	62	208
60+	Males	1,961	85	78	124	74	242
	Females	1,436	76	58	117	52	186

RDA = Recommended Daily Allowance; CHO = carbohydrate.

Adapted from the USDA (United States Department of Agriculture), Agricultural Research Service, 1999, "Food and nutrient intakes by children, 1994-96, 1998" and the USDA, Agricultural Research Service, 1998, "Data tables: Food and nutrient intakes by race, 1994-96" (Washington, DC: US Government Printing Office).

Summary

- Caloric consumption can be computed by using a dietary recall log to record all food consumed.
- If the total grams of protein, fat, and carbohydrate are known, the percentage of each of these macronutrients consumed in the diet can be computed.

Testing Descriptions

While this is a book of data it is important to know how to test your athletes or students so that you can compare their scores to the data. The following testing descriptions are provided for your convenience:

Muscular Strength Testing

The following test descriptions correspond with data from chapter 3.

Bench Press

1. The individual being tested lies supine on the bench, with feet flat on the floor, back straight, and eyes below the edge of the weight supports. He grasps the bar with a closed, pronated grip, with the hands slightly wider than shoulder-width apart.

2. The individual removes the bar from the rack and places it over the chest with or without the assistance of the spotter. He lowers the bar to touch the chest at approximately nipple level, keeping his wrists rigid and directly above his elbows (see photo *a*).

3. Once making contact with the chest, the individual pushes the bar upward until his elbows are fully extended, keeping his back flat on the bench without arching it or raising his chest (see photo *b*). Upon completing the repetition, he returns the bar to the rack.

4. The load and recovery format should be followed as described in the protocol for assessing a 1RM on page 34.

1RM Squat

1. The individual grasps the bar with his hands in a closed, pronated position (width will depend on the bar position and the individual's comfort).

2. The individual steps under the bar, keeping his feet parallel to each other.

3. The bar can be placed in either a low bar (see figure *a*) or a high bar position (see figure *b*). In the low bar position, the individual places the bar across the posterior deltoid, with the bar resting across the middle of the trapezius. In the high bar position, the individual places the bar above the posterior deltoid, with the bar resting at the base of the neck. In the low bar position the hands are wider than shoulder-width apart, while in the high bar position the hands are slightly wider than shoulder-width apart.

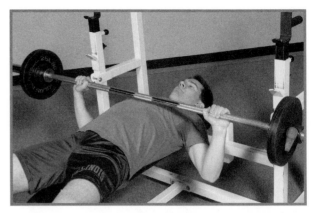

a

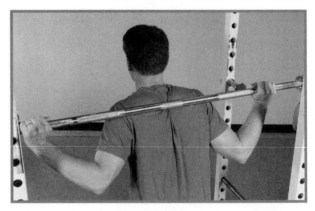

b

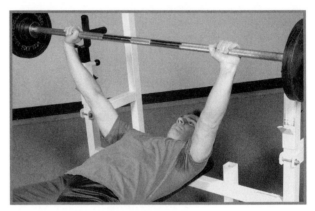

a

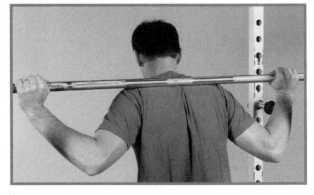

b

4. The individual lifts his elbows upward to create a shelf for the bar. The individual's chest is held up and out, scapulae are adducted, and head is tilted slightly up (see photo *c*).

5. The individual removes the bar from the rack and takes a couple of steps backward, placing his feet at least shoulder-width apart, with the toes pointed outward.

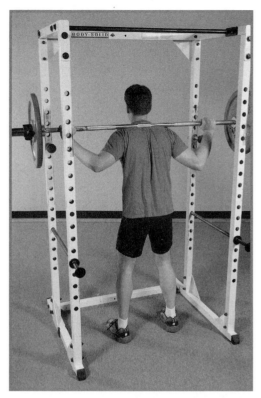

c

6. During the downward movement, the individual slowly flexes his hips and knees, keeping his torso-to-floor angle relatively constant. His back remains flat, with chest out and elbows high. Heels remain on the floor, and his knees are positioned over his toes. The hips and knees continue to flex until the thighs are parallel to the floor (see photo *d*).

7. Once the individual reaches the parallel position, his hips and knees are extended. He maintains body position (head, back, chest, legs) throughout the lift. His hips and knees are extended until he reaches the starting position. The bar is then racked.

8. The load and recovery format should be followed as described in the protocol for assessing a 1RM on page 34.

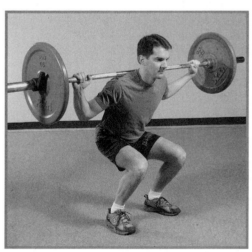

d

Power Clean

1. The individual stands with his feet approximately shoulder-width apart and his toes pointed slightly outward. His knees and hips are flexed so that his hips are lower than his shoulders. He grasps the bar, placing his hands slightly wider than shoulder-width apart and in a closed, pronated position.

2. His feet are flat on the floor and the bar is approximately 1 in. (2.5 cm) in front of his shins and over the balls of his feet.

3. His back is flat or slightly arched, his chest is up and out, and his scapulae are adducted. His head is aligned with the vertebral column or slightly hyperextended. His shoulders are over or slightly in front of the bar and his eyes are focused straight ahead or upward (see photo *a*).

4. The individual lifts the bar off the floor by forcefully contracting his hip and knee extensors. This lift is known as the *first pull*, and during this phase the torso-to-floor angle remains constant and the elbows remain fully extended. The back stays flat and the bar maintains its distance from the shins. The hips should not rise before the shoulders (see photo *b*).

5. As the individual raises the bar above his knees, he thrusts hips forward and slightly flexes his knees to get his thighs under the bar. This movement is known as the *scoop* phase (see photo *c*).

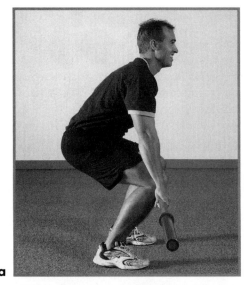

a

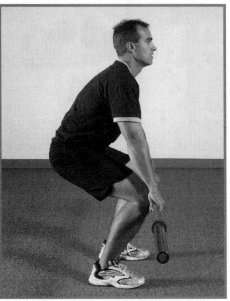

b

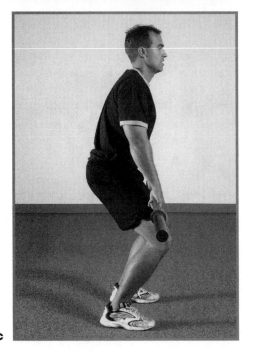

c

6. The next phase is the *second pull*. The individual forcefully extends his hips and knees and plantar-flexes his ankles. He keeps the bar close to his body, his back flat, and his elbows extended as long as possible. When his lower body is fully extended, he shrugs his shoulders (see photo *d*). When his shoulders reach their final elevation, he flexes his elbows, pulling his body under the bar. This action is continued for as long as possible. During this phase the torso remains erect or slightly hyperextended. The heels may lose contact with the floor.

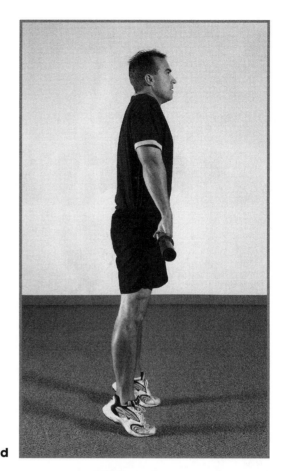

d

7. After the body is fully extended and the bar has reached maximum height, the individual pulls his body under the bar and rotates his arms around and under the bar. The hips and knees are flexed into a quarter-squat position. Once his arms are under the bar, he lifts his elbows so that his upper arms are parallel to the floor. This phase is known as the *catch* phase. The bar is racked across the clavicles and anterior deltoids (see photo *e*). The individual then extends both his knees and hips so that he stands fully upright.

8. The load and recovery format should be followed as described in the protocol for assessing a 1RM on page 34.

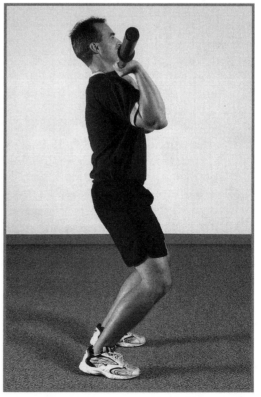

e

Muscular Endurance Testing

The following descriptions correspond with data presented in chapter 4.

Bent-Knee Sit-Up

1. The individual starts on her back with her knees bent and her hands interlocked behind her neck. The backs of her hands are touching the floor or mat. The individual's partner holds her feet with his hands to keep them firmly on the ground (see photo *a*).

2. On the command (stopwatch begins), the individual raises her upper body off the floor until her elbows touch her thighs (see photo *b*).

3. The individual lowers herself until the upper portion of her back touches the floor or mat. Her head, hands, arms, and elbows do not need to touch the floor.

4. The partner counts the number of repetitions performed in 1 min.

Partial Curl-Up

1. With masking tape or string, two parallel lines are placed 10 cm apart on a mat or floor.

2. The individual starts on her back with her knees bent and arms straight and fully extended at her sides. Her palms are flat on the ground, with her fingers contacting the top line (see photo *a*).

3. On the command, the individual curls her upper back so that both her middle fingers reach the 10 cm mark (second line). During each curl-up, her palms and feet remain in contact with the floor or mat (see photo *b*).

4. The individual performs as many curl-ups as possible in 1 min or curls in time to a metronome set for 40 beats/min (20 curl-ups per minute). No contact or support by a partner is permitted.

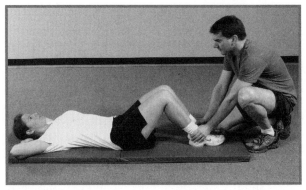

a

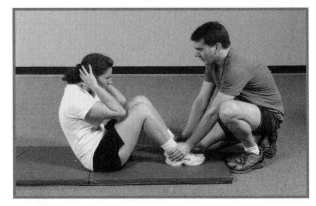

b

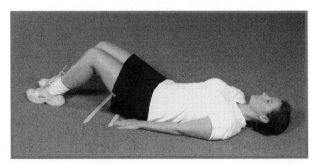

a

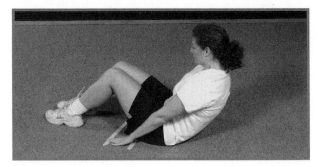

b

Pull-Up or Chin-Up

1. The individual starts by hanging from the bar with his arms straight and his hands in an overhand position for the pull-up or in an underhand position for the chin-up. His thumbs are wrapped around the bar for both hand positions (see photo *a*).

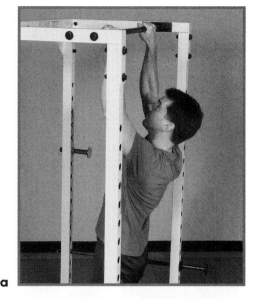

a

2. The individual pulls his body upward until his chin reaches above the bar (see photo *b*).

3. After each pull-up, the individual returns to the starting position.

4. Swinging movements should be avoided.

5. The number of repetitions performed until exhaustion is counted.

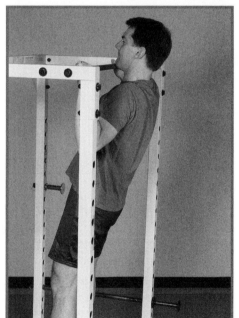

b

Push-Up

1. The individual assumes the up position with his body rigid and straight. The hands are slightly wider than shoulder-width apart and the fingers are pointing forward (see photo *a*).

2. A partner places a fist on the floor beneath the individual's chest.

3. The individual lowers himself to the fist and raises himself back to the starting position.

4. Throughout each push-up, the individual maintains a rigid back.

5. The partner counts the total number of push-ups performed either to exhaustion or in 1 min.

6. The female performs the push-up from the bent-knee position (see photo *b*).

7. Her hands should be placed slightly ahead of her shoulders so that in the lowered position her hands are directly under her shoulders.

8. If her partner is a male, a 3 in. (7.6 cm) sponge should be placed under her sternum to substitute for the fist.

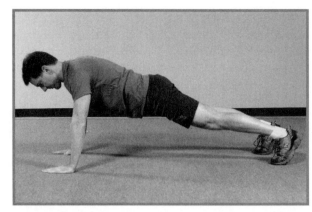

a

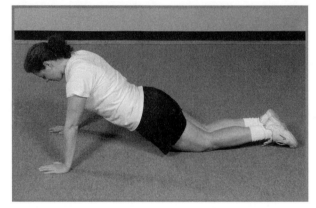

b

Flexed-Arm Hang

1. The bar should be higher than the individual's standing height.

2. An overhand grip should be used, with the thumbs wrapped around the bar.

3. With assistance from spotters, the individual is raised so that her chin is above the bar but not touching the bar. Her arms are flexed and her chest is close to the bar.

4. The individual hangs with no support. The time in seconds is recorded from the moment that the spotters release their support to the moment that the individual's chin touches the bar or falls below the bar.

Parallel Bar Dips

1. The individual begins the exercise with the arms and upper legs straight and the knees flexed at 90° (see photo *a*).

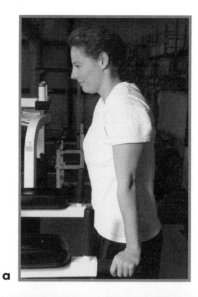

a

2. The individual lowers herself until the elbows are at 90° and the upper arms are parallel to the floor (see photo *b*).
3. The individual returns to the starting position. The return to starting position marks one complete repetition.
4. The number of repetitions performed until exhaustion is recorded.

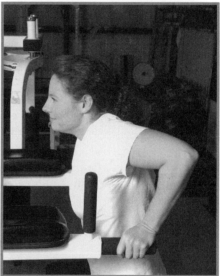

b

YMCA Bench Press

1. Using an adjustable barbell and weight plates, set the resistance at 80 lbs (36.3 kg) for males and at 35 lbs (15.9 kg) for females.
2. Set a metronome at 60 beats/min to establish a rate of 30 repetitions per minute.
3. The individual, with her arms extended and her hands shoulder-width apart on the barbell, lowers the bar to her chest. Without pausing, she raises the bar until her arms are fully extended.
4. The individual continues lifting and lowering the barbell until she is unable to maintain the cadence of the metronome.

Anaerobic Power Testing

The following test descriptions correspond with data from chapter 5.

Wingate Anaerobic Power Test

1. The subject sits comfortably on the cycle ergometer and warms up for 4 to 5 min at a comfortable pace (60-70 rpm) against a resistance equal to 20% of that calculated for the subsequent test.

2. The subject performs two to four 5 s sprints at the end of each minute of the warm-up.

3. At the conclusion of the warm-up the subject is given a minute to stretch before starting the test. This time can also be used for further instruction and for any last-minute adjustments to the equipment (e.g., securing the toe clips).

4. Upon the command, the subject pedals as fast as possible, and as the subject reaches full speed the tester applies the resistance (0.075 kg · kg body mass^{-1} for tests performed on a Monark cycle ergometer). The resistance may change depending on the cycle ergometer being used. Some laboratories record the maximal pedaling rate (rpm$_{max}$) during the warm-up (Hoffman et al. 2000). If this information is available, resistance should be applied when the subject attains 75% of the previously recorded rpm$_{max}$.

5. Pedaling begins at zero resistance to help the subject overcome the initial inertia. Only when resistance is applied does the 30 s count begin.

Margaria-Kalmen Test

1. The height of each step is measured and the elevation from the 3rd to 9th step is calculated (6 × step height).

2. Following a warm-up and several practice attempts, the athlete sprints toward the stairs from a standing start 20 ft (6 m) away from the base of the stairs.

3. The athlete sprints up the stairs 3 steps at a time (3rd to 6th to 9th) as quickly as possible.

4. The time from the 3rd to 9th step is calculated using the timing system.

5. Power is calculated by the following formula:

$$P \text{ (kg} \cdot m \cdot s^{-1}) = (W \times H) / t,$$

$$P \text{ (watts)} = P \text{ (kg} \cdot m \cdot s^{-1}) \times 9.807,$$

where P = power, W = weight of the athlete in kg, H = height between the 3rd and 9th steps, and t = time in s.

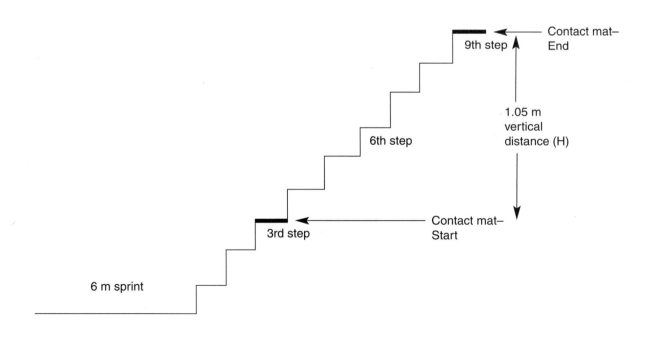

Standing Long Jump

1. Using masking tape and a tape measure that is at least 10 ft (3.0 m) long, construct the test station by taping the tape measure to the floor and placing a starting line at 0 in. (or 0 cm). A gym floor, artificial turf or grass field, or track with or without a sand pit can be used as a surface.

2. The athlete straddles the tape measure, with his feet parallel and about shoulder-width apart.

3. The athlete performs a countermovement and jumps as far horizontally (along the tape measure) as possible.

4. The athlete should land straddling the tape measure.

5. The floor at the edge of the athlete's heel is marked and the distance between the starting line and the mark is measured as the jump distance.

6. The best of three trials is recorded to the nearest 0.5 in. or 0.5 cm.

Vertical Jump

The following description uses a wall and chalk to test vertical jump height.

1. In a room with a smooth wall and a tall ceiling, rub chalk on the athlete's dominant hand.

2. The athlete stands with her dominant shoulder approximately 6 in. (15 cm) from the wall. With both feet flat on the floor, she reaches as high as possible with her dominant hand and makes a chalk mark on the wall. This mark represents her reach.

3. Without taking any step, the athlete lowers herself in a countermovement (flexes the knees and hips, brings the trunk forward, and swings the arms backward) and jumps as high as she can.

4. At the highest point in the jump, the athlete reaches up with her dominant hand and makes a second chalk mark on the wall.

5. The difference between the two marks is vertical jump height.

6. The best of three trials is recorded to the nearest 0.5 in. or 1.0 cm.

The following description uses a commercial Vertec device to test vertical jump height.

1. The tester adjusts the height of the Vertec so that the reach height falls within the colored horizontal vanes. The athlete stands so that when his dominant hand reaches straight upward, it is directly below the center of the vanes. The highest vane that can be reached is the athlete's reach.

2. The tester raises the column of vanes to a height that accommodates the jumping ability of the athlete.

3. As in step 3 in the previous description of the vertical jump, the athlete performs a countermovement jump without taking a step.

4. At the highest point of the jump the athlete reaches up with his dominant hand and taps the highest possible vane.

5. The difference between the height of the highest vane tapped and the reach height is the vertical jump height.

6. The best of three trials is recorded to the nearest 0.5 in. or 1.0 cm.

Adapted from Harman et al., 2000.

300 Yd (274.3 m) Shuttle Run

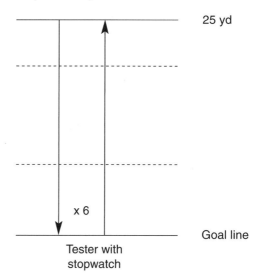

1. Following an adequate warm-up the athlete lines up at the starting point. On the tester's signal the athlete sprints to a point 25 yd (22.8 m) away and returns to the starting line. She performs a total of six round-trips (12 × 25 yd = 300 yd).

2. As the athlete crosses the line on the final sprint her time is recorded to the nearest 0.1 s and she begins a 5 min rest.

3. Following the 5 min rest the athlete repeats the 300 yd (274.3 m) shuttle.

4. The average of the two times is recorded.

Line Drill

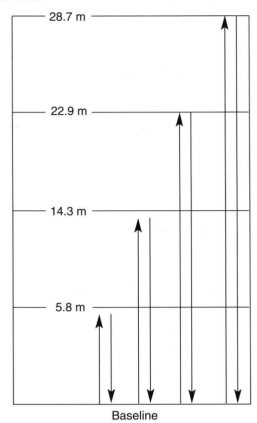

Baseline

1. Typically the line drill is performed on a regulation-size basketball court. However, it can be performed in any outdoor or indoor facility with similar space capabilities.

2. The athlete begins from a standing position and sprints from the baseline to 4 separate cones placed at the near-foul line (5.8 m), half-court line (14.3 m), far-foul line (22.9 m), and far baseline (28.7 m). As athlete arrives at each cone, she sprints back to

original baseline and then sprints on to the next cone.

3. When performing this test in an outdoor facility such as a football field, yard lines can be used as markers. For instance, the goal line is used as the starting point and cones are placed at the 10, 20, 30, and 40 yd (9.1, 18.3, 27.4, and 36.6 m) lines. The sprint procedure is the same as if performed indoors.

4. The athlete must touch each cone with her hand or she is disqualified.

Aerobic Power and Endurance Testing

The following descriptions correspond with data in chapter 6.

YMCA Submaximal Cycle Ergometer Test

1. Set the initial workload at 150 kg · m/min (0.5 kp).

2. Each stage lasts 3 min.

3. The workload for the second stage depends on the heart rate in the last minute of the first stage.

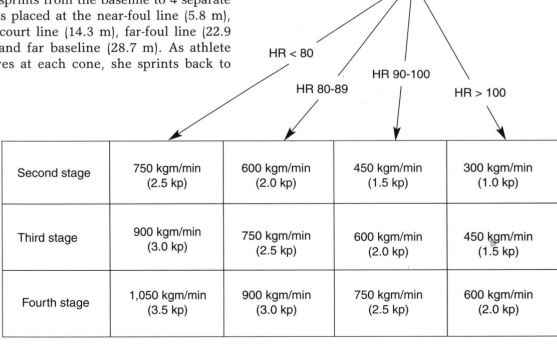

	HR < 80 750 kgm/min (2.5 kp)	HR 80-89 600 kgm/min (2.0 kp)	HR 90-100 450 kgm/min (1.5 kp)	HR > 100 300 kgm/min (1.0 kp)
Second stage	750 kgm/min (2.5 kp)	600 kgm/min (2.0 kp)	450 kgm/min (1.5 kp)	300 kgm/min (1.0 kp)
Third stage	900 kgm/min (3.0 kp)	750 kgm/min (2.5 kp)	600 kgm/min (2.0 kp)	450 kgm/min (1.5 kp)
Fourth stage	1,050 kgm/min (3.5 kp)	900 kgm/min (3.0 kp)	750 kgm/min (2.5 kp)	600 kgm/min (2.0 kp)

4. The heart rate measured during the last minute in each stage is plotted against work rate. The resulting line is extrapolated to the individual's age-predicted maximal heart rate (line a), and a perpendicular line (b) is dropped to the x-axis to determine the work rate that would have been achieved if the person had worked to maximum.

5. The work rate in kg · m · min⁻¹ is converted to watts (W) with the following formula:

Work rate (W) = work rate (kg · m · min⁻¹) / 6.12.

6. Using the individual's body weight (BW) in kg (BW in lb / 2.2046), $\dot{V}O_2$max (in ml/min) is calculated with the formula

$\dot{V}O_2$max = (10.8 × work rate) / BW + 7.

Åstrand-Rhyming Cycle Ergometer Test

1. This test is a single stage lasting 6 min.

2. The pedaling cadence is set at 50 rpm.

3. The work rate is based on gender and fitness level.

Gender	Fitness level	Work rate
Male	Unfit	300 or 600 kg · m · min⁻¹
Male	Fit	600 or 900 kg · m · min⁻¹
Female	Unfit	300 or 450 kg · m · min⁻¹
Female	Fit	450 or 600 kg · m · min⁻¹

Adapted, by permission, from J.T. Cramer and J.W. Coburn, 2004, Fitness testing protocols and norms. In *NSCA's Essentials of Personal Training*, edited by R.W. Earle and T.R. Baechle (Champaign, IL: Human Kinetics), 231.

4. Following 2 min of exercise the heart rate is measured. If the heart rate is ≥120 beats/min, the individual continues at the selected work rate throughout the 6 min test. If the heart rate is ≤120 beats/min, the work rate is raised to the next highest increment or until the heart rate is ≥120 beats/min after riding at a constant work rate.

5. Heart rates are measured at the end of the 5th and 6th min and averaged. This average is used to estimate $\dot{V}O_2$max in L/min from table 6.3 for men and table 6.4 for women.

6. Once $\dot{V}O_2$max is estimated, it must be corrected for the age of the individual.

The estimated $\dot{V}O_2$max is multiplied by the appropriate correction factor in table 6.5.

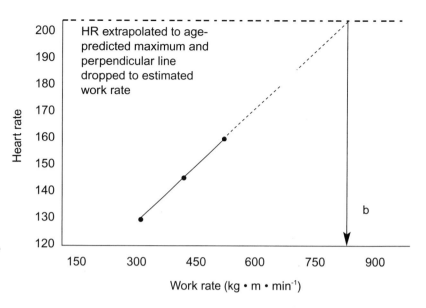

7. The $\dot{V}O_2$max in L · min⁻¹ can be converted into relative terms (ml · kg · min⁻¹) by the following formula:

$\dot{V}O_2$max (ml · kg · min⁻¹) = ($\dot{V}O_2$max (L · min⁻¹) × 1000) / BW (kg).

8. Obtained values can be compared to normative values specific to this test, which are listed in table 6.6.

Speed and Agility Testing

The following descriptions correspond with data in chapter 9.

40 Yd (36.6 m) Sprint

1. The test is generally performed on a football field, but it may also be performed on a track or on marked flat ground.

2. The athlete begins in a 3- or 4-point stance with his hand(s) on the starting line. He runs through the end line 40 yd (36.6 m) away and does not slow down or stop until crossing the line.

3. The tester stands on the end line with a stopwatch in hand (the protocol for electronic measuring devices is performed according to the manufacturer's specifications).

4. Upon the initial movement of the athlete, the tester starts the stopwatch. As the athlete crosses the finish line, the tester stops the stopwatch.

5. The best of three attempts is recorded. Time is recorded to nearest 0.01 s.

T-Test (Seminick 1990)

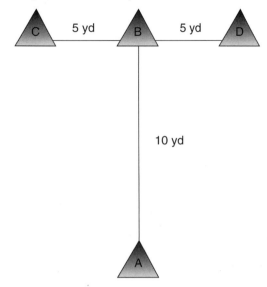

1. Arrange 4 cones as shown in the figure. Cones A and B are 10 yd (9.1 m) apart, and cones C and D are 5 yd (4.6 m) from cone B on either side.

2. Following a warm-up, the athlete stands at cone A.

3. On the command, the athlete sprints to cone B and touches the base of the cone with her hand.

4. The athlete shuffles either to the left toward cone C or to the right toward cone D and touches the cone with her closest hand. The athlete faces forward at all times and cannot cross her feet. Crossing of the feet results in disqualification.

5. Upon touching cone C or D, the athlete shuffles to the other far cone and touches it with her closest hand. The athlete does *not* touch cone B as she crosses to the other cone.

6. The athlete shuffles back to cone B and touches its base. The athlete runs backward to cone A, and at the moment she crosses the cone the time is stopped.

7. If the athlete fails to touch a cone she is disqualified.

Edgren Side Step Test (Harman, Garhammer, and Pandorf 2000)

1. Divide a 12 ft (3.7 m) wide gymnasium floor into four 3 ft (0.9 m) segments (see figure).

2. Following a warm-up, the athlete stands astride the centerline. On the command he sidesteps to the right until his right foot touches or crosses the outside line.

3. The athlete then sidesteps to the left until his left foot touches or crosses the left outside line.

4. The athlete sidesteps back and forth to the outside lines as rapidly as possible for 10 s.

5. The number of lines crossed during the 10 s is recorded. Any time the athlete crosses his feet, a single line, or point, is subtracted from his score.

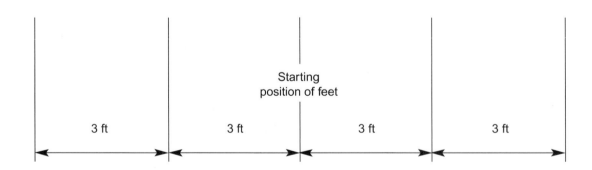

Hexagon Agility Test (Harman, Garhammer, and Pandorf 2000)

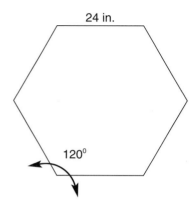

1. Using adhesive tape, create a hexagon (on a gym floor) with 24 in. (61 cm) sides meeting to form a 120° angle.

2. Following a warm-up, the athlete stands in the middle of the hexagon. On the command she begins double-leg hopping from the center of the hexagon to one side and back to the center again. She hops from the center to each side in a continuous clockwise direction until all 6 sides are covered 3 times (she completes 3 revolutions).

3. The athlete faces the same direction throughout the test.

4. If the athlete lands on a line, loses her balance, takes an extra step, or changes the direction she is facing, the trial is stopped and restarted.

5. The stopwatch begins with the athlete's initial movement and stops when the athlete lands back in the middle of the hexagon following the final repetition.

3-Cone Drill

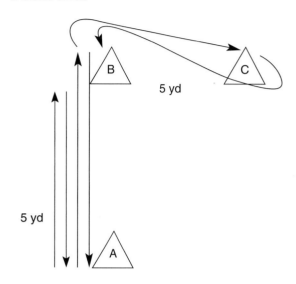

1. Three cones are placed in an upside-down L configuration. Each cone is 5 yd (4.6 m) apart from the others.

2. The athlete begins at cone A from behind the starting line. He sprints as fast as possible to cone B, which is 5 yd (4.6 m) directly in front of cone A, and touches the cone. He then returns to cone A and without stopping changes directions, corners cone B, and sprints directly to cone C, which is 5 yd (4.6 m) lateral to cone B on the athlete's right-hand side. The athlete circles cone C to his left, returns to cone A by cornering cone B, and sprints at full speed past cone A.

3. Time is recorded to the nearest 0.01 sec.

Pro Agility Test

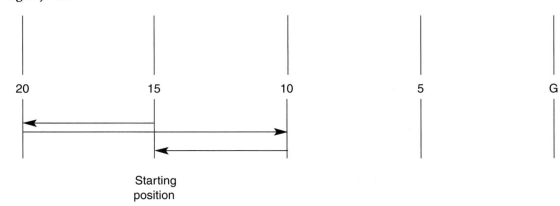

Starting
position

1. The pro agility test is also known as the 20 yd (18.3 m) shuttle run.

2. The test is performed on a football field or may be performed on a marked field. The athlete straddles the 15 yd (13.7 m) line and sprints to the 20 yd (18.3 m) line. She then changes direction and sprints to the 10 yd (9.1 m) line and again changes direction and returns to the 15 yd (13.7 m) line.

3. The stopwatch begins on the athlete's initial movement and stops when the athlete crosses the 15 yd (13.7 m) line.

References

ACSM. *See* American College of Sports Medicine.

Adams, W.C., K. Deck-Côté, and K.M. Winters. 1992. Anthropometric estimation of bone mineral content in young adult females. *American Journal of Human Biology* 4:767-774.

Ainsworth, B.E., W.L. Haskell, M.C. Whitt, M.L. Irwin, A.M Swartz, S.J. Strath, W.L. O'Brien, D.R. Bassett Jr., K.H. Schmitz, P.O. Emplaincourt, D.R. Jacobs Jr., and A.S. Leon. 2000. Compendium of physical activities: An update of activity codes and MET intensities. *Medicine and Science in Sports and Exercise* 32:S498-S504.

American College of Sports Medicine. 1995. *Guidelines for exercise testing and prescription.* Ed. W.L. Kenney. Philadelphia: Lippincott Williams & Wilkins.

American College of Sports Medicine. 2000. *Guidelines for exercise testing and prescription.* Ed. B.A. Franklin. Philadelphia: Lippincott Williams & Wilkins.

Anderson, M.A., J.B. Gieck, D. Perrin, A. Weltman, R. Rutt, and C. Denegar. 1991. The relationships among isometric, isotonic and isokinetic quadriceps and hamstring force and three components of athletic performance. *Journal of Orthopedic Sports Physical Therapy* 14:114-120.

Andreoli, A., M. Monteleone, M. Van Loan, L. Promenzio, U. Tarantino, and A. De Lorenzo. 2001. Effects of different sports on bone density and muscle mass in highly trained athletes. *Medicine and Science in Sports and Exercise* 33:507-511.

Armstrong, L.E., C.M. Maresh, M.Whittlesey, M.F. Bergeron, C. Gabaree, and J.R. Hoffman. 1994. Longitudinal exercise-heat tolerance and running economy of collegiate distance runners. *J. Strength and Cond. Res.* 8:192-197.

Åstrand, P.O. 1960. Aerobic capacity in men and women with special reference to age. *Acta Physiologica Scandinavica* Suppl. no. 49:45-60.

Austin, M.A., J.E. Hokanson, and K.L. Edwards. 1998. Hypertriglyceridemia as a cardiovascular risk factor. *American Journal of Cardiology* 81:7B-12B.

Ayalon, A., O. Inbar, and O. Bar-Or. 1974. Relationships among measurements of explosive strength and anaerobic power. In *Biomechanics IV,* Vol. 1 of *International Series on Sport Sciences,* ed. Nelson and Morehouse, 527-532. Baltimore: University Park Press.

Baker, D., and S. Nance. 1999. The relation between running speed and measures of strength and power in professional rugby players. *Journal of Strength and Conditioning Research* 13:230-235.

Ballard, T.P., L. Fafara, and M.D. Vukovich. 2004. Comparison of Bod Pod and DXA in female collegiate athletes. *Medicine and Science in Sports and Exercise* 36:731-735.

Bar-Or, O. 1987. The Wingate anaerobic test: An update on methodology, reliability and validity. *Sports Medicine* 4:381-394.

Bar-Or, O. 1993. Importance of differences between children and adults for exercise testing and prescription. In *Exercise testing and exercise prescription for special cases.* 2nd ed., ed. J.S. Skinner, 57-74. Baltimore: Williams & Wilkins.

Bar-Or, O., R. Dotan, O. Inbar, A. Rotstein, J. Karlsson, and P. Tesch. 1980. Anaerobic capacity and muscle fiber type distribution in man. *International Journal of Sports Medicine* 1:89-92.

Bassey, E.J., and S.J. Ramsdale. 1994. Increase in femoral bone density in young women following high impact exercise. *Osteoporosis International* 4: 72-75.

Bemben, M.G., B.H. Massey, R.A. Boileau, and J.E. Misner. 1992. Reliability of isometric force-time curve parameters for men aged 20 to 79 years. *Journal of Applied Sport Science Research* 6:158-164.

Bennell, K.L., S.A. Malcom, K.M. Khan, S.A. Thomas, S.J. Reid, P.D. Brukner, P.R. Eberling, and J.D. Wark. 1997. Bone mass and bone turnover in power athletes, endurance athletes and controls: A 12-month longitudinal study. *Bone* 20:477-484.

Berg, K., R.W. Latin, and T. Baechle. 1990. Physical and performance characteristics of NCAA division I football players. *Research Quarterly* 61:395-401.

Bergeron, M.F., C.M. Maresh, W.J. Kraemer, A. Abraham, B. Conroy, and C. Gabaree. 1991. Tennis: A physiological profile during match play. *International Journal of Sports Medicine* 12:474-479.

Blair, S.N., and S. Brodney. 1999. Effects of physical inactivity and obesity on morbidity and mortality: Current evidence and research issues. *Medicine and Science in Sports and Exercise* Suppl. no. 31: S646-S662.

Blimkie, C. 1989. Age- and sex-associated variation in strength during childhood: Anthropometric, morphological, neurological, biomechanical, endocrinologic, genetic and physical activity correlates. In *Perspectives in exercise science and sports,* ed. G. Gisolfi and D. Lamb, 99-163. Indianapolis: Benchmark Press.

Boddington, M.K., M.I. Lambert, and M.R. Waldeck. 2004. Validity of a 5-meter multiple shuttle run test for assessing fitness of women field hockey players. *Journal of Strength and Conditioning Research* 18:97-100.

Boot, A.M., M.A. de Ridder, H.A.P. Pols, E.P. Krenning, and S.M.P.F. de Muinck Keizer-Schrama. 1997. Bone mineral density in children and adolescents: Relation to puberty, calcium intake, and physical activity. *Journal of Clinical Endocrinology and Metabolism* 82:57-62.

Bosco, C., P. Mognoni, and P. Luhtanen. 1983. Relationship between isokinetic performance and ballistic movement. *European Journal of Applied Physiology* 51:357-364.

Boulay, M.R., O. Serresse, N. Almeras, and A. Tremblay. 1994. Energy expenditure measurement in male cross-country skiers: Comparison of two field methods. *Medicine and Science in Sports and Exercise* 26:248-253.

Bracko, M.R., and J.D. George. 2001. Prediction of ice skating performance with off-ice testing in women's ice hockey players. *Journal of Strength and Conditioning Research* 15:116-122.

Bray, G.A., and D.S. Gray. 1988. Obesity part I—Pathogenesis. *Western Journal of Medicine* 149:432-441.

Brown, D.A., and W.C. Miller. 1998. Normative data for strength and flexibility of women throughout life. *European Journal of Applied Physiology* 78:77-82.

Bruce, R.A., F. Kusumi, and D. Hosmer. 1973. Maximal oxygen uptake and nomographic assessment of functional aerobic impairment in cardiovascular disease. *American Heart Journal* 85:546-562.

Brzycki, M. 1993. Strength testing: Predicting a one-rep max from reps to fatigue. *Journal of Health, Physical Education, Recreation and Dance* 64:88-90.

Burkett, L.N. 1970. Causative factors in hamstring strains. *Medicine and Science in Sports* 2:39-42.

Callan, S.D., D.M. Brunner, K.L. Devolve, S.E. Mulligan, J. Hesson, R.L. Wilber, and J.T. Kearney. 2000. Physiological profiles of elite freestyle wrestlers. *Journal of Strength and Conditioning Research* 14: 162-169.

Callister, R., R.J. Callister, S.J. Fleck, and G.A. Dudley. 1990. Physiological and performance responses to overtraining in elite judo athletes. *Medicine and Science in Sports and Exercise* 22:816-824.

Canadian standardized test of fitness operations manual. 3rd ed. 1986. Ottawa, Ontario: Fitness Canada and Fitness Amateur Sport Canada.

Caterisano, A., B.T. Patrick, W.L. Edenfield, and M.J. Batson. 1997. The effects of a basketball season on aerobic and strength parameters among college men: Starters vs. reserves. *Journal of Strength and Conditioning Research* 11:21-24.

Christ, C.B., M.H. Slaughter, R.J. Stillman, J. Cameron, and R.A. Boileau. 1994. Reliability of select parameters of isometric muscle function associated with

testing 3 days × 3 trials in women. *Journal of Strength and Conditioning Research* 8:65-71.

Chu, D.A. 1996. *Explosive power and strength.* Champaign, IL: Human Kinetics.

Clark, R.R., J.C. Sullivan, C. Bartok, and D.A. Schoeller. 2003. Multicomponent cross-validation of minimum weight predictions for college wrestlers. *Medicine Science in Sports and Exercise* 35:342-347.

Cohen, J.L., and K.R. Segal. 1985. Left ventricular hypertrophy in athletes: An exercise-echocardiographic study. *Medicine and Science in Sports and Exercise* 17:695-700.

Colan, S.D., S.P. Sanders, D. MacPherson, and K. Borow. 1985. Left ventricular diastolic function in elite athletes with physiologic cardiac hypertrophy. *Journal of American College of Cardiology* 6:545-549.

Coleman, A.E., and L.M. Lasky. 1992. Assessing running speed and body composition in professional baseball players. *Journal of Applied Sport Science Research* 6:207-213.

Collins, M.A., M.L. Millard-Stafford, P.B. Sparling, T.K. Snow, L.B. Rosskopf, S.A. Webb, and J. Omer. 1999. Evaluation of the Bod Pod for assessing body fat in collegiate football players. *Medicine and Science in Sports and Exercise* 31:1350-1356.

Conroy, B.P., W.J. Kraemer, C.M. Maresh, S.J. Fleck, M.H. Stone, A.C. Fry, P.D. Miller, and G.P. Dalsky. 1993. Bone mineral density in elite junior Olympic weightlifters. *Medicine and Science in Sports and Exercise* 23:1103-1109.

Cook, E.E., V.L. Gray, E. Savinar-Nogue, and J. Medeiros. 1987. Shoulder antagonistic strength ratios: A comparison between college-level baseball pitchers and nonpitchers. *The Journal of Orthopaedic and Sports Physical Therapy* 8:451-60.

Costill, D.L. 1966. Use of a swimming ergometer in physiological research. *Research Quarterly* 37: 564-567.

Costill, D.L., and E.L. Fox. 1969. Energetics of marathon running. *Medicine and Science in Sport* 1:81-86.

Cote, K.D., and W.C. Adams. 1993. Effect of bone density on body composition estimates in young adult black and white women. *Medicine and Science in Sports and Exercise* 23:290-296.

Cramer, J.T., and J.W. Coburn. 2004. Fitness testing protocols and norms. In *NSCA's essentials of personal training,* ed. R.W. Earle and T.R. Baechle, 217-264. Champaign, IL: Human Kinetics.

Crielaard, J.M., and F. Pirnay. 1981. Anaerobic and aerobic power of top athletes. *European Journal of Applied Physiology* 47:295-300.

Cunningham, D.A., and J.A. Faulkner. 1969. The effect of training on aerobic and anaerobic metabolism during a short exhaustive run. *Medicine and Science in Sports* 1:65-69.

Deligiannis, A., E. Zahopoulou, and K. Mandroukas. 1988. Echocardiographic study of cardiac dimensions and function in weight lifters and body builders. *Journal of Sports Cardiology* 5:24-32.

Delistraty, D.A., B.J. Noble, and J.G. Wilkinson. 1990. Treadmill and swim bench ergometry in triathletes, runners and swimmers. *Journal of Applied Sport Science Research* 4:31-36.

Devereux, R.B., E.M. Lutas, P.N. Casale, P. Kligfield, R.R. Eisenberg, I.W. Hammon, D.H. Miller, G. Reis, M.H. Alderman, and J.H. Laragh. 1984. Standardization of M-mode echocardiographic left ventricular anatomic measurements. *Journal of American College of Cardiology* 4:1222-1230.

Dishman, R.K., R.A. Washburn, and G.W. Heath. 2004. *Physical activity epidemiology.* Champaign, IL: Human Kinetics.

Dook, J.E., C. James, N.K. Henderson, and R.I. Price. 1997. Exercise and bone mineral density in mature female athletes. *Medicine and Science in Sports and Exercise* 29:291-296.

Douglas, P.S., M.L. O'Toole, S.E. Katz, and G.S. Ginsburg. 1997. Left ventricular hypertrophy in athletes. *American Journal of Cardiology* 80:1384-1388.

Durnin, J.V.G.A., and J. Womersley. 1974. Body fat assessment from total body density and its estimation from skinfold thickness: Measurements on 481 men and women aged 16-72 years. *British Journal of Nutrition* 32:77-97.

Dyson, K., C.J.R. Blimkie, K.S. Davison, C.E. Webber, and J.D. Adachi. 1997. Gymnastic training and bone density in preadolescent females. *Medicine and Science in Sports and Exercise* 29:443-450.

Ebbeling, C.B., A. Ward, E.M. Puleo, J. Widrick, and J.M. Rippe. 1991. Development of a single-stage submaximal treadmill walking test. *Medicine and Science in Sports and Exercise* 23:966-973.

Ellenbecker, T.S. 1991. A total arm strength isokinetic profile of highly skilled tennis players. *Isokinetic Exercise Science* 1:9-21.

Epley, B. 1985. Poundage chart. Lincoln, NE: *Boyd Epley Workout.*

Faigenbaum, A., L. Milliken, and W. Westcott. 2003. Maximal strength testing in healthy children. *Journal of Strength and Conditioning Research* 17:162-166.

Falk, B., Y. Weinstein, R. Dotan, D.R. Abramson, D. Mann-Segal, and J.R. Hoffman. 1996. A treadmill test of sprint running. *Scandinavian Journal of Medicine and Science in Sports* 6:259-264.

Farrel, M., and J.G. Richards. 1986. Analysis of the reliability and validity of the kinetic communicator exercise device. *Medicine and Science in Sports and Exercise* 18:44-49.

Filaire, E., X. Bernain, M. Sagnol, and G. Lac. 2001. Preliminary results on mood state, salivary testosterone:cortisol ratio and team performance in a professional soccer team. *European Journal of Applied Physiology* 86:179-184.

Filaire, E., C. Le Scanff, P. Duche, and G. Lac. 1999. The relationship between salivary adrenocortical hormone changes and personality in elite female athletes during handball and volleyball competition. *Research Quarterly for Exercise and Sport* 70:297-302.

Filaire, E., and G. Lac. 1999. Dehydroepiandrostenedione (DHEA) rather than testosterone shows saliva androgen responses to exercise in elite female handball players. *International Journal of Sports Nutrition* 20:17-20.

Findley, B.W., L.E. Brown, M. Whitehurst, R. Gilbert, and S.A. Apold. 1995. Age-group performance and physical fitness in male firefighters. *Journal of Strength and Conditioning Research* 9:259-260.

Fisman, E.Z., P. Embon, A. Pines, A. Tenenbaum, Y. Drory, I. Shapira, and M. Motro. 1997. Comparison of left ventricular function using isometric exercise Doppler echocardiography in competitive runners and weightlifters versus sedentary individuals. *American Journal of Cardiology* 79:355-359.

Fleck, S.J., and W.J. Kraemer. 2004. *Designing resistance training programs.* 3rd ed. Champaign, IL: Human Kinetics.

Flynn, M.G., F.X. Pizza, J.B. Boone, F.F. Andres, T.A. Michaud, and J.R. Rodriguez-Zayas. 1994. Indices of training stress during competitive running and swimming seasons. *International Journal of Sports Medicine* 15:21-26.

Fornetti, W.C., J.M. Pivarnik, J.M. Foley, and J.J. Fliechtner. 1999. Reliability and validity of body composition measures in female athletes. *Journal of Applied Physiology* 87:1114-1122.

Fox, E.L., and D.K. Mathews. 1981. *The physiological basis of physical education and athletics.* 3rd ed. Philadelphia: Saunders.

Fry, A.C., W.J. Kraemer, C.A. Weseman, B.P. Conroy, S.E. Gordon, J.R. Hoffman, and C.M. Maresh. 1991. The effects of an off-season strength and conditioning program on starters and non-starters in women's intercollegiate volleyball. *Journal of Applied Sport Science Research* 5:174-181.

Fry, A.C., and D.R. Powell. 1987. Hamstring/quadriceps parity with three different weight training methods. *Journal of Sports Medicine* 27:362-367.

Fry, A.C., B.K. Schilling, R.S. Staron, F.C. Hagerman, R.S. Hikida, and J.T. Thrush. 2003. Muscle fiber characteristics and performance correlates of male Olympic style weightlifters. *Journal of Strength and Conditioning Research* 17:747-754.

Fry, R.W., A.R. Morton, and D. Keast. 1991. Overtraining in athletes. *Sports Medicine* 12:32-65.

Funato, K., T. Yanagiya, and T. Fukunaga. 2001. Ergometry for estimation of mechanical power output in sprinting in humans using a newly developed self-driven treadmill. *European Journal of Applied Physiology* 84:169-173.

Garstecki, M.A., R.W. Latin, and M.M. Cuppett. 2004. Comparison of selected physical fitness and performance variables between NCAA Division I and II football players. *Journal of Strength and Conditioning Research* 18:292-297.

Gettman, L.R. 1993. Fitness testing. In *ACSM's resource manual for guidelines for exercise testing and prescription.* 2nd ed., ed. J.L. Durstine, A.C. King, P.L. Painter, J.L. Roitman, and L.D. Zwiren, 229-246. Philadelphia: Williams & Wilkins.

Gillam, G.M. 1983. 300 yard shuttle run. *National Strength and Conditioning Association Journal* 5:46.

Golding, L.A., C.R. Myers, and W.E. Sinning. 2000. *YMCA fitness testing and assessment manual.* 4th ed. Champaign, IL: Human Kinetics.

Granier, P., B. Mercier, J. Mercier, and F. Anselme. 1995. Aerobic and anaerobic contribution to Wingate test performance in sprint and middle-distance runners. *European Journal of Applied Physiology* 70:58-65.

Grant, J.A., A.N. Joseph, and P.D. Campagna. 1999. The prediction of $\dot{V}O_2$max: A comparison of 7 indirect tests of aerobic power. *Journal of Strength and Conditioning Research* 13:346-352.

Greendale, G.A., M.H. Huang, Y. Wang, J.S. Finkelstein, M.E. Danielson, and B. Sternfeld. 2003. Sport and home physical activity are independently associated with bone density. *Medicine and Science in Sports and Exercise* 35:506-512.

Guidetti, L., A. Musulin, and C. Baldari. 2002. Physiological factors in middleweight boxing performance. *Journal of Sports Medicine and Physical Fitness* 42:309-314.

Hagerman, F.C., L.M. Starr, and T.F. Murray. 1989. Effects of a long-term fitness program on professional baseball players. *The Physician and Sports Medicine* 17:101-119.

Hakkinen, K. 1993. Changes in physical fitness profile in female basketball players during the competitive season including explosive type strength training. *The Journal of Sports Medicine and Physical Fitness* 33:19-26.

Hakkinen, K., A. Pakarinen, M. Alen, H. Kauhanen, and P.V. Komi. 1987. Relationships between training volume, physical performance capacity, and serum hormone concentration during prolonged training in elite weightlifters. *International Journal of Sports Medicine* Suppl. no. 8:61-65.

Harman, E., J. Garhammer, and C. Pandorf. 2000. Principles of test selection and administration. In *Essentials of strength and conditioning*, ed. T. Baechle and R. Earle, 275-286. Champaign, IL: Human Kinetics.

Harman, E.A., M.T. Rosenstein, P.N. Frykman, R.M. Rosenstein, and W.J. Kraemer. 1991. Estimation of human power output from vertical jump. *Journal of Applied Sport Science Research* 5:116-120.

Harris, R.C., R.H.T. Edwards, E. Hultman, L.O. Nordesjo, B. Nylind, and K. Sahlin. 1976. The time course of phosphorylcreatine resynthesis during recovery of the quadriceps muscle in man. *Pflugers Archives* 367:137-142.

Heinonen, A. 2001. Biomechanics. In *Physical activity and bone health*, ed. K. Khan, H. McKay, D. Bailey, J. Wark, and K. Bennell, 23-34. Champaign, IL: Human Kinetics.

Heinonen, A., P. Kannus, H. Sievanen, P. Oja, M. Pasanen, M. Rinne, K. Uusi-Rasi, and I. Vuori. 1996. Randomized controlled trial of effect of high-impact exercise on selected risk factors for osteoporotic fractures. *Lancet* 348:1343-1347.

Heinonen, A., P. Oja, P. Kannus, H. Sievanen, A. Manttari, and I. Vuori. 1993. Bone mineral density of female athletes in different sports. *Bone and Mineral* 23:1-14.

Hennessy, L., and J. Kilty. 2001. Relationship of the stretch-shortening cycle to sprint performance in trained female athletes. *Journal of Strength and Conditioning Research* 15:326-331.

Henriksen, E., J. Landelius, T. Kangro, T. Jonason, P. Hedberg, L. Wessien, C.N. Rosander, C. Rolf, I. Ringqvist, and G. Friman. 1999. An echocardiographic study of right and left ventricular adaptation to physical exercise in elite female orienteers. *European Heart Journal* 20:309-16.

Henry, W.L., J.M. Gardin, and J.H. Ware. 1980. Echocardiographic measurements in normal subjects from infancy to old age. *Circulation* 62:1054-1061.

Heyward, V.H. 2002. *Advanced fitness assessment and exercise prescription.* Champaign, IL: Human Kinetics.

Heyward, V.H., and L.M. Stolarczyk. 1996. *Applied body composition assessment.* Champaign, IL: Human Kinetics.

Hinkle, D.E., W. Wiersma, and S.G. Jur. 1988. *Applied statistics for the behavioral sciences.* Boston: Houghton Mifflin.

Hodgdon, J.A. 1999. *A history of the U.S. Navy physical readiness program from 1976 to 1999.* Office of Naval Research technical document no. 99-6F.

Hoeger, W.W.K., and S.A. Hoeger. 2000. *Lifetime physical fitness and wellness.* Englewood, CO: Morton Publishing.

Hoeger, W.W.K., S.L. Barette, D.F. Hale, and D.R. Hopkins. 1987. Relationship between repetitions and selected percentages of one repetition maximum. *Journal of Applied Sports Science Research* 1:11-13.

Hoeger, W.W.K., D.R. Hopkins, S.L. Barette, and D.F. Hale. 1990. Relationship between repetitions and selected percentages of one repetition maximum: A comparison between untrained and trained males and females. *Journal of Applied Sports Science Research* 4:47-54.

Hoff, J., and B. Almasbakk. 1995. The effects of maximum strength training on throwing velocity and muscle strength in female team-handball players. *Journal of Strength and Conditioning Research* 9: 255-258.

Hoffman, J.R. 2002. *Physiological aspects of sport training and performance.* Champaign, IL: Human Kinetics.

Hoffman, J.R., J. Cooper, M. Wendell, J. Im, and J. Kang. 2004. Forthcoming. Effects of β-hydroxy β-methylbutyrate on power performance and indices of muscle damage and stress during high intensity training. *Journal of Strength and Conditioning Research* 18:747-752.

Hoffman, J.R., S. Epstein, M. Einbinder, and Y. Weinstein. 1999. The influence of aerobic capacity on anaerobic performance and recovery indices in basketball players. *Journal of Strength and Conditioning Research* 13:407-411.

Hoffman, J.R., S. Epstein, M. Einbinder, and Y. Weinstein. 2000. A comparison between the Wingate anaerobic power test to both vertical jump and line drill tests in basketball players. *Journal of Strength and Conditioning Research* 14:261-264.

Hoffman, J.R., A.C. Fry, R. Howard, C.M. Maresh, and W.J. Kraemer. 1991. Strength, speed and endurance changes during the course of a Division I basketball season. *Journal of Applied Sport Science Research* 5:144-149.

Hoffman, J.R., and M. Kaminsky. 2000. Use of performance testing for monitoring overtraining in elite youth basketball players. *Strength and Conditioning* 22:54-62.

Hoffman, J.R., and J. Kang. 2003. Strength changes during an in-season resistance-training program for football. *Journal of Strength and Conditioning Research* 17:109-114.

Hoffman, J.R., W.J. Kraemer, A.C. Fry, M. Deschenes, and M. Kemp. 1990. The effect of self-selection for frequency of training in a winter conditioning program for football. *Journal of Applied Sport Science Research* 3:76-82.

Hoffman, J.R., C.M. Maresh, and L.E. Armstrong. 1992. Isokinetic and dynamic constant resistance strength testing: Implications for sport. *Physical Therapy Practice* 2:42-53.

Hoffman, J.R., C.M. Maresh, L.E. Armstrong, and W.J. Kraemer. 1991. Effects of off-season and in-season resistance training programs on a collegiate male basketball team. *Journal of Human Muscle Performance* 1:48-55.

Hoffman, J.R., G. Tenenbaum, C.M. Maresh, and W.J. Kraemer. 1996. Relationship between athletic performance tests and playing time in elite college basketball players. *Journal of Strength and Conditioning Research* 10:67-71.

Hoffman, R.J., and T.R. Collingwood. 2005. *Fit for duty.* 2nd ed. Champaign, IL: Human Kinetics.

Hopkins, D.R., and W.W.K. Hoeger. 1992. A comparison of the sit-and-reach test and the modified sit-and-reach test in the measurement of flexibility for males. *Journal of Applied Sport Science Research* 6:7-10.

Housh, T.J., G.O. Johnson, D.J. Housh, J.R. Stout, D.B. Smith, and K.T. Ebersole. 1997. Isokinetic peak torque and estimated muscle cross-sectional area in high school wrestlers. *Journal of Strength and Conditioning Research* 11:45-49.

Housh, T.J., G.O. Johnson, L. Marty, G. Eichen, C. Eishen, and D. Housh. 1988. Isokinetic leg flexion and extension strength of university football players. *Journal of Orthopedic and Sports Physical Therapy* 9:365-369.

Huck, S.W., W.H. Cormier, and W.G. Bounds. 1974. *Reading statistics and research.* New York: Harper & Row.

Hughes, S.S., B.C. Lyons, and J.J. Mayo. 2004. Effect of grip strength and grip strengthening exercises on instantaneous bat velocity of collegiate baseball players. *Journal of Strength and Conditioning Research* 18:298-301.

Hunter, G.R., J. Hilyer, and M. Forster. 1993. Changes in fitness during 4 years of intercollegiate basketball. *Journal of Strength and Conditioning Research* 7:26-29.

Inbar, O., O. Bar-Or, and J.S. Skinner. 1996. *The Wingate anaerobic test.* Champaign, IL: Human Kinetics.

Jackson, A., K. Der Weduwe, R. Schick, and R. Sanchez. 1990. An analysis of the validity of the three-mile run as a field test of aerobic capacity in college males. *Research Quarterly in Exercise and Sport* 61: 233-237.

Jackson, A.S., and M.L. Pollock. 1978. Generalized equations for predicting body density of men. *British Journal of Nutrition* 40:497-504.

Jackson, A.S., and M.L. Pollock. 1985. Practical assessment of body composition. *The Physician and Sports Medicine* 13:76-90.

Jackson, A.S., M.L. Pollock, and A. Ward. 1980. Generalized equations for predicting body density of women. *Medicine and Science in Sports and Exercise* 12:175-182.

Johnson, B.L., and J.K. Nelson. 1979. *Practical measurement for evaluation in physical education.* Minneapolis: Burgess Publishing.

Jorgensen, H.L., L. Warming, N.H. Bjarnason, P.B. Anderson, and C. Hassager. 2001. How does quantitative ultrasound compare to dual x-ray absorptiometry at various skeletal sites in relation to the WHO diagnosis categories? *Clinical Physiology* 21:51-59.

Karlsson, M.K., O. Johnell, and K.J. Obrant. 1993. Bone mineral density in weightlifters. *Calcified Tissue International* 52:212-215.

Katch, V., A. Weltman, R. Martin, and L. Gray. 1977. Optimal test characteristics for maximal anaerobic work on the bicycle ergometer. *Research Quarterly* 48:319-327.

Khan, K., H. McKay, D. Bailey, J. Wark, and K. Bennell. 2001. *Physical activity and bone health.* Champaign, IL: Human Kinetics.

Kin, K., J.H. Lee, K. Kushida, D.J. Sartoris, A. Ohmura, P.L. Clopton, and T. Inoue. 1993. Bone density and body composition on the Pacific rim: A comparison between Japan-born and U.S.-born Japanese-American women. *Journal of Bone Mineral Research* 8:861-869.

Kinosian, B., H. Glick, and G. Garland. 1994. Cholesterol and coronary heart disease: Predicting risks by levels and ratios. *Annals of Internal Medicine* 121:641-647.

Kirkendall, D.T., 2000. Physiology of soccer. In *Exercise and sport science,* ed. W.E. Garrett and D.T. Kirkendall, 875-84. Philadelphia: Lippincott Williams & Wilkins.

Kline, G.M., J.P. Porcari, R. Hintermeister, P.S. Freedson, A. Ward, R.F. McCarron, J. Ross, and J.M. Rippe. 1987. Estimation of $\dot{V}O_2$max from a one-mile track walk, gender, age, and body weight. *Medicine and Science in Sports and Exercise* 19:253-259.

Knapik, J.J., C.L. Bauman, B.H. Jones, J.M. Harris, and L. Vaughan. 1991. Preseason strength and flexibility imbalances associated with athletic injuries in female collegiate athletes. *American Journal of Sports Medicine* 19:76-81.

Komi, P., H. Rusko, J. Vos, and V. Vihko. 1977. Anaerobic performance capacity in athletes. *Acta Phsyiological Scandinavia* 100:107-114.

Kraemer, W.J., D.N. French, N.J. Paxton, K. Hakkinen, J.S. Volek, W.J. Sebastianelli, M. Putukian, R.U. Newton, M.R. Rubin, A.L. Gomez, J.D. Vescovi, N.A. Ratamess, S.J. Fleck, J.M. Lynch, and H.G. Knuttgen. 2004. Changes in exercise performance and hormonal concentrations over a big ten soccer season in starters and nonstarters. *Journal of Strength and Conditioning Research* 18:121-128.

Kraemer, W.J., A.C. Fry, M.R. Rubin, T. Triplett-McBride, S.E. Gordon, P. Koziris, J.M. Lynch, J.S. Volek, D.E. Meuffels, R.U. Newton, and S.J. Fleck. 2001. Physiological and performance responses to tournament wrestling. *Medicine and Science in Sports and Exercise* 33:1367-1378.

Kraemer, W.J., and L.A. Gotshalk. 2000. Physiology of American football. In *Exercise and sport science*, ed. W.E. Garrett and D.T. Kirkendall, 795-813. Philadelphia: Lippincott Williams & Wilkins.

Kraemer, W.J., K. Hakkinen, T. Triplett-McBride, A.C. Fry, L.P. Koziris, N.A. Ratamess, J.E. Bauer, J.S. Volek, T. McConnell, R.U. Newton, S.E. Gordon, D. Cummings, J. Hauth, F. Pullo, J.M. Lynch, S.A. Mazzetti, and H.G. Knuttgen. 2003. Physiological changes with periodized resistance training in women tennis players. *Medicine and Science in Sports and Exercise* 35:157-168.

Kraemer, W.J., J. Patton, S.E. Gordon, E.A. Harmon, M.R. Deschenes, K. Reynolds, R.U. Newton, N.T. Triplett, and J.E. Dziados. 1995. Compatibility of high intensity strength and endurance training on hormonal and skeletal muscle adaptations. *Journal of Applied Physiology* 78:976-989.

Krauss, R.M. 1998. Atherogenicity of triglyceride-rich lipoproteins. *American Journal of Cardiology* 81: 13B-17B.

LaMonte, M.J., J.T. McKinney, S.M. Quinn, C.N. Bainbridge, and P.A. Eisenman. 1999. Comparison of physical and physiological variables for female college basketball players. *Journal of Strength and Conditioning Research* 13:264-270.

Landers, J. 1985. Maximum based on reps. *National Strength and Conditioning Association Journal* 6: 60-61.

Latin, R.W., K. Berg, and T. Baechle. 1994. Physical and performance characteristics of NCAA Division I male basketball players. *Journal of Strength and Conditioning Research* 8:214-218.

Lee, C.D., S.N. Blair, and A.S. Jackson. 1999. Cardiorespiratory fitness, body composition, and all-cause and cardiovascular disease mortality in men. *American Journal of Clinical Nutrition* 69:373-380.

Lee, E.J., K.A. Long, W.L. Risser, H.B.W. Poindexter, W.E. Gibbons, and J. Goldzieher. 1995. Variations in bone status of contralateral and regional sites in young athletic women. *Medicine and Science in Sports and Exercise* 27:1354-1360.

Leveritt, M., and P.J. Abernethy. 1999. Acute effects of high-intensity endurance exercise on subsequent resistance activity. *Journal of Strength and Conditioning Research* 13:47-51.

Lewington, S., R. Clarke, N. Qizilbash, R. Peto, and R. Collins. 2002. Age-specific relevance of usual blood pressure to vascular mortality: A meta-analysis of individual data for one million adults in 61 prospective studies. *Lancet* 14:1903-1913.

Linn, S., R. Fulwood, M. Carroll, J.G. Brook, C. Johnson, W.D. Kalsbeek, and B.M. Rifkind. 1991. Serum total cholesterol: HDL cholesterol ratios in US white and black adults by selected demographic and socioeconomic variables (HANES II). *American Journal of Public Health* 81:1038-1043.

Lohman, T.G. 1981. Skinfolds and body density and their relation to body fatness: A review. *Human Biology* 53:181-225.

Lohman, T., S. Going, R. Pamenter, M. Hall, T. Boyden, L. Houtkooper, C. Ritenbaugh, L. Bare, A. Hill, and M. Aickin. 1995. Effects of resistance training on regional and total bone mineral density in premenopausal women: A randomized prospective study. *Journal of Bone and Mineral Research* 10:1015-1024.

Longhurst, J.C., A.R. Kelly, W.J. Gonyea, and J.H. Mitchell. 1980. Echocardiographic left ventricular masses in distance runners and weight lifters. *Journal of Applied Physiology: Respiration, Environmental Exercise Physiology* 48:154-162.

Lusiani, L., G. Ronsisvalle, A. Bonanome, A. Visona, V. Castellani, C. Macchia, and A. Pagnan. 1986. Echocardiographic evaluation of the dimensions and systolic properties of the left ventricle in freshman athletes during physical training. *European Heart Journal* 7:196-203.

Mackinnon, L.T. 1999. *Advances in exercise immunology.* Champaign, IL: Human Kinetics.

Magnusson, S.P., G.W. Gleim, and J.A. Nicholas. 1994. Shoulder weakness in professional baseball pitchers. *Medicine and Science in Sports and Exercise* 26: 5-9.

Malina, R.M., J.C. Eisenmann, S.P. Cumming, B. Ribeiro, and J. Aroso. 2004. Maturity-associated variation in the growth and functional capacities of youth football (soccer) players 13-5 years. *European Journal of Applied Physiology* 91:555-562.

Mangine, R.E., F.R. Noyes, M.P. Mullen, and S.D. Baker. 1990. A physiological profile of the elite soccer athlete. *Journal of Orthopedic Sports Physical Therapy* 12:147-152.

Margaria, R., P. Aghemo, and E. Rovelli. 1966. Measurement of muscular power (anaerobic) in man. *Journal of Applied Physiology* 21:1662-1664.

Maud, P.J., and M.Y.Cortez-Cooper. 2002. Static techniques for the evaluation of joint range of motion.

In *Physiological assessment of human fitness,* ed. P.J. Maud and C. Foster, 221-243. Champaign, IL: Human Kinetics.

Maud, P.J., and B.B. Shultz. 1989. Norms for the Wingate anaerobic test with comparison to another similar test. *Research Quarterly* 60:144-151.

Maughan, R.J. 1991. Fluid and electrolyte loss and replacement. *Journal of Sport Sciences* 9:117-142.

Mayhew, J.L., T.E. Ball, and J.C. Bowen. 1992. Prediction of bench press lifting ability from submaximal repetitions before and after training. *Sports Medicine, Training and Rehabilitation* 3:195-201.

Mayhew, J.L., F.C. Piper, T.M. Schwegler, and T.E. Ball. 1989. Contributions of speed, agility and body composition to anaerobic power measurements in college football players. *Journal of Applied Sport Science Research* 3:101-106.

Mayhew, J.L., J.S. Ware, M.G. Bemben, B. Wilt, T.E. Ward, B. Farris, J. Juraszek, and J.P. Slovak. 1999. The NFL-225 test as a measure of bench press strength in college football players. *Journal of Strength and Conditioning Research* 13:130-134.

Maynard, L.M., S.S. Guo, W.C. Chumlea, A.F. Roche, W.A. Wisemandle, C.M. Zeller, B. Towne, and R.M. Stervogel. 1998. Total-body and regional bone mineral content and areal bone mineral density in children aged 8-18 y: The Fels longitudinal study. *American Journal of Clinical Nutrition* 68:1111-1117.

McArdle, W.D., F.I. Katch, and V.L. Katch. 1996. *Exercise physiology. Energy, nutrition, and human performance.* 4th ed. Baltimore: Williams & Wilkins.

McClanahan, B.S., K. Harmon-Clayton, K.D. Ward, R.C. Klesges, C.M. Vukadinovich, and E.D. Cantler. 2002. Side to side comparisons of bone mineral density in upper and lower limbs of collegiate athletes. *Journal of Strength and Conditioning Research* 16:586-590.

McGee, K.J., and L.N. Burkett. 2003. The National Football League combine: A reliable predictor of draft status? *Journal of Strength and Conditioning Research* 17: 6-11.

McMaster, W.C., S.C. Long, and V.J. Caiozzo. 1991. Isokinetic torque imbalances in the rotator cuff of the elite water polo player. *American Journal of Sports Medicine* 19:72-75.

Meir, R., R. Newton, E. Curtis, M. Fardell, and B. Butler. 2001. Physical fitness qualities of professional rugby league football players: Determination of positional differences. *Journal of Strength and Conditioning Research* 15:450-458.

Menapace, F.J., W.J. Hammer, T.F. Ritzer, K.M. Kessler, H.F. Warner, J.F. Spann, and A.A. Bove. 1982. Left ventricular size in competitive weight lifters: An echocardiographic study. *Medicine and Science in Sports and Exercise* 14:72-75.

Millard-Stafford, M., P.B. Sparling, L.B. Rosskopf, and L.J. DiCarlo. 1991. Differences in peak physiological responses during running, cycling and swimming. *Journal of Applied Sport Science Research* 5: 213-218.

Minkler, S., and P. Patterson. 1994. The validity of the modified sit-and-reach test in college-age students. *Research Quarterly for Exercise and Sport* 65:189-192.

Morganroth, J., B.J. Maron, W.L. Henry, and S.E. Epstein. 1975. Comparative left ventricular dimensions in trained athletes. *Annals of Internal Medicine* 82: 521-524.

Morrow, J.R., A. Jackson, J. Disch, and D. Mood. 2000. *Measurement and evaluation in human performance.* 2nd ed. Champaign, IL: Human Kinetics.

National Cholesterol Education Program. 2002. *Third report. Detection, evaluation, and treatment of high blood cholesterol in adults (Adult treatment panel III).* Final report. Bethesda, MD: National Institute of Health.

National Institute of Health, and National Heart, Lung and Blood Institute. 1998. *Clinical guidelines on the identification, evaluation, and treatment of overweight and obesity in adults (executive summary).* NIH publication 98-4083.

NCEP. *See* National Cholesterol Education Program.

Neumayr, G., H. Hoertnagl, R. Pfister, A. Koller, G. Eibi, and E. Raas. 2003. Physical and physiological factors associated with success in professional alpine skiing. *International Journal of Sports Medicine* 24: 571-575.

Nichols, J.F., J.E. Palmer, and S.S. Levy. 2003. Low bone mineral density in highly trained male master cyclists. *Osteoporosis International* 14:644-649.

Nieman, D.C. 1999. *Exercise testing and prescription.* 4th ed. Mountain View, CA: Mayfield.

Noel, M.B., J.L. VanHeest, P. Zaneteas, and C.D. Rodgers. 2003. Body composition in Division I football players. *Journal of Strength and Conditioning Research* 17:228-237.

Norkin, C.C., and D.J. White. 1995. *Measurement of joint motion: A guide to goniometry.* Philadelphia: Davis.

Nowacki, P.E., D.Y. Cai, C. Bihi, and U. Krummelbein. 1988. Biological performance of German soccer players (professional and juniors) tested by special ergometry and treadmill methods. In *Science and football,* ed. T. Reilly, A. Lees, K. Davids, and W.J. Murphy, 145-157. London: E & FN Spon.

Nyland, J.A., D.N.M. Caborn, J.A. Brosky, C.L. Kneller, and G. Freidhoff. 1997. Anthropometric, muscular fitness, and injury history comparison by gender of youth soccer teams. *Journal of Strength and Conditioning Research* 11:92-97.

Oberg, B., M. Moller, J. Gillquist, and J. Ekstrand. 1986. Isokinetic torque levels for knee extensors and knee flexors in soccer players. *International Journal of Sports Medicine* 7:50-53.

Ogden, C.L., C.D. Fryar, M.D. Carroll, and K.M. Flegal. 2004. Mean body weight, height, and body mass index, United States 1960-2002. Advance data from vital and health statistics; no. 347. Hyattsville, MD: National Center for Health Statistics.

Osbahr, D.C., D.L. Cannon, and K.P. Speer. 2002. Retroversion of the humerus in the throwing shoulder of college baseball pitchers. *The American Journal of Sports Medicine* 30:347-353.

Osbeck, J.S., S.N. Maiorca, and K.W. Rundell. 1996. Validity of field testing to bobsled start performance. *Journal of Strength and Conditioning Research* 10:239-245.

O'Toole, ML., P.S. Douglas, and W.D.B. Hiller. 1989. Applied physiology of a triathlon. *Sports Medicine* 8:201-225.

Paffenbarger, R.S., and R.T. Hyde. 1980. Exercise as protection against heart attack. *New England Journal of Medicine* 302:1026-1027.

Paffenbarger, R.S., R.T. Hyde, A.L. Wing, and C.C. Hsieh. 1986. Physical activity, all-cause mortality and longevity of college alumni. *New England Journal of Medicine* 314:605-613.

Paffenbarger, R.S., A.L. Wing, and R.T. Hyde. 1978. Physical activity as an index of heart attack risk in college alumni. *American Journal of Epidemiology* 108:161-175.

Parr, R.B., R. Hoover, J.H. Wilmore, D. Bachman, and R.K. Kerlan. 1978. Professional basketball players: Athletic profiles. *The Physician and Sports Medicine* 6:77-84.

Parker, M.G., R.O. Ruhling, D. Holt, E. Bauman, and M. Drayna. 1983. Descriptive analysis of quadriceps and hamstring muscle torque in high school football players. *Journal of Orthopaedic and Sports Physical Therapy* 5:2-6.

Pate, R.R., M.L. Burgess, J.A. Woods, J.G. Ross, and T. Baumgartner. 2003. Validity of field tests of upper body muscular strength. *Research Quarterly in Exercise and Sport* 64:17-24.

Pate, R.R., M. Pratt, S.N. Blair, W.L. Haskell, C.A. Macera, C. Bouchard, D. Buchner, W. Ettinger, G.W. Heath, A.C. King, A. Kriska, A.S. Leon, B.H. Marcus, J. Morris, R.S. Paffenbarger Jr., K. Patrick, M.L. Pollock, J.M. Rippe, J. Sallis, and J.H. Wilmore. 1995. Physical activity and public health—A recommendation from the Centers for Disease Control and Prevention and the American College of Sports Medicine. *Journal of American Medical Association* 273:402-407.

Pauole, K., K. Madole, J. Garhammer, M. Lacourse, and R. Rozenek. 2000. Reliability and validity of the T test as a measure of agility, leg power, and leg speed in college-aged men and women. *Journal of Strength and Conditioning Research* 14:443-450.

Pearson, A.C., M. Schiff, D. Mrosek, A.J. Labovitz, and G.A. Williams. 1986. Left ventricular diastolic function in weight lifters. *American Journal of Cardiology* 58:1254-1259.

Pelliccia, A., F. Culasso, F.M. DiPaolo, and B.J. Maron. 1999. Physiologic left ventricular cavity dilatation in elite athletes. *Annals of Internal Medicine* 130:23-31.

Pelliccia, A., B.J. Maron, A. Spataro, M.A. Proschan, and P. Spirito. 1991. The upper limit of physiologic cardiac hypertrophy in highly trained elite athletes. *New England Journal of Medicine* 324:295-301.

Pelliccia, A., A. Spataro, G. Caselli, and B.J. Maron. 1993. Absence of left ventricular wall thickening in athletes engaged in intense power training. *America Journal of Cardiology* 72:1048-1054.

Pearce, M.E., D.A. Cunningham, A.P. Donner, P.A. Rechnitzer, G.M. Fullerton, and J.H. Howard. 1983. Energy cost of treadmill and floor walking at self-selected paces. *European Journal of Applied Physiology and Occupational Physiology* 52:15-119.

Pipes, T.V. 1978. Variable resistance versus constant resistance strength training in adult males. *European Journal of Applied Physiology and Occupational Physiology* 39:27-35.

Pluim, B.M., H.J. Lamb, H.W.M. Kayser, F. Leujes, H.P. Beyerbacht, A.H. Zwinderman, A. van der Laarse, H.W. Vliegen, A. de Roos, E.E. van der Wall. 1998. Functional and metabolic evaluation of the athlete's heart by magnetic resonance imaging and dobutamine stress magnetic resonance spectroscopy. *Circulation* 97:666-672.

Pollock, M.L., J.H. Wilmore, and S.M. Fox. 1978. *Health and fitness through physical activity.* New York: Wiley.

Potteiger, J.A., H.N. Williford, D.L. Blessing, and J. Smidt. 1992. Effect of two training methods on improving baseball performance variables. *Journal of Applied Sport Science Research* 6:2-6.

President's Council for Physical Fitness. *President's Challenge normative data spreadsheet.* www.presidents challenge.org. Accessed May 3, 2004.

Prior, B.M., C.M. Modlesky, E.M. Evans, M.A. Sloniger, M.J. Saunders, R.D. Lewis, and K.J. Cureton. 2001. Muscularity and the density of the fat-free mass in athletes. *Journal of Applied Physiology* 90:1523-1531.

Public Health Service. 1985. Summary of findings from National Children and Youth Fitness study. *Journal of Physical Education, Recreation and Dance* January:44-90.

Raglin, J.S., D.M. Koceja, J.M. Stager, and C.A. Harms. 1996. Mood, neuromuscular function, and performance during training in female swimmers. *Medicine and Science in Sports and Exercise* 28:372-377.

Reed, M.T.F., and M.J. Bellamy. 1990. Comparison of hamstring/quadriceps isokinetic strength ratios and power in tennis, squash, and track athletes. *British Journal of Sports Medicine* 24:178-182.

Rivera, M.A., A.M. Rivera-Brown, and W. Frontera. 1998. Health related physical fitness characteristics of elite Puerto Rican athletes. *Journal of Strength and Conditioning Research* 12:199-203.

Roetart, E.P., G.E. Garrett, S.W. Brown, and D.N. Camaione. 1992. Performance profiles of nationally ranked junior tennis players. *Journal of Applied Sport Science Research* 4:225-231.

Sargeant, A.J., E. Hoinville, and A. Young. 1981. Maximum leg force and power output during short-term dynamic exercise. *Journal of Applied Physiology* 26: 188-194.

Sawyer, D.T., J.Z. Ostarello, E.A. Suess, and M. Dempsey. 2002. Relationship between football playing ability and selected performance measures. *Journal of Strength and Conditioning Research* 16:611-616.

Schannwell, C.M., M. Schneppenheim, G. Plehn, R. Marx, and B.E. Strauer. 2002. Left ventricular diastolic function in physiologic and pathologic hypertrophy. *American Journal of Hypertension* 15:513-517.

Schmidt, W.D. 1999. Strength and physiological characteristics of NCAA Division III American football players. *Journal of Strength and Conditioning Research* 13:210-213.

Schmidt-Trucksass, A., A. Schmid, C. Haussler, G. Huber, M. Huonker, and J. Keul. 2000. Left ventricular wall motion during diastolic filling in endurance-trained athletes. *Medicine and Science in Sports and Exercise* 33:189-195.

Seiler, S., M. Taylor, R. Diana, J. Layes, P. Newton, and B. Brown. 1990. Assessing anaerobic power in collegiate football players. *Journal of Applied Sport Science Research* 4:9-15.

Seminick, D. 1990. The T-test. *National Strength and Conditioning Association Journal* 12:36-37.

Seminick, D. 1994. Testing protocols and procedures. In *Essentials of strength training and conditioning,* ed. T. Baechle, 258-273. Champaign, IL: Human Kinetics.

Sharratt, M.T., A.W. Taylor, and T.M. Song. 1986. A physiological profile of elite Canadian freestyle wrestlers. *Canadian Journal of Applied Sport Science* 11:100-105.

Shimokata, H., J.D. Tobin, D.C. Muller, D. Elahi, P.J. Coon, and R. Andres. 1989. Studies in the distribution of body fat: I. Effects of age, sex, and obesity. *Journal of Gerontology* 44:66-73.

Singer, B., B. Palmer, B. Rogers, and J. Smith. 2002. *Military services physical fitness and weight management database: A review and analysis.* U.S. Army medical research document no. HSIAC-RA-2002-001.

Sjogaard, G. 1986. Water and electrolyte fluxes during exercise and their relation to muscle fatigue. *Acta Physiologica Scandinavica* Suppl. no. 128:129-136.

Slaughter, M.H., T.G. Lohman, R.A. Boileau, C.A. Horswill, R.J. Stillman, M.D. Van Loan, and D.A. Bemben. 1988. Skinfold equations for estimation of body fatness in children and youth. *Human Biology* 60:709-723.

Smith, D.J., and D. Roberts. 1991. Aerobic, anaerobic and isokinetic measures of elite Canadian male and female speed skaters. *Journal of Applied Sport Science Research* 5:110-115.

Smith, D.J., H.A. Quinney, R.D. Steadward, H.A. Wenger, and J.R. Sexsmith. 1982. Physiological profiles of the Canadian Olympic Hockey Team (1980). *Canadian Journal of Applied Sport Science* 7:142-146.

Smith, H.K., and S.G. Thomas. 1991. Physiological characteristics of elite female basketball players. *Canadian Journal of Sport Science* 16:289-295.

Smith, R., and O.M. Rutherford. 1993. Spine and total body bone mineral density and serum testosterone levels in male athletes. *European Journal of Applied Physiology* 67:330-334.

Smolander, J., V. Louhevaara, T. Hakola, E. Ahonen, and T. Klen. 1989. Cardiorespiratory strain during walking in snow with boots of different weights. *Ergonomics* 32 (1): 3-13.

Snow, T.K., M. Millard-Stafford, and L.B. Rosskopf. 1998. Body composition profile of NFL football players. *Journal of Strength and Conditioning Research* 12: 146-149.

Spirito, P., A. Pelliccia, M. Proschan, M. Granata, A. Spataro, P. Bellone, G. Caselli, A. Biffi, C. Vecchio, and B.J. Maron. 1994. Morphology of the "athlete's heart" assessed by echocardiography in 947 elite athletes representing 27 sports. *American Journal of Cardiology* 74:802-806.

Staron, R.S., M.J. Leonardi, D.L. Karapondo, E.S. Malicky, J.E. Falkel, F.C. Hagerman, and R.S. Hikida. 1991. Strength and skeletal muscle adaptations in heavy resistance trained women after detraining and retraining. *Journal of Applied Physiology* 70 (2): 631-640.

Steiner, G., L. Schwartz, S. Shumak, and M. Poapst. 1987. The association of increased levels of intermediate-density lipoproteins with smoking and with coronary artery disease. *Circulation* 75:124-230.

Stewart, A.D., and J. Hannon. 2000. Total and regional bone density in male runners, cyclists and controls. *Medicine and Science in Sports and Exercise* 32:1373-1377.

Stoessel, L., M.H. Stone, R. Keith, D. Marple, and R. Johnson. 1991. Selected physiological, psychological and performance characteristics of national-caliber United States women weightlifters. *Journal of Applied Sport Science Research* 5:87-95.

Stuempfle, K.J., F.I. Katch, and D.F. Petrie. 2003. Body composition relates poorly to performance tests in NCAA Division III football players. *Journal of Strength and Conditioning Research* 17:238-244.

Taaffe, D.R., L. Pruitt, B. Lewis, and R. Marcus. 1995. Dynamic muscle strength as a predictor of bone mineral density in elderly women. *Journal of Sports Medicine and Physical Fitness* 35:136-142.

Teegarden, D., W.R. Proulx, B.R. Martin, J. Zhao, G.P. McCabe, R.M. Lyle, M. Peacock, C. Slemenda, C.C. Johnston, and C.M. Weaver. 1995. Peak bone mass in young women. *Journal of Bone and Mineral Research* 5:711-715.

Terbizan, D.J., M. Walders, P. Seljevold, and D.J. Schweigert. 1996. Physiological characteristics of masters women fastpitch softball players. *Journal of Strength and Conditioning Research* 10:157-160.

Theoharopoulos, A., G. Tsitskaris, M. Nikopoulou, and P. Tsaklis. 2000. Knee strength of professional basketball players. *Journal of Strength and Conditioning Research* 14:457-463.

Thorstensson, A., and J. Karlson. 1976. Fatigability and fiber composition of human skeletal muscle. *Acta Physiologica Scandinavica* 98:318-322.

Tucker, K.L., H. Chen, M.T. Hannan, L.A. Cupples, P.W.F. Wilson, D. Felson, and D.P. Kiel. 2002. Bone mineral density and dietary patterns in older adults: The Framingham osteoporosis study. *American Journal of Clinical Nutrition* 76:245-252.

United States Department of Agriculture. Agricultural Research Service. 1999a. *Food and nutrient intakes by children 1994–96, 1998.* Washington, DC: U.S. Government Printing Office.

United States Department of Agriculture. Agricultural Research Service. 1999b. *Food and nutrient intakes by race 1994–96.* Washington, DC: U.S. Government Printing Office.

United States Department of Agriculture. 2002. *Nutritive value of foods.* Home and Garden Bulletin no. 72. Washington, DC: U.S. Government Printing Office.

United States Department of Health and Human Services. 2000. *Healthy people 2010: Understanding and improving health.* Washington, DC: U.S. Government Printing Office.

United States Department of Health and Human Services. 2003. *The seventh report of the Joint National Committee on prevention, detection, evaluation, and treatment of high blood pressure.* Washington, DC: U.S. Government Printing Office.

USDA. *See* United States Department of Agriculture.

USDHHS. *See* United States Department of Health and Human Services.

Vanderford, M.L., M.C. Meyers, W.A. Skelly, C.C. Stewart, and K.L. Hamilton. 2004. Physiological and sport-specific skill response of Olympic youth soccer athletes. *Journal of Strength and Conditioning Research* 18:334-342.

Van der Sluis, I.M., M.A.J. de Ridder, A.M. Boot, E.P. Krenning, S.M.P.F. Muinck Keizer-Schrama. 2002. Reference data for bone density and body composition measured with dual energy x-ray absorptiometry in white children and young adults. *Archives of Disease in Childhood* 87:341-347.

Vescovi, J.D., L. Hildebrandt, W. Miller, R. Hammer, and A. Spiller. 2002. Evaluation of the Bod Pod for estimating percent fat in female collegiate athletes. *Journal of Strength and Conditioning Research* 16: 599-605.

Vescovi, J.D, S.L. Zimmerman, W.C. Miller, L. Hildebrandt, R.L. Hammer, and B. Fernhall. 2001. Evaluation of the Bod Pod for estimating percentage body fat in a heterogenous group of adult humans. *European Journal of Applied Physiology* 85:326-332.

Vincent, W.J. 2005. *Statistics in kinesiology.* 3rd ed., 1-17. Champaign, IL: Human Kinetics.

Viru, A., and M. Viru. 2001. *Biochemical monitoring of sport training.* Champaign, IL: Human Kinetics.

Visser M., T. Fuerst, T. Lang, L. Salamone, and T. Harris. 1999. Validity of fan-beam dual-energy x-ray absorptiometry for measuring fat-free mass and leg muscle mass. *Journal of Applied Physiology* 87:1513-1520.

Volkov, N., E. Shirkovets, and V. Borilkevich. 1975. Assessment of aerobic and anaerobic capacity of athletes in treadmill running tests. *European Journal of Applied Physiology* 34:121-130.

Ware, J.S., C.T. Clemens, J.L. Mayhew, and T.J. Johnston. 1995. Muscular endurance repetitions to predict bench press and squat strength in college football players. *Journal of Strength and Conditioning Research* 9:99-103.

Wathen, D. 1994. Load assignment. In *Essentials of strength training and conditioning,* ed. T. Baechle, 435-46. Champaign, IL: Human Kinetics.

Whaley, M.H., L.A. Kaminsky, G.B. Dwyer, L.H. Getchell, and J.A. Norton. 1992. Predictors of over- and underachievement of age-predicted maximal heart rate. *Medicine and Science in Sports and Exercise* 24:1173-1179.

Williford, H.N., W.J. Duey, M.S. Olson, R. Howard, and N. Wang. 1999. Relationship between fire fighting suppression tasks and physical fitness. *Ergonomics* 42:1179-1186.

Wilmore, J.H., J.S. Green, P.R. Stanford, J. Gagnon, T. Rankinin, A.S. Leon, D.C. Rao, J.S. Skinner, and C. Bouchard. 2001. Relationship of changes in maximal and submaximal aerobic fitness to changes in cardiovascular disease and non-insulin-dependent diabetes mellitus risk factors with endurance training: The Heritage Family study. *Metabolism* 11:1255-1263.

Wilson, G.J., A.D. Lyttle, K.J. Ostrowski, and A.J. Murphy. 1995. Assessing dynamic performance: A comparison of rate of force development tests. *Journal of Strength and Conditioning Research* 9: 176-181.

Wisloff, U., J. Helgerud, and J. Hoff. 1998. Strength and endurance of elite soccer players. *Medicine and Science in Sports and Exercise* 30:462-467.

World Health Organization. 1994. *Assessment of fracture risk and its application to screening for postmenopausal osteoporosis.* WHO technical report series no. 843. Geneva: WHO.

Worrel, T.W., D.H. Perrin, B.M. Gansneder, and J. Gieck. 1991. Comparison of isokinetic strength and flexibility measures between hamstring injured and noninjured athletes. *Journal of Orthopedic Sports Physical Therapy* 13:118-125.

Wroble, R.R., and D.P. Moxley. 2001. The effect of winter sports participation on high school football players: Strength, power, agility, and body composition. *Journal of Strength and Conditioning Research* 15: 132-135.

YMCA of the USA. 2000. *YMCA fitness testing and assessment manual.* 4th ed. Champaign, IL: Human Kinetics.

Zabukovec, R., and P.M. Tiidus. 1995. Physiological and anthropometric profile of elite kickboxers. *Journal of Strength and Conditioning Research* 9:240-242.

Index

Note: The italicized *f* and *t* following page numbers refer to figures and numbers, respectively.

About the Author

Jay Hoffman, PhD, is a professor and the chair of the department of health and exercise science at the College of New Jersey. Long recognized as an expert in the field of exercise physiology, Hoffman has more than 75 publications to his credit on human performance in refereed journals, book chapters, and books. He also has more than 17 years of experience coaching at the collegiate and professional levels. This combination of the practical and the theoretical provides him with a unique perspective to write for both coaches and academic faculty.

Hoffman was voted to the National Strength and Conditioning Association (NSCA) Board of Directors, for which he serves as vice president, and was awarded the 2005 Outstanding Kinesiological Professional Award by the Neag School of Education at the University of Connecticut. He also was awarded the 2000 Outstanding Junior Investigator Award by the NSCA. He is a fellow of the American College of Sports Medicine. He is also the author of *Physiological Aspects of Sport Training and Performance* (Human Kinetics, 2002).

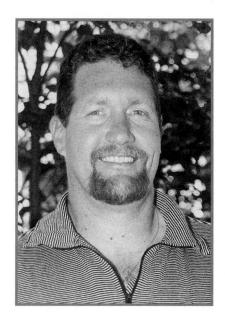

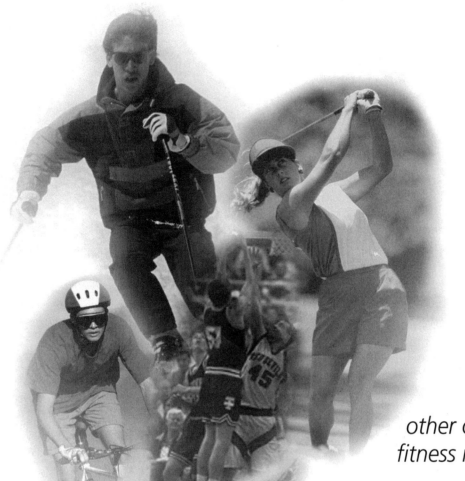